ABHANDLUNGEN
DER AKADEMIE DER WISSENSCHAFTEN DER DDR
Abteilung Mathematik – Naturwissenschaften – Technik
Jahrgang 1989 · Nr. 1 N

# Interactions in Protein Systems

Proceedings
of the
3rd Symposium on Food Proteins organized by
the Central Institute of Nutrition, Potsdam-Rehbrücke,
of the Academy of Sciences of the GDR
Reinhardsbrunn / GDR, May 17–20, 1988

Edited by
Klaus Dieter Schwenke
Barbara Raab

AKADEMIE-VERLAG BERLIN 1989

Herausgegeben im Auftrage des Präsidenten
der Akademie der Wissenschaften der DDR
von Vizepräsident Prof. Dr. Heinz Stiller

Die Beiträge dieser Abhandlung wurden nach den Originalmanuskripten der Autoren reproduziert.

ISBN 3-05-500595-3
ISSN 0138-1059

Erschienen im Akademie-Verlag Berlin, Leipziger Straße 3–4, Berlin, DDR - 1086

Lizenznummer: 202 · 100/370/89
Printed in the German Democratic Republic
Gesamtherstellung: IV/2/14 VEB Druckerei „G. W. Leibniz", 4450 Gräfenhainichen · 7147
LSV 1315
Bestellnummer: 763 905 5 (2001/89/1N)
04800

## PREFACE

The 3rd Symposium on Food Proteins continues the fruitfull tradition of Protein Symposia organized by the Central Institute of Nutrition. Starting in 1974 with the symposium entitled "Charakterisierung, Bewertung und Verarbeitung von Proteinen für Nahrungzwecke", held at the Wartburg Hotel in Eisenach, we tried to cover the most important aspects of protein research in food and nutrition. Therefore, the main sections of the programme were devoted to analytical problems including chemical, structural and nutritional evaluation and to the more practical problems of food protein preparation and processing. We needed 10 years - in 1984 we organized the second symposium, held in Reinhardsbrunn Castle, Friedrichroda, from november 27 to 30. Increase in the knowledge of food proteins had become exponential in the meantime, so to cover all aspects of basic and applied food protein research was not possible. We decided to focus the programme on some of the most current, chemical and physical topics. "Functional properties" had gained importance in evaluating food protein quality, especially for new proteins from plant origin. The symposium, subtitled "Structure, Modification and Functional Properties of Proteins for Human Food", summarized through contributions from leading specialists from different countries the recent research on food protein structure and their chemical and enzymatic modification for an intended alteration of functional properties.

The good resonance on the second symposium encouraged us to organize the third one four years later. The intimate atmosphere of Reinhardsbrunn Castle which promoted the climate of scientific discussion determined us to chose this place again for a symposium which was held from May 17 to 20 1988.

This third symposium was devoted mainly to problems of "Interactions in Protein Systems" as a central phenomenon in food protein functionality, the understanding of which is a basis for the preparation of more complex protein systems thus having practical significance. In preparing the programme we felt it necessary to consider progress in the research of protein structure, too. Moreover, in the poster session, we gave our colleagues working on very different fields of applied research the possiblity to present actual results on protein isolation, characterization and processing. Therefore, we hope to have taken into consideration the main aspects in recent food protein research in this symposium, too.

Although a formal separation into different topics was not taken up, the arrangement of the papers - corresponding mainly to the sequence of the contributions in the programme - provided a certain grouping according to special themes. Starting with different aspects of protein-protein interactions including multicomponent systems and interactions on interfaces, we find a number of main papers and poster contributions devoted to protein interactions with non-protein compounds such as polyanions, procyanidins, carbohydrates, lipids and others, Some of them are concerned with more complex systems of practical significance such as meat or bread dough. For special biochemical or biotechnological interest are papers dealing with the protein-dye interaction as a tool for protein purification, protein-inhibitor interactions and interactions between lectins and microorganims.

Insight into recent food protein structure research provided papers on legumeseed storage proteins and their proteolytic degradation as well on low-molecular mass proteins from oilseeds including attempts to predict their structure and to find structural similaries between proteins of different botanical species. The molden globule as a special state of partially unfolded structure of globular proteins was also presented and the fluorescence technique to follow the denaturation of a plant seed globulin was discussed.

All the contributions of the Proceedings of the Second and the Third Symposium are a major basis of comprehensive information for many scientists working on food proteins. Offset printing was chosen to edit the Proceedings of the 3$^{th}$ Food Protein Symposium as rapidly as possible. The papers were published in the author's version who are the only responsibles concerning content, language and figures of their contributions. Semitone figures as electron microphotos or electrophoretograms are printed on special paper in an appendix of the volume.

The Academy of Sciences of the GDR and the Director of the Central Institute of Nutrition, Prof. Dr. habil. H. Schmandke, gave invaluable support in the preparation of the Symposium. The editors want to express their gratitude to all those who contributed to the success of the Symposium, especially Dr. Ch. Schneider for the technical organization, as well as Mrs. H. Beyer and Mrs. Jäger.

The support and patience of Mr. K. Abel of the Academy-Verlag, the publishing house of the Academy of Sciences of the GDR, is greatly appreciated as well as the assistance of Miss A. Neumann and Dr. R. Mothes during the preparation of the papers for printing.

The editors

CONTENTS

Oral Contributions

Poster contributions

Role of protein-protein interactions in surface functional properties

Akio Kato, Department of Agricultural Chemistry, Yamaguchi University, Yamaguchi 753, Japan

## Introduction

Recently many attempts to develop new functional food proteins have been done by food researchers to meet the world's protein needs. In order to elucidate the molecular basis of protein functionality, many food chemists have studied on the relationships between the structural and functional properties of proteins. Much emphasis has been placed on the surface properties such as foaming and emulsifying properties, because of critical elements in developing new food proteins. If we can know the relationships between the structural and functional properties, we can make design of functional proteins. However, our understanding of the determinants of protein functional properties is still limited. We have proposed that the surface hydrophobicity and the flexibility or stability of proteins are the important structural factors governing the functional properties. In addition to these factors, this paper describes the importance of protein-protein interaction in air-water and oil-water interfaces.

## Methodology to study the functional properties of proteins

A quantitative method is required to investigate the relationship between the structural and functional properties of proteins. Pearce and Kinsella have developed the turbidity method to measure the emulsifying properties.[1] We have developed the conductivity method to measure the foaming properties.[2] These methods were used to determine the emulsifying and foaming properties, because of simple, exact and quantitative methods. The surface hydrophobicity of proteins was determined by fluorometric method using *cis*-parinaric acid.[3] The flexibility of proteins was estimated by protease susceptibility method.[4] The stability of proteins was estimated by measuring free energy change of unfolding ($\Delta G$).

## Relationship between structural and functional properties of proteins

Table 1 summarizes the relationships between structural and functional properties of proteins which have been elucidated by our group. The emulsifying properties are distinguished between emulsifying activity and emulsion stability whose structural factors are related with each other but main factors are different. Similarly, foaming properties are distinguished between foaming power and foam stability. The surface hydrophobicity is the determinant of emulsifying activity.[3] Protein stability or flexibility are the determinants of foaming power.[4] The protein-protein interaction is an

obtained between the stability and both surface properties, foaming power and emulsifying activity.

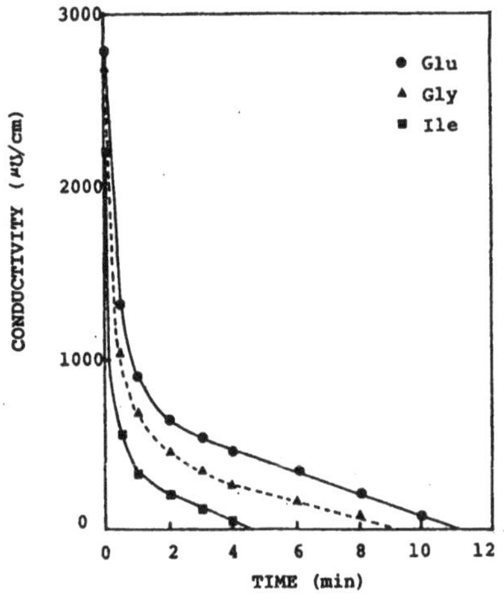


Fig.3. Foaming Property of Wild-Type and Mutant α-Subunit of Tryptophan Synthase Substituted at the Same Position 49 by Site-Directed Mutagenesis. ●, wild-type (glu); ▲, mutant substituted by glycine; ■, mutant substituted by isoleucine.

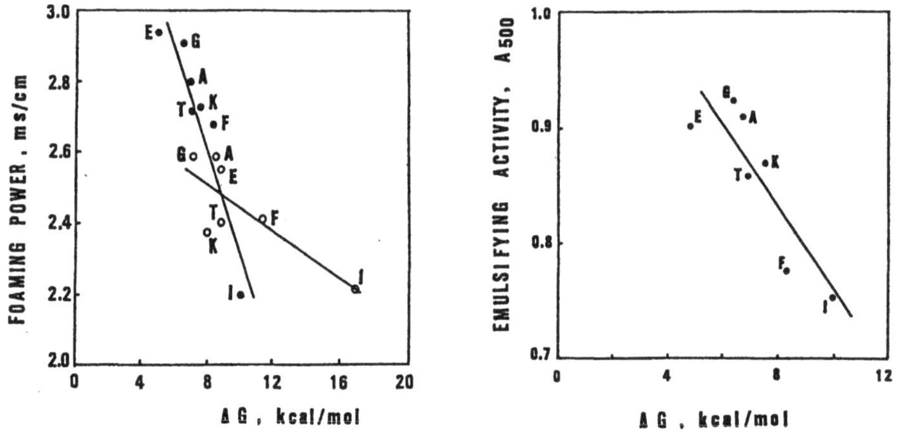


Fig.4. Relationships between Free Energy of Unfolding and Foaming Power or Emulsifying Activity of α-Subunits of Tryptophan Synthase Substituted at Position 49 at pH 7 (o) and pH 9 (●). Amino acids designated by single letter code indicate the mutant proteins substituted at position 49. A, alanine; E, glutamic acid (wild-type); F, phenylalanine; G, glycine; I, isoleucine; T, threonine. The values of ΔG are cited from Reference 15.

The correlation coefficient of the surface functional properties with the stability (ΔG) and surface hydrophobicity ($S_0$) of α-subunits of tryptophan synthase were summarized in Table 2. The correlation coefficient of ΔG with foaming properties was higher than that with emulsifying properties, while that of $S_0$ with foaming properties was lower than that with emulsifying activity. Thus, the conformational stability (ΔG) is deduced to be the important determinant for the functional properties, especially for the foaming properties.

TABLE 2 Correlation Coefficients of Surface Properties at pH 9 with the Structural Parameter, $\Delta G$ and $S_0$, of Tryptophan Synthase α-Subunits.

| Surface properties | ΔG | $S_0$ |
|---|---|---|
| surface tension | 0.90 | -0.92 |
| foaming power | -0.93 | 0.72 |
| foam stability | -0.95 | 0.81 |
| emulsifying activity | -0.83 | 0.83 |

Importance of protein-protein interaction in surface properties

In addition to the factors mentioned above, the importance of protein-protein interaction in surface functional properties is described below.

First, to investigate the effect of protein association on the surface properties, the foaming and emulsifying properties of various polymeric forms of ovomucin were measured and correlated with their molecular weight.[6] Soluble ovomucin is a polymeric form (8300 kD) of heterogeneous subunits consisting of α- and β-ovomucin, and is dissociated with sonication or reduction into smaller units of molecular weight of 1100 kD and 400 kD, respectively. As shown in Table 3, good correlations were observed between polymerization and foaming properties, while the emulsifying properties showed a good correlation with the surface hydrophobicity not with the polymerization.

TABLE 3 Structural and Functional Properties of Various Ovomucin.[6]

| | Ovomucin | | |
|---|---|---|---|
| | soluble | sonicated | reduced |
| molecular weight(kD) | 8300 | 1100 | 400 |
| surface hydrophobicity($S_0$) | 22 | 48 | 90 |
| foaming power(μ℧/cm) | 1174 | 465 | 373 |
| foam stability(%) | 95 | 60 | 54 |
| emulsifying activity($OD_{500}$) | 1.09 | 1.25 | 1.40 |
| emulsion stability(min) | 10 | 20 | 38 |

Similarly, various polymeric forms of ovalbumin aggregates were used to study the effect of protein association on the surface properties. Fig 5 shows changes in the surface functional properties of ovalbumin soluble aggregates during standing at room temperature. When ovalbumin is heated at controlled condition (at 80°C, pH 7.4), it forms soluble aggregates. The average molecular weight increased with prolonged standing at room temperature after heat-treatment,[7] as shown in Fig.5. The molecular weight was determined by the small-angle laser light scattering technique combined with HPLC. The foam stability was increased with increase of the molecular weight of soluble aggregates, while the other properties were not changed. From these results, it is suggested that protein association was an important structural factor governing the foaming property, while it is independent of the emulsifying property.

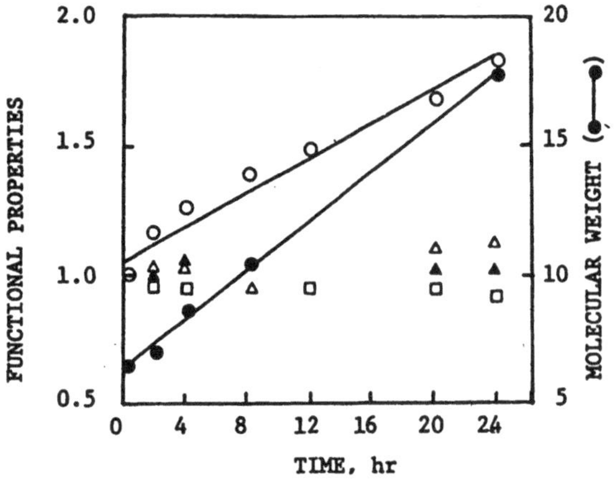


Fig.5. Changes in the Molecular Weight and Functional Properties of Heat-Denatured Ovalbumin during Standing at Room Temperature. O, foam stability; □, foaming power; ▲, emulsifying activity; △, emulsion stability.

Illustration of the role of protein-protein interaction in the surface properties was also achieved when polyanion-type proteins were used which inhibit the interaction at interface. Ovomucin and phosvitin were used as polyanion-type proteins. Fig.6 shows the effect of terminal sialic acid residues on the emulsifying and foaming properties of ovomucin.[8] The terminal sialic acid was removed by sialidase. Removal of sialic acids greatly affected the functional properties. The emulsifying properties of ovomucin were greatly decreased by the removal of sialic acid, suggesting that sialic acid plays an important role for the emulsifying properties. On the other hand, the foaming properties of ovomucin were increased by the removal of sialic acid. This may be because the decrease in negatively charged sialic acids enhance the interaction of ovomucin molecules at air-water interface which subsequently strengthen the foam film. Fig.7 shows the effect of phosphate residues on the emulsifying properties of phosvitin.[9] The emulsifying properties were greatly decreased by removal of phosphate by phosphatase. The foaming properties of phosvitin was too poor to study its changes. Thus, removal of sialic acid and phosphate from ovomucin and phosvitin, respectively, affected greatly on their functional properties. The foaming properties of these proteins were increased by the removal of polyanions. On the other hand, the emulsifying properties of these proteins were commonly decreased by the removal of polyanions. Accordingly,these results reveal the importance of electrostatic repulsive force to stabilize the emulsion droplets.

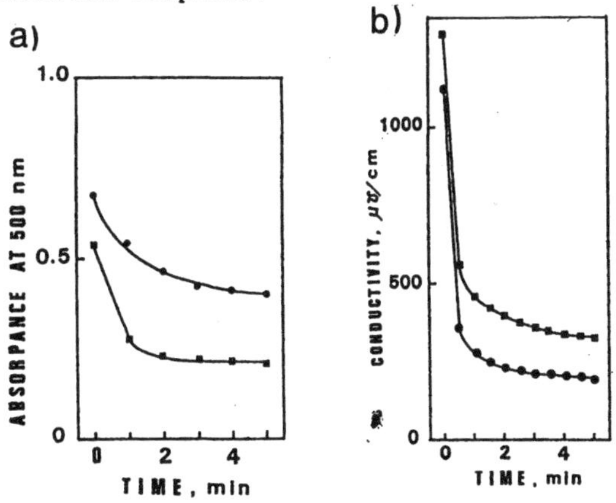


Fig.6. Effects of Sialic Acid Residues on the Emulsifying (a) and Foaming (b) Properties of Ovomucin. ●, untreated; ■, treated with sialidase.

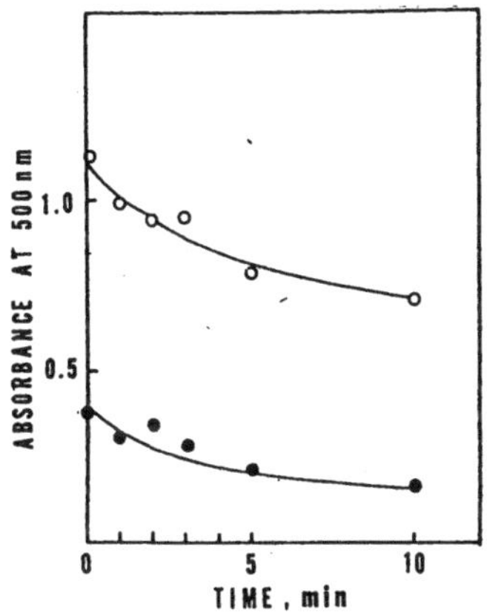


Fig.7. Effect of Phosphate Residues on the Emulsifying Properties of Phosvitin. o , untreated; ● , treated with phosphatase.

How to design new functional proteins

Thus, we have obtained the information on the relationship between structural and functional properties of proteins. Summarizing these results, good emulsifying properties of proteins are obtained by endowing the following three structural factors. First one is increasing protein hydrophobicity to endow amphiphilic properties, second one is enhancing protein flexibility to make easy to unfold at interface, third one is strengthening the electrostatic repulsion in hydrophilic region of proteins to stabilize emulsion droplets. On the other hand, good foaming properties of proteins are obtained by enhancing protein flexibility and strengthening protein-protein interaction. By using these information, we have developed the new methods to make new functional proteins.

Various enzymatic and chemical modifications of food proteins have been attempted to improve the functional properties. These will offer the possibility for food application of unutilized protein sources, if the safety for food use is solved. We have studied the deamidation of proteins as the most promising method to improve the solubility and surface properties.[10-14] The deamidation of proteins is expected to cause increases in the electrostatic repulsion and flexibility due to an increase in the negative charge of proteins.

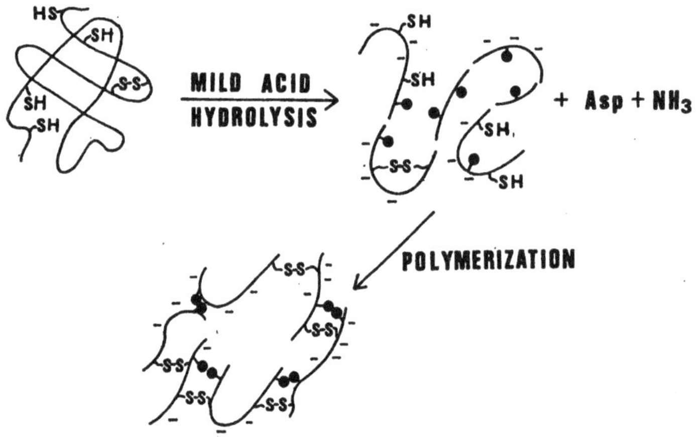


Fig.8. Scheme of Polymerization of Ovalbumin Peptides Deamidated by Mild Acid Hydrolysis. (-) negative charge, (●) hydrophobic residue.

The mild acid treatment to deamidate proteins was very effective to improve their functional properties. Fig 8 shows scheme of the deamidation of ovalbumin.[12] The mild acid treatment causes not only deamidation but also limited cleavage of peptide bond. Free sulfhydryl-rich proteins such as ovalbumin are polymerized by disulfide bond after deamidation. Therefore, deamidation of ovalbumin may cause both increase in protein-protein interaction and negative charges. As shown in Table 4, the emulsifying and foaming properties of ovalbumin were greatly improved by deamidation. This is the same with other food proteins such as soy proteins and wheat gluten.[10), 11]

TABLE 4 Improvement of Surface Properties of Ovalbumin by Mild Acid Hydrolysis (in 0.03 N HCl at 115 °C for 30 min)[12].

| ovalbumin | emulsifying activity($OD_{500}$) | emulsion stability (min) | foaming power( μΩ/cm) | foam stability(min) |
|---|---|---|---|---|
| untreated | 0.25 | 0.6 | 110 | 0.02 |
| treated | 0.92 | 4.1 | 1350 | 0.25 |

Recently, we found that proteases have the deamidation activity of proteins in an alkaline pH region where is scarcely subject to proteolysis. Table 5 shows the effect of proteolytic deamidation on the structural and functional properties of proteins.

TABLE 5 Effects of Proteolytic Deamidation on the Structural and Functional Properties of Various Proteins.

| proteins | surface hydrophobicity | digestion velocity (%/min) | foaming power (μ℧/cm) | foam stability (min) | emulsifying activity ($OD_{500}$) |
|---|---|---|---|---|---|
| ovalbumin | | | | | |
| native | 10 | 0.23 | 82 | 2.0 | 0.220 |
| deamidated | 20 | 0.34 | 208 | 6.5 | 0.450 |
| lysozyme | | | | | |
| native | 10 | 0.20 | 54 | 1.0 | 0.150 |
| deamidated | 52 | 0.31 | 96 | 3.5 | 0.230 |
| 7S globulin(soybean) | | | | | |
| native | 99 | 2.93 | 1250 | 7.7 | 0.420 |
| deamidated | 183 | 3.53 | 2550 | 10.2 | 0.540 |
| 11S globulin | | | | | |
| native | 44 | 2.53 | 1300 | 9.8 | 0.390 |
| deamidated | 153 | 4.70 | 2250 | 11.4 | 0.600 |

Increases in the surface hydrophobicity and digestion velocity (flexibility) were observed in deamidated proteins. An increase in several carboxyl residues due to deamidation may cause flexible conformation and may expose the hydrophobic residues from inside of molecules. Thus, protein deamidation may result in the improvement of

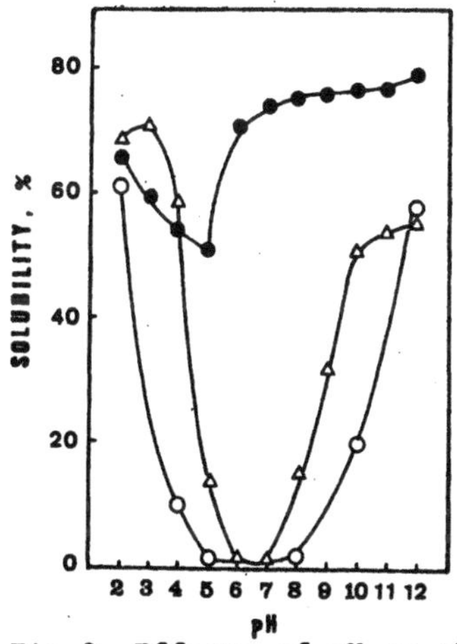


Fig.9. Effects of pH on the Solubility of Gluten by Proteolytic Deamidation. ○, untreated; △, treated without chymotrypsin; ●, treated with chymotrypsin.

functional properties. The effects of proteolytic deamidation on the functional properties were especially remarkable for wheat gluten containing a high content of glutamine and asparagine. Fig.9 shows the effect of proteolytic deamidation on the solubility of gluten at various pH.[15] Although untreated gluten is insoluble in the range of pH 5 to 8, the solubility is greatly increased by proteolytic deamidation. In the condition used here, proteolysis was not observed and deamidation rate was around 20 percents. Fig.10 shows the effects

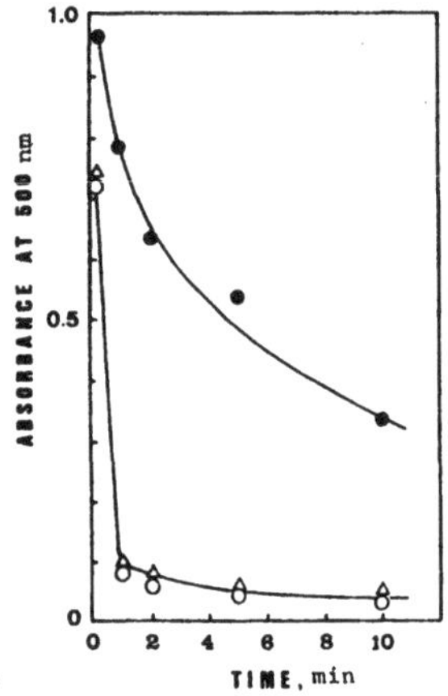


Fig.10, Effect of Proteolytic Deamidation on the Emulsifying Properties of Gluten. o , untreated; Δ , treated without chymotrypsin; ●, treated with chymotrypsin.

of proteolytic deamidation on the emulsifying properties of gluten.[15] A remarkable improvement was observed as shown in figure. Thus, proteolytic deamidation by chymotrypsin can be used as a useful method to improve the functional properties of proteins. Since deamidation of proteins causes an increase in solubility, this method may contribute to a larger effect for proteins poor in solubility. Alkaline treatment of proteins is generally used for food application to improve the functional properties such as solubility, emulsifying and foaming properties. However, excessive alkaline treatment results in undesirable effects on food proteins such as lysinoalanine formation and racemization of amino acid. On the other hand, proteolytic deamidation in a mild alkaline condition is a favorable method for food application, because of no degradation of amino acids.

As described above, the structural determinants of emulsifying and foaming properties of proteins have been considerably elucidated. As the relationship between structural and functional properties could be more demonstrated, we will be able to design more easily new functional proteins by using safe chemical and enzymatic modification, and protein engineering technique.

## References


(1) Pearce,K.N. and Kinsella,J.E. J. Agric. Food Chem.(1978) 26, 716-723.

(2) Kato,A.; Takahashi,A.; Matsudomi,N. and Kobayashi,K. J. Food Sci. (1983) 48, 62-65.

(3) Kato,A. and Nakai,S. Biochim. Biophys. Acta (1980) 624, 13-20.

(4) Kato,A.; Komatsu,K.; Fujimoto,K. and Kobayashi,K. J. Agric. Food Chem. (1985) 33, 931-934.

(5) Kato,A. and Yutani,K. Protein Engineering (1988) in press.

(6) Kato,A.; Oda,S.; Yamanaka,Y.; Matsudomi,N. and Kobayashi,K. Agric. Biol. Chem. (1985) 49, 3501-3504.

(7) Kato,A.; Nagase,Y.; Matsudomi,N. and Kobayashi,K. Agric. Biol. Chem. (1983) 47, 1829-1834.

(8) Kato,A.; Miyachi,N.; Matsudomi,N. and Kobayashi,K. Agric. Biol. Chem. (1987) 51, 641-645.

(9) Kato,A.; Miyazaki,S.; Kawamoto,A. and Kobayashi,K. Agric. Biol. Chem. (1987) 51, 2989-2994.

(10) Matsudomi,N.; Kato,A. and Kobayashi,K. Agric. Biol. Chem. (1982) 46, 1583-1586.

(11) Matsudomi,N.; Sasaki,T.; Kato,A. and Kobayashi,K. Agric. Biol. Chem. (1985) 49, 1251-1256.

(12) Matsudomi,N.; Sasaki,T.; Tanaka,A.; Kobayashi,K. and Kato,A. J. Agric. Food Chem. (1985) 33, 738-742.

(13) Kato,A.; Tanaka,A.; Matsudomi,N. and Kobayashi,K. J. Agric. Food Chem. (1987) 35, 224-227.

(14) Kato,A.; Tanaka,A.; Lee,Y.; Matsudomi,N. and Kobayashi,K. J. Agric. Food Chem. (1987) 35, 285-288.

(15) Yutani,K.; Ogasahara,K.; Tsujita,T. and Sugino,Y. Proc. Natl. Acad. Sci. USA (1987) 84, 4441-4444.

## SURFACE PROPERTIES IN RELATION TO THE SELF-ASSOCIATION (MICELLIZATION) OF AN ISOLATED FABABEAN (VICIA FABA) PROTEIN

M.A.H. Ismond, S.D. Arntfield and E.D. Murray[1]

### Background to the Micellization Concept

Protein-protein interactions are of major importance to food proteins, in terms of both isolation procedures and utilization in food products. In this respect, both covalent (particularly disulfide bridges) and noncovalent reactions must be considered, although the contribution of noncovalent forces appears to have a greater impact on the utilization of plant proteins. This impact has been realized in one recently developed technique for isolating plant proteins which involves the self-association of the protein into a micelle conformation, in which noncovalent interactions, and in particular hydrophobic interactions, have a dominant role. [1,2]

The basic steps in this procedure are outlined in Figure 1. In this study system using fababeans, protein is solubilized by a salt extraction with no pH adjustment and separated from the insoluble material by centrifugation. Upon dilution in cold water, a cloudy precipitate forms, which settles into a cohesive mass after sitting for a period of time. This precipitate, referred to as a micelle protein isolate tends to be very viscous in nature and can be recovered by simply decanting the supernatant. The micelle protein isolate contains a high percentage protein (96% - N X 5.85) which tends to be in a highly native state. [2] Furthermore, most of the problematic antinutritional factors commonly associated with fababean protein isolates are eliminated. [3]

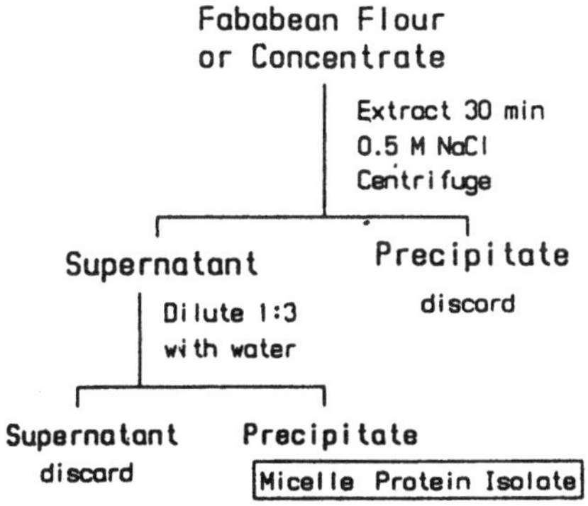


**Figure 1.** Schematic diagram of the procedure for the preparation of a micelle protein isolate from fababean (Vicia faba).

Examination of the structures developed during this process using light microscopy lead to some interesting observations. Upon dilution, the protein precipitates as discrete spheres, reminiscent of starch granules, yet showing no birefringent properties. This sphere-like configuration was attributed to the thermodynamic stability obtained by the burial of hydrophobic residues in the interior of the structure, while the majority of the charged groups remain on the surface. The

---

1). Food Science Department, University of Manitoba, Winnipeg, Manitoba, CANADA R3T 2N2

similarity of this structure to the better known detergent micelle has lead to the adoption of the term "protein micelle" and hence a "micelle protein isolate".

**Variations in the Protein Micelle Response**

Further investigations into this phenomenon have shown that the conditions under which micelles will form are limited and even within this range there is a great deal of variation in the response. In addition to differences in terms of the size of micelles produced, interactions between micelles can vary resulting in a range of interaction products. Therefore, a visual rating scale (MR - micelle rating) has been established in order to provide a semi-quantitative comparison of micelle responses (Fig.2). These photomicrographs were obtained by dilution of a vicilin sample (approximately 25 mg/ml) with an equal volume of distilled water on the microscope slide; post dilution structures were monitored with a Zeiss Universal Research microscope. The variation in micelle response is associated with the solvent used to dissolve the vicilin sample prior to dilution. The minimum micelle response (MR = 1) involves the formation of isolated tiny micelles ($< 2$ µm in diameter). If there is some degree of surface attraction, yet no coalescence then a granular network can result (MR = 2). Under the right conditions, the smaller micelles actually coalesce to give larger micelles which seem to be able to maintain their spherical shape (MR = 3). Further coalescence leads to larger aggregated products (MR =4) and eventually to the formation of extensive networks or protein sheets (MR =5).

The extent of micelle coalescence and interaction is important to optimizing of the recovery of proteins with this isolation technique as well as establishing a network which has potential value as a functional food ingredient. In fact, in some preliminary studies, a micelle protein isolate has been used to replace gluten in bread with only minimal loss in loaf volume.

With the recognition of this micelle response as both a valuable product in protein isolation and a usable network for structural integrity in food products, the necessity of understanding the exact nature of the protein-protein interactions is apparent. In order to predict or even manipulate this response, the forces promoting intermolecular association in the micelles are of fundamental concern.

**Parameters Involved in Micelle Response Characterization**

As an initial step in achieving this goal, a single storage protein, vicilin, isolated from the fababean micelle protein isolate has been used. By using a single purified protein, changes in both the surface properties and thermal behavior can be monitored as a function of environment and related to the micelle response. In this respect, the micelle ratings (Fig. 2) have served as a basis for comparison between different environmental effects. An assessment of surface hydrophobicity (So) provides an indication of variation in the surface profile of the molecule. This parameter can be determined using two different fluorescent probes. Cis-parinaric acid (CPA) can be used to estimate the hydrophobicity associated with aliphatic residues [5] while 1-anilino-8-naphthalene sulfonate (ANS) is used as an indicator of aromatic hydrophobicity [6]. With both these probes the relative fluorescence intensity is recorded as a function of protein concentration and the initial slope of this relationship is reported as the surface hydrophobicity (So).

The thermal properties of vicilin in various environments determined using differential scanning calorimetry, (DSC) provide some insight into conformational changes in the molecule. The temperature associated with the thermal denaturation of the protein (Td) is an indicator of the stability of the molecule. The enthalpy of denaturation (ΔH) measures the enthalpy required for thermal denaturation. Any unfolding of the protein due to the solvent will result in a lower ΔH value during thermal analysis. [7] One additional parameter that can be obtained form thermal curves is an assessment of the degree of cooperativity as measured by the width of the peak at half height (1/2 bw). An increase in this value reflects a decrease in cooperativity of unfolding, such as that resulting from a distortion in subunit association within the multimeric molecule. The inclusion of these thermal properties gives perspective to the observed changes in So and consequently the significance of these changes in terms of intermolecular associations.

**Effect of pH on Protein Micelle Formation**

Due to the limited range in which micelles will form, variations in pH were considered between pH 6.0 and 8.0 only. Phosphate buffers (0.1 M) were used to maintain these pH values. It can be seen that as the pH is increased beyond pH 6.5, there is a sharp decrease in the micelle response (MR) such that the highly interactive networks obtained at pH 6.0 and 6.5 are reduced to small non-interactive micelles at the higher pH values (Fig. 3). This reduced micelle response is accompanied by a reduction in both Td and So values. The 1/2 bw, on the other hand, tends to increase. It should be noted that there is very little variation in ΔH values over this range. [4] As a result, there do not appear to be any major structural alterations in this pH range; however, the decrease in Td and the corresponding increase in 1/2 bw may reflect a gradual distortion in the subunit association. Interestingly, the So values do not increase as would be characteristic of protein unfolding. The increased values obtained suggested an increase burial of hydrophobic residues. It is possible that this results from the distorted subunit association at the quaternary level.

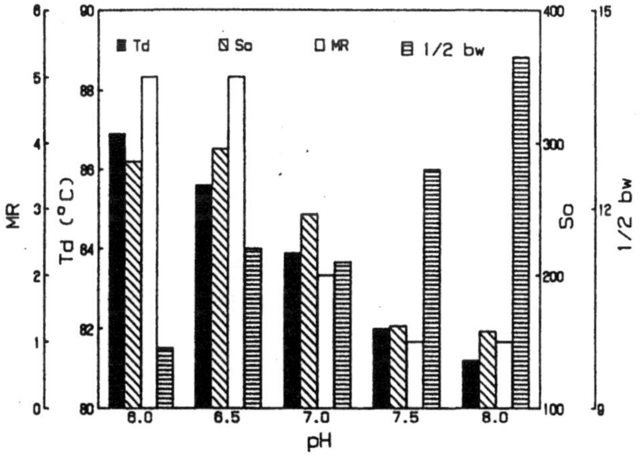


**Figure 3.** Thermal properties (Td, 1/2 bw), aliphatic surface hydrophobicity (So-CPA) and micelle rating (MR) for vicilin exposed to a series of 0.1 M phosphate buffers ranging in pH form 6.0 to 8.0. [4]

Due to the low ionic strength used in this study, an increase in pH away from the isoelectric point (for vicilin - pH 5.0 [8]) would be expected to increase the overall negativity of the molecule. This increase in the repulsive negative surface charge may be responsible for the induced conformational change within the molecule. Furthermore, the increased surface charge, in conjunction with reduced So values results in a progressive decrease in the inter-micelle interactions. Increased negativity may exert a significant surface repulsion among established micelles. The importance of hydrophobic interactions, believed to be important to the establishment of the original micelle structure may also be key to interactions of the micelles. The reduced So values at higher pH values may reflect a decrease in the attractive hydrophobic forces.

**Effect of Anions of Sodium Salts on Protein Micelle Response**

In view of the relative importance of hydrophobic interactions in the micelle response, the use of environments which result in manipulation of the So value should provide additional information on the nature of the interactions between micelles. Salts provide such a tool; protein conformation can be affected by both the concentration and the type of salt included. For a given cation (e.g. sodium), the identity of the anion can have a significant impact on this response. Essentially, there are two factors which contribute to the influence of salt environments. At low electrolyte concentrations ( $\mu < 0.5$), electrostatic influences related to the polyionic nature of the protein are dominant. [9] At higher concentrations, the position of anions in the Hofmeister or lyotropic series becomes important. The capacity of anions to exert a stabilizing influence at these concentration has been related to its ability to increase the surface tension of the aqueous protein environment [10] as well as cause preferential hydration of the protein molecule [11]. In fact, a correlation exists between the stability of a protein and the molal surface tension increment ($\sigma$) of the salt [10]; hence the $\sigma$ value can be used to define the position of an anion (or cation) in the lyotropic series.

For vicilin, the first evidence of the lyotropic influence can be seen at a concentration of 0.2 M (Fig. 4). The increase in $\sigma$ is generally accompanied by a increase in Td values. Only Td values have been used to assess thermal properties; there were no differences in $\Delta H$ values for these salts at a concentration of 0.2 M. Variation in Td for acetate, bromide and chloride are not significantly different nor are those between sulfate and citrate. [12] The So values for these anions (except iodide and bromide, whose values could not be determined due to quenching effects) tend to decrease with increasing $\sigma$; however, the values for acetate, chloride and sulfate were not significantly different. Basically this supports the general concept of a lyotropic stabilizing influence. The increased stability (increased Td values) results from increased burial of hydrophobic residues due to the increase in surface tension in the aqueous protein environment.

The micelle response, however does not follow the same trend. A strong micelle response (MR = 5) is obtained only with the anions in the middle of the series, including iodide, which tends to destabilize the protein, and the stabilizing univalent anions (acetate, bromide and chloride). The low micelle rating for the thiocyanate anion seems to be associated with molecular destabilization as evidenced by a significant decrease in Td and increase in So values. At the other end of the lyotropic series, which includes the highly stabilizing multivalent anions sulfate and citrate, a similar decrease in micelle response is observed (MR = 1). The sulfate response may be related to the multivalent nature of the anion as So values and thermal properties are comparable to those for chloride and acetate; with citrate, the reduced MR is associated with reduced So values and a high degree of thermal stability.

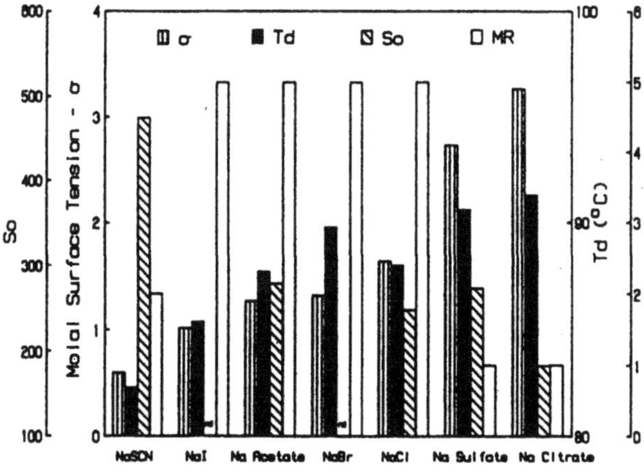


**Figure 4.** Micelle ratings (MR), aliphatic surface hydrophobicities (So - CPA) and denaturation temperatures (Td) for vicilin exposed to a series of 0.2 M sodium salts with different molal surface tension increments ( $\sigma$- $10^{-3}$ dyn g $cm^{-1}$ $mol^{-1}$). So values designated nd were not determined due to quenching effect of these anions. [12]

The differences in protein conformation and micelle response due to this lyotropic influence are more pronounced at a salt concentration of 0.5 M (Fig. 5). In fact, the increase in Td as a function of $\sigma$ can be defined as a linear relationship (Td = 7.21$\sigma$ + 80.3) with a correlation coefficient of 0.9241. [12] Similarly, a linear relationship exists between the So value and $\sigma$ (So = -132.4$\sigma$ + 517; r = 0.8463). [12] Once again, the low Td and high So values associated with the destabilizing salts NaSCN and NaI were not conducive to good micelle interactions. The high Td and low So values observed with sulfate and citrate did not even allow the formation of the very small non interacting micelles required for a micelle rating of one.

The importance of both electrostatic and lyotropic affects to the formation and interaction of vicilin micelles can be seen from these relationships. At low salt concentrations, stabilization is related to the general electrostatic influence. Sudden dilution of a concentrated vicilin solution in this situation results in a physical disturbance of the electrical double layer around the protein molecule. In response, hydrophobic associations are thermodynamically favored. It would also appear that electrostatic influences on the micelle surface are minimized, thus promoting further inter-micelle associations.

The destabilization by NaSCN and NaI, even at these low concentrations, has been related to the binding of the anions to the protein. If this binding persists after dilution, then a charge repulsion may be created among established micelles. Although the So value observed for vicilin in NaSCN would appear ideal for hydrophobic associations and hence micelle formation, the exposure of internal hydrophobic sidechains to this extent may disturb the orientation of the hydrophobic - hydrophilic residues such that micelle formation is no longer favored. These two factors seem to be responsible for the low micelle rating for NaSCN at both concentrations examined (0.2 and 0.5 M) and may also be effective in terms of the response observed with the other destabilizing anion, iodide.

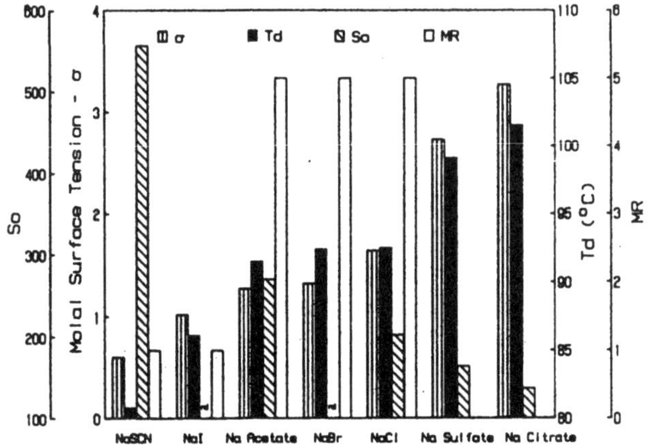


**Figure 5.** Micelle ratings (MR), aliphatic surface hydrophobicities (So - CPA) and denaturation temperatures (Td) for vicilin exposed to a series of 0.5 M sodium salts with different molal surface tension increments ($\sigma \cdot 10^{-3}$ dyn g $cm^{-1}$ $mol^{-1}$). So values designated nd were not determined due to the quenching effect of the anions.

The dominating lyotropic influence is seen for salts at the higher salt concentrations as evidenced by the dependency of Td and So on the molal surface tension increment. For moderately stabilizing anions (acetate, bromide and chloride), however, this resulted in optimum micelle response. The preferential hydration of the protein in the pre-dilution state and post-dilution electrostatic interactions are not prohibitive for inter-micelle associations. These conditions actually promote coalescence and aggregation. The increase in So in these environments increased the potential for attractive hydrophobic associations while the change in charge profile is not sufficient to create significant electrostatic repulsion. The balance between these two forces is key to micellization.

With the more stabilizing salts, sulfate and citrate, this balance is shifted such that micelle formation is inhibited. The reduced surface hydrophobicity, resulting from the preferential hydration of the protein, is inadequate to promote extensive hydrophobic associations. Interestingly, further increases in salt concentration to 1.0 M result in suppression of the micelle response for all salt environments except NaSCN where small non interactive micelles persist. [12] The change in So values at this higher concentration (compared to those at 0.5 M) are minimal, indicating that anion protein interactions may represent an additional destabilizing influence responsible for the deterioration of protein interactions.

As a result, it appears that a hydrophilic - hydrophobic balance is important to the micelle response. Distortion of this balance, either by the creation of a repulsive electrostatic profile (despite high So values) or a decrease in the number of exposed hydrophobic residues is detrimental to intermolecular interactions.

**Effect of Cations on Micelle Formation**

Cations can also be considered in terms of their position in a lyotropic series. The impact of this series on the overall conformation and micelle forming capacity of vicilin is not as dramatic as was seen with the anions. For chloride-associated cations (lithium, potassium and sodium), strong interactive micelle responses are observed for all environments at 0.2 and 0.5 M concentrations (Fig.6). This is despite somewhat random variations in both Td and So values. At 1.0 M concentration, however, an interesting difference occurs. For LiCl and KCl, a stable static population of various sized micelles is observed (MR =3), whereas with NaCl, the initial formation of micelles is transitory, and with post-dilution protein chloride binding resulting in destabilization of the aggregated molecules. As the $\sigma$ values for these salts are fairly close (Fig. 6), the preferential hydration of the pre-dilution vicilin would be comparable for all three salts. However, in contrast to NaCl, the cationic components, lithium and potassium, may exhibit binding to the protein [11,13] resulting in incomplete exclusion of the salt from the surface. As vicilin in this environment has an overall negative charge, a protein-cation association may promote a stabilizing influence. However, the electrostatic field eventually established at the protein surface, appears to set up a basic repulsive force among the individual micelles and further interaction was prohibited.

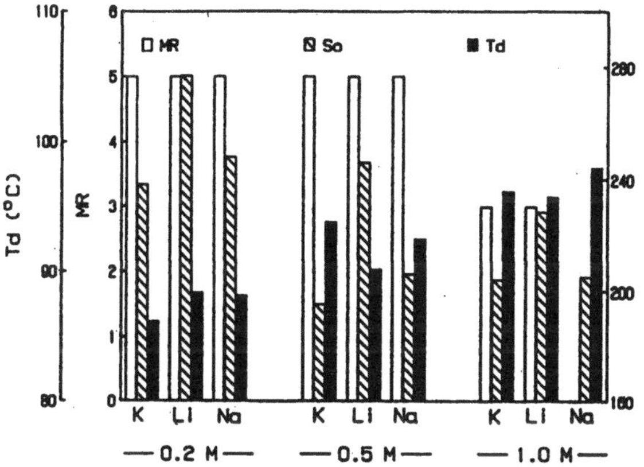


**Figure 6.** Micelle ratings (MR), aliphatic surface hydrophobicity (So - CPA) and denaturation temperatures (Td) for vicilin exposed to 0.2, 0.5 and 1.0 M levels of three chloride salts. Salts are listed in order of increasing molal surface tension increment ( $\sigma$- $10^{-3}$ dyn g $cm^{-1}$ $mol^{-1}$); the $\sigma$ values for these three salts are: KCl - 1.49; LiCl - 1.63 and NaCl - 1.64.

The different micelle response for vicilin exposed to the sulfate - associated cations (in comparison with the chloride salts) emphasizes the influence of the anionic salt component (Fig. 7). For both $Li_2SO_4$ and $Na_2SO_4$ strong interactive micelle systems are established at concentrations as low as 0.1 M. At this concentration the physical disturbance of the electrical double layer by the dilution procedure in combination with post-dilution reduced salt concentrations appears to minimize the electrostatic influence of the sulfate anion. With $K_2SO_4$, the micelle response is reduced (MR = 2), presumably due to the high So value and the resulting disturbance of the hydrophobic-hydrophilic balance. This behavior is analogous to that observed for the NaSCN environment.

At a higher salt level (0.2 M), the micelle response for the three cations varies (Fig. 7). The poor MR value for $Na_2SO_4$ and the lack of a micelle response for $Li_2SO_4$ may be attributed to the pre- and post-dilution electrostatic influence of the sulfate anion. The high So value for vicilin in $K_2SO_4$ may be beneficial in this situation in that it offsets the repulsive electrostatic interactions associated with sulfate, thus explaining the highly interactive micelle response. The high So value for $Na_2SO_4$ in comparison to that for $Li_2SO_4$ may account for the limited micelle response that was observed for sodium but not lithium. In this respect the position of the cations may have an influence on the micelle response, but the effect of the anion, and particularly if it binds to the protein and disrupts the balance of noncovalent forces, appears to be a more influential factor in these systems.

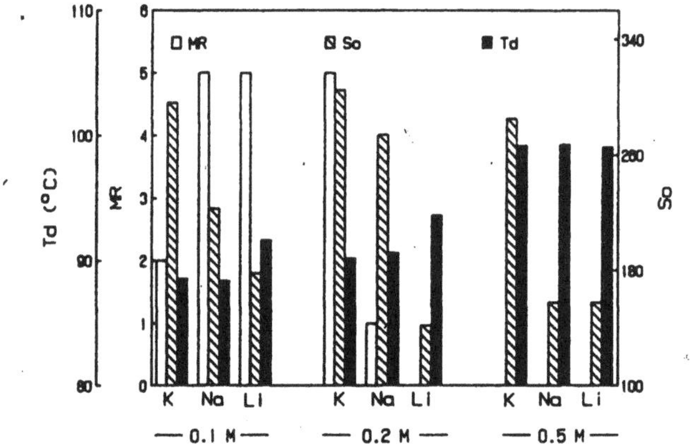


**Figure 7.** Micelle ratings (MR), aliphatic surface hydrophobicities (So - CPA) and denaturation temperatures (Td) for vicilin exposed to 0.1, 0.2 and 0.5 M levels of three chloride salts. Salts are listed in order of increasing molal surface tension increment ($\sigma$ - $10^{-3}$ dyn g $cm^{-1}$ $mol^{-1}$); the $\sigma$ values for these three salts are: $K_2SO_4$ - 2.58, $Na_2SO_4$ - 2.73, and $Li_2SO_4$ - 2.78.

This anion affect is even more evident for salts at the 0.5 M concentration, where the environment is not appropriate for micelle formation with any of the sulfate salts. With the sodium and lithium salts, this may be a reflection of the low So values expected from the preferential hydration phenomenon, whereas the So value for $K_2SO_4$ was relatively high. In this situation the disturbed hydrophobic - hydrophilic balance may be the dominant factor contributing to the lack of micelle formation.

**Effect of Denaturants on Micelle Formation**

Due to the dramatic impact of denaturants such as guanidine hydrochloride (GdnHcl) and urea on the conformation and therefore, surface properties of proteins, it was felt that additional information on the properties contributing to self-association of vicilin could be obtained through the use of these compounds. Exposure of vicilin to increasing concentrations of GdnHCl results in a linear decrease in the Td values up to a concentration of 2.0 M, indicating progressive destabilization of the molecule (Fig. 8). A decrease in $\Delta H$ values in this range reinforces the concept of progressive denaturation. [14] The lack of Td values beyond this concentration reflects the lack of an endotherm on the thermal curves; in other words, the protein has been completely denatured. Changes in aromatic So progressively decrease at low GdnHCl concentrations and level off when complete denaturation according to the thermal properties is obtained. Aliphatic So values tend to be fairly constant at the lower GdnHCl concentrations and decrease as concentrations required for complete protein denaturation are achieved. The micelle response is reasonably stable (MR =5) at the low GdnHCl concentrations (< 0.2 M) and produces small, but somewhat unreactive micelles (MR = 2) at higher concentrations which do not completely denature the protein. Complete denaturation of the protein and subsequent change in hydrophobic - hydrophilic balance is detrimental to micelle formation.

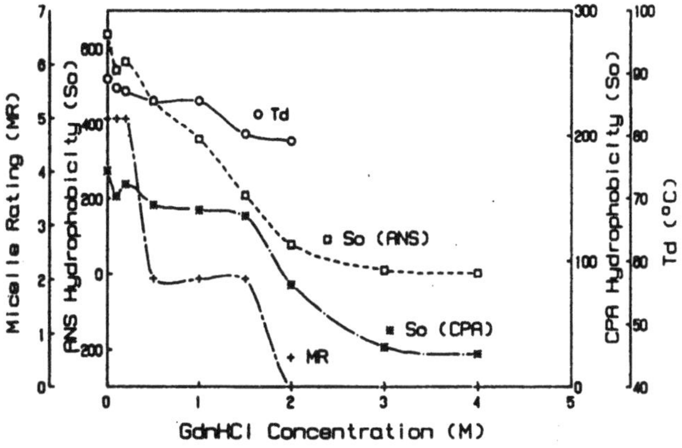


**Figure 8.** Effect of GdnHCl concentration (M) on the denaturation temperature (Td), surface hydrophobicity (both ANS and CPA) and micelle rating (MR) of vicilin. [14]

A similar effect is seen when urea is used as the denaturant, only the concentration associated with complete denaturation is higher (> 3.0 M), and consequently so is that for the final reduction in aliphatic surface hydrophobicity and micelle rating. Unlike GdnHCl, however, even very low concentrations of urea adversely affect the micelle response; a micelle rating of 2 is obtained with only 0.1 M urea. This reflects the different mechanism of denaturation for urea. This rating does not change until complete protein denaturation occurs.

The addition of denaturants to vicilin results in conformational disturbances at concentrations as low as 0.5 M for GdnHCl and 1.0 M for urea. This is evidenced by decreases in both thermal stability and So values. The decreases for both aliphatic and aromatic hydrophobicities, however, were unexpected as an unfolding of the protein should be parallelled by an increase in the exposure of hydrophobic residues. These decreased values may reflect intermolecular aggregation as the presence of urea or GdnHCl has no quenching effect on ANS or CPA fluorescence. [14] With GdnHCl, this change in surface properties and conformation results in a decrease in the micelle response, while for urea, the micelle response deteriorates even before there are indications of conformational change. The direct influence of urea on the potential for hydrophobic interactions appears to have an additional effect on micelle interactions.

Micelle formation was totally suppressed when vicilin was completely denatured. This is most likely related to a critical decrease in availabe/exposed hydrophobic residues due to intermolecular aggregation prior to micelle formation. [14] In addition, electrostatic repulsion associated with the unfolded protein may be prohibitive to micelle formation.

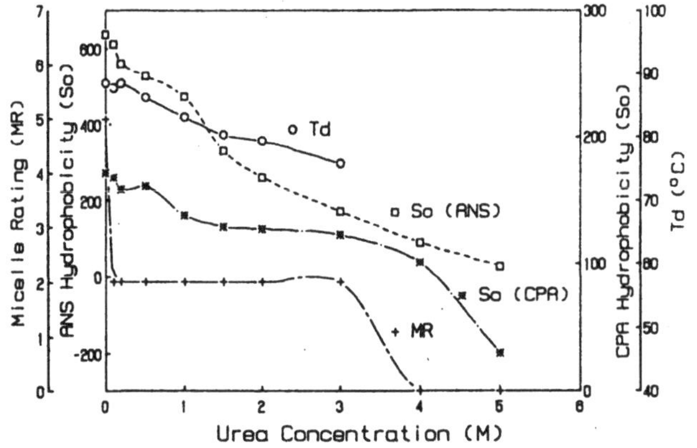


**Figure 9.** Effect of urea concentration (M) on the denaturation temperature (Td), surface hydrophobicity (So; both ANS and CPA) and micelle rating (MR) of vicilin. [14]

**Effect of Sucrose on Micelle Formation**

In contrast to the denaturants, sucrose has a stabilizing effect on vicilin (Fig. 10), as seen by a direct increase in Td values. Furthermore, even low levels of sucrose have an impact on both the aliphatic and aromatic So values as would be expected if the stabilization is a consequence of the preferential hydration of vicilin. This effect is similar to that associated with the stabilizing anions in the lyotropic series. Interestingly, increased sucrose levels do not result in any further change in the overall surface hydrophobicity (aliphatic or aromatic) yet there is a decline in the micelle response. In this case, an increase in solvent cohesive force as a result of preferential hydration, rather than increased burial of hydrophobic residues may be responsible for the observed micelle response.

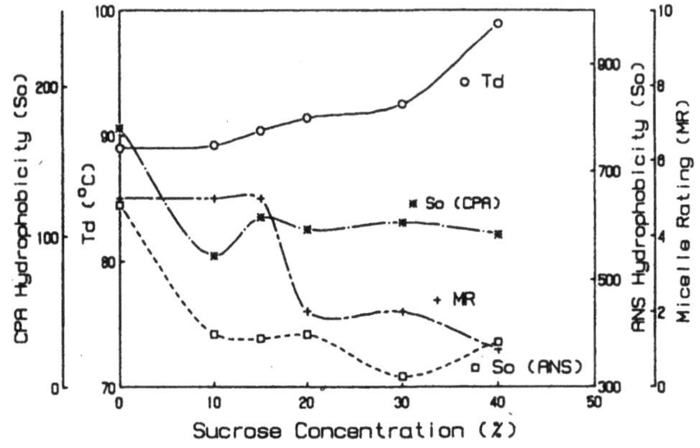


**Figure 10.** Effect of sucrose concentration (%) on the denaturation temperature (Td), surface hydrophobicity (So; with both ANS and CPA) and micelle rating of vicilin.

Overall, a balance between attractive hydrophobic associations and repulsive electrostatic interactions in food proteins is critical to micelle formation and network development due to micelle interaction. Distortion of this balance through changes in protein conformation will impair this micelle response. Destabilization through anion binding increases surface hydrophobicity and the charge on the molecule; denaturants result in reduced So values. In either case, micelle response is reduced. Stabilization of vicilin by salts is related to increased burial of hydrophobic residues, which is again detrimental to micelle formation. There appears to be a range of So values optimum for micelle interaction; yet even this is complicated by the preferential hydration effect which does not alter the surface properties, as was seen with sucrose. The importance of the surface properties to micellization is clear and a delicate balance of these forces is required for an optimal response in the formation of this imprortant intermediate when food protein networks are being established.

**References**


[1] Murray, E.D., C.D. Myers and L.D. Barker: Protein product and process for preparing same. Can Patent #1,028,522. 1978.

[2] Murray, E.d., C.D. Myers, L.D. Barker and T.J. Maurice: Functional attributes of proteins - A noncovalent approach to processing and utilizing proteins. In: Utilization of Protein Resources. D.W. Stanley, E.D. Murray and D.H. Lees (Eds.). pp. 158-176. Food and Nutr. Press, Inc., Westport, CT. 1981.

[3] Arntfield, S.D., M.A.H. Ismond and E.D. Murray: The fate of antinutritional factors during the preparation of a fababean protein isolate using a micellization technique. Can. Inst. Food Sci. Technol. J. 18 (1985) 137-143.

[4] Ismond, M.A.H., E.D. Murray and S.D. Arntfield: The role of non-covalent forces in micelle formation by vicilin form Vicia faba. The effect of pH variations on protein interactions. Food Chem. 20 (1986) 305-318.

[5] Kato, A. and S. Nakai: Hydrophobicity determined by a fluorescent probe method and its correlation with surface properties of proteins. Biochim. Biophys. Acta 624 (1980) 13-20.

[6] Hayakawa, S. and S. Nakai: Relationships of hydrophobicity and net charge to the solubility of milk and soy proteins. J. Food Sci. 50 (1985) 486-491.

[7] Arntfield, S.D. and E.D. Murray: The influence of processing parameters on food protein functionality. I. Differential scanning calorimetry as an indicator of protein denaturation. Can. Inst. Food Sci. Technol. J. 14 (1981) 289-291.

[8] Ismond, M.A.H.: The role of noncovalent forces on food protein interactions - A study system using the legume storage protein vicilin. PhD Thesis, University of Manitoba. 1984.

[9] von Hippel, P.H. and T. Schleich: The effects of neutral salts on the structure and conformational stability of macromolecules. S.N. Timasheff and G.D. Fasman (Eds.). pp. 417-453. Marcel Dekker Inc. New York. 1969.

[10] Melander, W. and C. Horvath: Salt effects on hydrophobic interactions in precipitation and chromatography of proteins; An interpretation of the lyotropic series. Arch. Biochem. Biophys. 183 (1977) 200-215.

[11] Arakawa, J. and S.N. Timasheff: Preferential interactions of protein with salts in concentrated solutions. Biochemistry 24 (1982) 6545-6552.

[12] Ismond, M.A.H., E.D. Murray and S.D. Arntfield: The role of non-covalent forces in micelle formation by vicilin from Vicia faba. II. The effect of stabilizing and destabilizing anions on protein interactions. Food Chem. 21 (1986) 27-46.

[13] Eagland, D.: Nucleic acids, peptides and proteins. In: Water: A Comprehensive Treatise, Vol. 4. F. Franks (Ed.) pp. 305-516. Plenum Press, New York. 1975.

[14] Ismond, M.A.H., E.D. Murray and S.D. Arntfield: The role of noncovalent forces in micelle formation from Vicia faba. III. The effect of urea, guanidine hydrochloride and sucrose on protein interactions. Accepted Food Chem. 1988.

# EFFECT OF ANIONS ON THE STABILITY OF FABABEAN (*VICIA FABA*) STORAGE PROTEINS

S.D. Arntfield, M.A.H. Ismond and E.D. Murray[1]

## Introduction

Conformational stability is a key factor to the utilization of protein in food systems. In fact, the high thermal stability associated with plant proteins in comparison to animal proteins has been cited as a factor limiting their incorporation into traditional food products.[1] As a result, an understanding of the mechanism responsible for this stability and how it varies in response to solvent manipulation is critical to the effective utilization of plant proteins.

The fababean storage proteins represent a good study system for the investigation of the influence of solvents, such as aqueous salt solutions, on thermal stability. Furthermore, the use of a micelle protein isolate [2,3] and purified proteins from this isolate (e.g. vicilin) provides starting materials in which protein conformation has not been severely influenced by processing conditions. This isolation technique is characterized by mild conditions during both the extraction (NaCl) and precipitation (dilution); hence protein denaturation, often encountered with the more traditional techniques which utilize alkaline extraction followed by isoelectric precipitation, is avoided.[4]

An investigation of the influence of salts on protein thermal stability can serve two purposes. First, salts are present in many food products and the influence of various salts and salt concentrations will have a direct influence on how the protein functions in any given environment. Secondly, the use of salt, and in particular salts in the Hofmeister or lyotropic series, provides a tool for examining the types of interactions associated with this conformational stability.

Key to these investigations is the assessment of the thermal stability. In this respect, differential scanning calorimetry (DSC) has proved to be a most valuable technique for purified proteins as well as the less soluble protein isolates and flours. The technique involves monitoring the heat flow to a protein in an aqueous system using a controlled heating regime. Protein denaturation is represented by a peak on the resulting thermal curve, the area of which is related to the enthalpy of protein denaturation ($\Delta H$) and the temperature associated with the peak (i.e. denaturation temperature - Td) is an indicator of protein stability. Both parameters are of value in an investigation of salt or anion effects. The Td value can be used as a direct assessment of stability and the $\Delta H$ value will indicate any major conformational changes (i.e. decreased $\Delta H$ value due to protein denaturation) associated with a given salt environment.

## Effect of Anions on the Stability of Purified Vicilin

The effects of a series of anions of sodium salts (sulfate, chloride, acetate, and thiocyanate) on the thermal properties of purified vicilin have been investigated over a concentration range from 0.2 to 1.0 M. By comparing the $\Delta H$ values, the distinction between the chaotropic (i.e. destabilizing) and non-chaotropic salts is readily

---

1). Food Science Department, University of Manitoba, Winnipeg, Manitoba, CANADA R3T 2N2

apparent at the higher salt levels (Fig. 1). With sulfate, chloride, and acetate, increasing the salt concentration results in no change or a slight increase in the ΔH value, suggesting no major conformational changes. The low ΔH value for the sodium thiocyanate at 1.0 M is a clear indication of conformational changes associated with that salt environment. At the lower concentrations (.2 and .5 M), differences in ΔH for the various salts are small (all between 10 and 15 J/g); the values for sulfate and chloride, however, are significantly higher than those of acetate and thiocyanate ($P \leq 0.05$). At a concentration of 1.0 M, however, the ΔH values can be ranked according to their position in the Hofmeister series: sulfate > chloride, acetate > thiocyanate. Changes in ΔH for some systems have been shown to be a function of Td, rather than the direct influence of the environment. This is related to the reduced potential for non-polar contacts at higher temperatures, which results in a reduction of the exothermic portion of the enthalpy value. As the net enthalpy is endothermic in nature, there is an increase in the resulting ΔH value.[5] For this reason, apart for noting that the thiocyanate ion actually results in a change in protein conformation, the Td values, rather than ΔH values will be used to follow thermal stability.

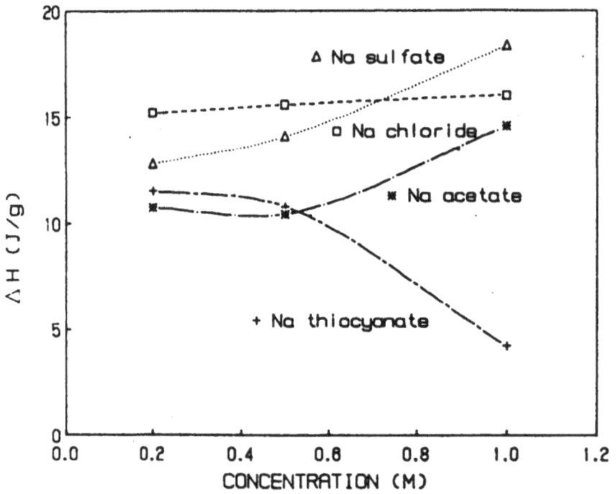


**Figure 1.** Influence of anions of sodium salts on the enthalpy of denaturation (ΔH) of vicilin as a function of concentration.[9]

The position of the salts in the lyotropic series has a significant impact on the Td values of vicilin, particularly at concentrations greater than or equal to 0.5 M (Fig.2). At lower concentrations, the salt effect does not discriminate as much with respect to anion type and is primarily related to electrostatic interactions based on the polar polyionic nature of the protein.[6] The destabilizing potential of the thiocyanate, however, is apparent even at these low concentrations as evidenced by significantly lower Td values. This has been attributed to the capacity of thiocyanate to exhibit non-specific binding to the polar sites on the protein.[7] The ranking of these salts in terms of their stabilizing effect at higher concentrations parallels that observed for the ΔH values, with sulfate > chloride, acetate > thiocyanate. The ability of a salt to stabilize protein structure appears to be related to its ability to increase surface tension of the aqueous environment. In fact, the molal surface tension increment ($\sigma$) has been used to describe the position of the various salts in the lyotropic series.[8] Theoretical studies have indicated that the correlation between the $\sigma$ and protein stabilization has been attributed to hydrophobic interactions. The relationship between $\sigma$ and Td values for vicilin (Fig. 2) indicates the dependence of the Td value on the position of the salt in the lyotropic series and emphasizes the importance of hydrophobic interactions to the quaternary structure of vicilin.

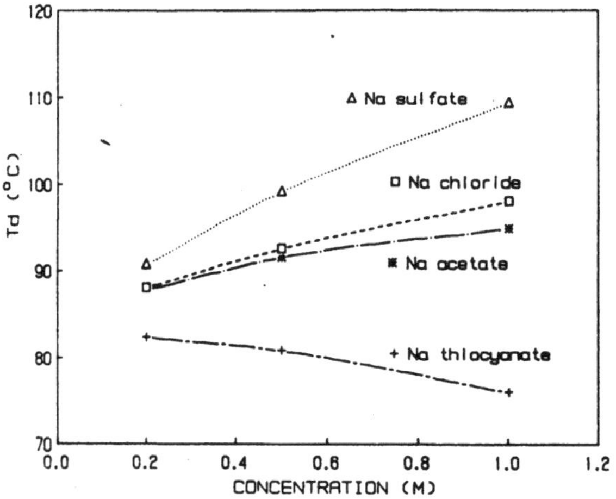


**Figure 2.** Influence of anions of sodium salts on the temperature of denaturation (Td) of vicilin as a function of concentration. Positions of the salts in the lyotropic series are related to the molal surface tension increment ($\sigma$ - $10^{-3}$ dyne g $cm^{-1}$ $mol^{-1}$); the $\sigma$ values for the salts are as follows: Na sulfate - 2.73, Na chloride - 1.64, Na acetate - 1.27, and Na thiocyanate - 0.60.[9]

__Role of Anions in Protein Structure Development for Vicilin__

This stabilization can have a significant impact on the ability of proteins to interact. The self-association of vicilin into a micelle configuration and interaction products thereof, is highly dependent on hydrophobic interactions and thus the response to different salt environments varies with the position of the salt in the lyotropic series. Both destabilizing conditions (eg. NaSCN) and very stabilizing conditions (eg. $Na_2SO_4$), in which surface hydrophobicity significantly decreases, are detrimental to good micelle interaction.[9] In addition, various anions in the lyotropic series can influence the networks which result from heat induced denaturation. Characterization of this type of network involves the use of dynamic rheological techniques or small amplitude oscillatory testing with a rheoemeter such as the Bohlin VOR rheometer. The sinusoidal nature of both the applied strain and the resulting stress measured in this technique result in three different parameters which can be used to describe a network. These are: G' - the storage or elastic modulus, G" - the loss or viscous modulus and tan delta (G"/G) - the loss tangent which is a measure of the energy lost to the energy stored during a deformation cycle.

Examination of heat induced vicilin networks prepared at varying NaCl concentration shows the relative significance of these parameters (Fig. 3). At low concentrations (0.1 and 0.2 M), G' is very high (1068 pascals at 0.1 M) compared to G" (168 pascals), thus giving a relatively low tan delta (.157). This represents an interactive system with a certain amount of crosslinking. As the concentration increases, there is a noticeable drop in G' and to a lesser extent G", resulting in a slight increase in tan delta. In other words, the interactions in the network, of both an elastic and viscous nature, are reduced and the resulting network is not as well structured as at lower concentrations.

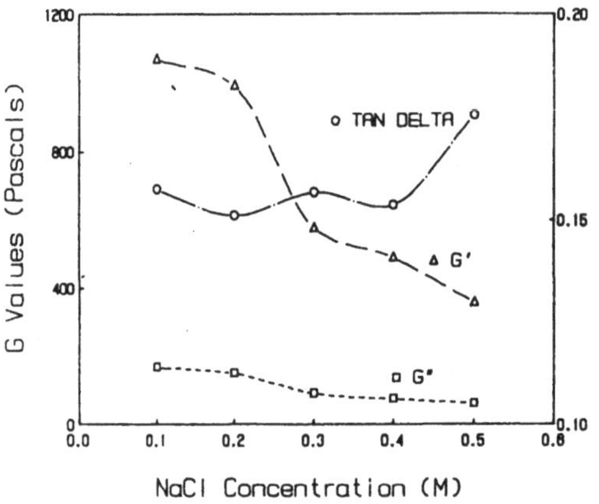


**Figure 3.** Effect of NaCl concentration on the dynamic rheological properties of heat set vicilin networks (pH 8.5). Rheological parameters determined using oscillatory testing in a Boohlin VOR rheometer.

Various anions of sodium salts also affect these parameters (Fig. 4). With thiocyanate, both G' and G" are very low, negligible in comparison to the values for the other anions. The high tan delta (.591) indicates a lack of structure in the resulting precipitate. In addition to destabilizing vicilin, the binding of thiocyanate to vicilin also inhibits good network formation.

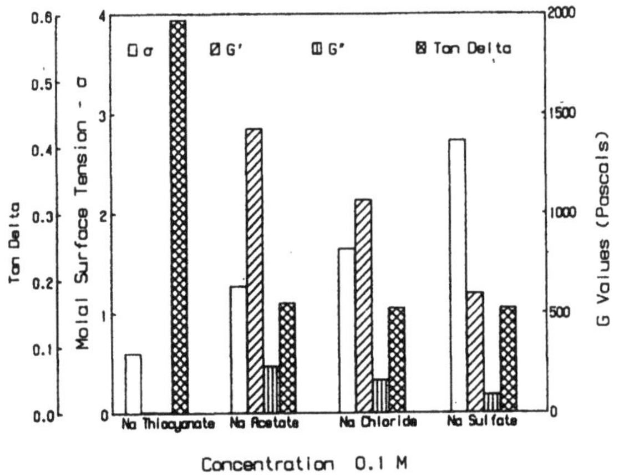


**Figure 4.** Effect of anions of sodium salts with varying molal surface tension increments ($\sigma - 10^{-3}$ dyne g $cm^{-1}$ $mol^{-1}$) on the rheological properties of heat set vicilin networks (pH 8.5, salt concentration = 0.1 M).

For the three non-chaotropic anions, an increase in σ results in a decrease in both G' and G" but does not have a significant impact on tan delta. It appears that even at these low salt concentrations the impact of the lyotropic series is sufficient to alter the degree of interactions in these heat induced networks (decreased G' and G" values). The relative proportions of these two variables (tan delta) remains the same, indicating that while the extent of interaction is decreased, the nature of the resulting network is essentially unchanged.

At higher salt concentrations (0.5 M), similar trends are observed (Fig. 5). The binding of the thiocyanate anion resulted in a soluble protein even after heat treatment. Both G' and G" decreased with increasing σ, as was seen with 0.1 M salt. With tan delta values, there is one major difference not seen at the lower concentration. The network in the presence of sulfate was characterized by both very low G values and a high tan delta, indicating minimal network formation. It appears that extensive stabilization through hydrophobic interactions, such as was observed for the native vicilin molecule, is not conducive to good network formation. Furthermore, this promotion of hydrophobic interactions results in an overall decrease in the degree of interaction between proteins and those which do occur, tend to result in a viscous product rather than an elastic gel-like structure.

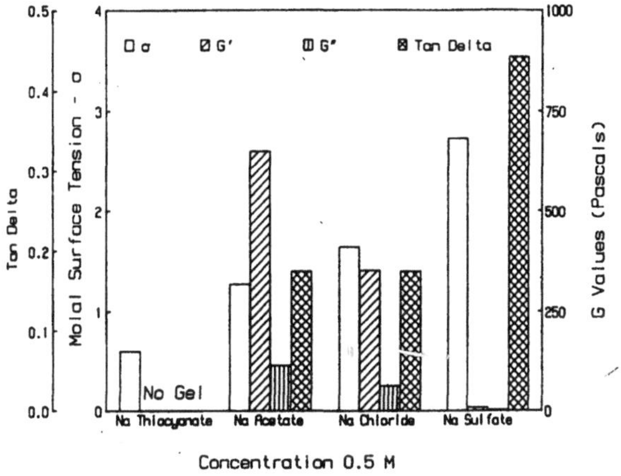


**Figure 5.** Effect of anions of sodium salts with varying molal surface tension increments ($\sigma - 10^{-3}$ dyne g $cm^{-1}$ $mol^{-1}$) on the rheological properties of heat set vicilin networks (pH 8.5, salt concentration = 0.5 M).

From these results, it is clear that the impact of anions in the lyotropic series on heat induced vicilin networks is similar to that for the micelle type interaction in that both highly destabilizing and highly stabilizing anions are not conducive to good interactions. Furthermore, comparison of the stability data to the rheological properties of the heat induced networks for the stabilizing salts indicates there is a linear relationship between Td and G' (Fig. 6). A similar relationship exists for G". It appears that regardless of the anion type and concentration, an increase in the Td value or overall stability results in a decrease in the elastic component. As a similar trend exists for G" values, it is clear that protein-protein interactions for the heat induced network are reduced if the stability of the native protein is increased. This would account for some of the problems associated with the use of plant proteins with high thermal stability. This also indicates that hydrophobic interactions are important to heat induced networks and changes in the overall stability (Td values) without major conformational changes (i.e. no decrease in the ΔH value) may serve as a technique for the prediction of the degree of interaction in such a network.

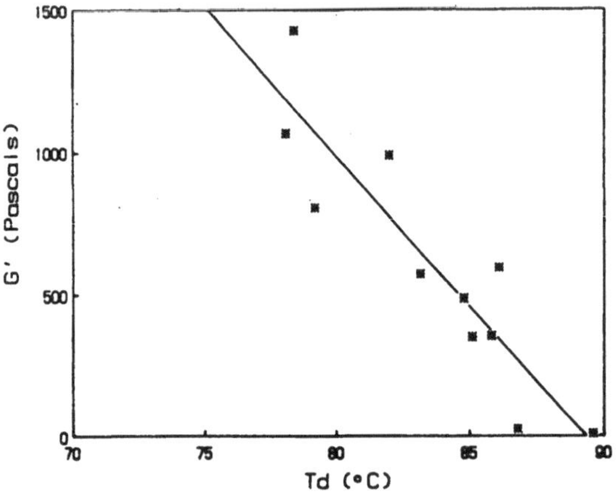


**Figure 6.** Relationship between storage modulus (G') and denaturation temperature (Td) for heat set vicilin gels in chaotropic sodium salts with various anions (sulfate, chloride, acetate, thiocyanate) and salt concentration (0.1 - 0.5 M). The relationship is described by the equation G' = 9013 - 100 Td; r = 0.9714).

**Effect of Anions on the Stability of a Micelle Protein Isolate from Vicilin**

The first step in the extension of this information to food systems requires examination of protein isolates in addition to purified proteins. A fababean micelle isolate is a proteinaceous product consisting primarily of two storage proteins - vicilin and legumin. In the presense of water, the thermal curve for this isolate is characterized by a single endotherm (Fig. 7).

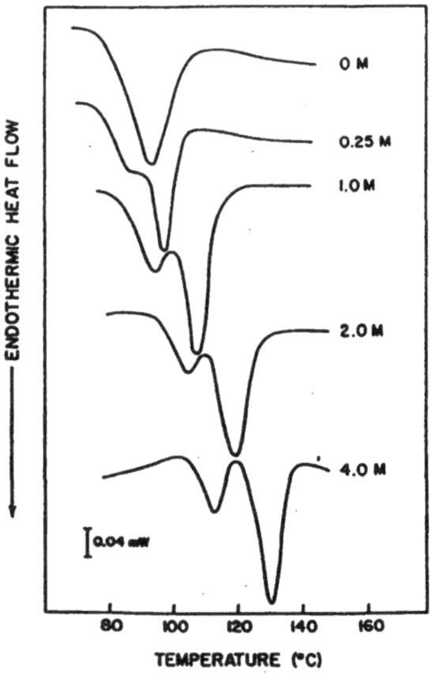


**Figure 7.** Influence of NaCl concentration on the DSC thermal curves of a micelle protein isolate from fababean. Sample concentration was 20% total solids and heating rate 5°C/min. [10]

The addition of NaCl, however, leads to the appearance of two endotherms, the separation of which increases with increasing salt level. These two endotherms have been attributed to vicilin (lower Td) and legumin (higher Td).[10] This behavior was also observed with other stabilizing salts, and represents a differential response for the two proteins to the effect of salt on hydrophobic interactions. This may be related to different levels of hydration associated with the two proteins and thus the level of a given salt required to promote a degree of stabilization.

Increasing concentrations of NaSCN also elicit differential responses for the two proteins as evidenced by a shoulder appearing on the main endotherm in the thermal curves (Fig. 8). In this situation, Td and $\Delta H$ values (area under curve) for the peak as well as the shoulder decrease with increasing concentration, reflecting denaturation of both proteins. The lack of an endotherm at a concentration of 4.0 M indicates complete denaturation of the proteins. As the denaturation of proteins in the presence of NaSCN has been related to binding of the anion to the protein, it is felt that the differential response in this environment reflects differences in the electrostatic profiles for the two proteins. With both stabilizing and destabilizing anions, however, it is possible to assess the changes associated with both vicilin and legumin in an isolate by simply examining Td values associated with the individual peaks.

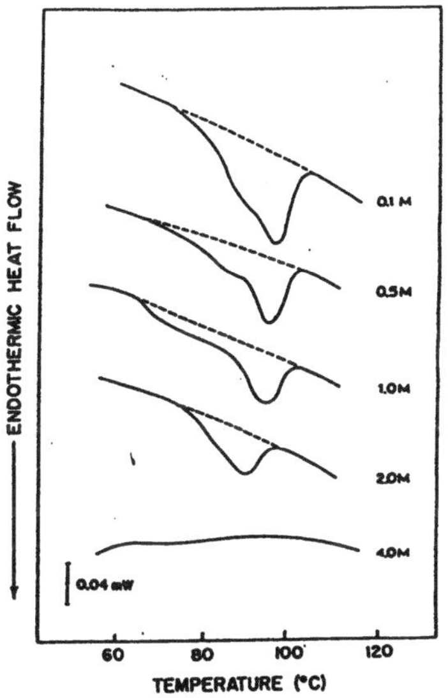


**Figure 8.** Influence of NaSCN concentration on the DSC thermal curves of a micelle protein isolate from fababean. Sample concentration was 20% total solids and heating rate was 5°C/min. [10]

With both vicilin and legumin in the isolate, there is an increase in the stability associated with increased salt concentration for the non-chaotropic anions (sulfate, acetate and chloride) similar to that observed for the purified vicilin. The behavior with NaSCN is also similar to that for the purified vicilin; Td values decrease with increasing NaSCN concentration due to binding of the thiocyanate ion (Figs. 9 and 10). The relative effectiveness of the stabilizing salts in terms of their positions in the lyotropic series also follows the same trend as the purified sample in that sulfate > acetate, chloride > thiocyanate. Interestingly, although the difference between acetate and chloride is not significant in either of the two proteins in the isolate or the purified vicilin fraction, the relative positions of the two curves for vicilin is reversed in comparison to those for the purified sample. This leads to the suggestion that the simple relationship between σ and Td observed with the pure protein may be complicated by other factors such as phenolic compounds in the isolate.

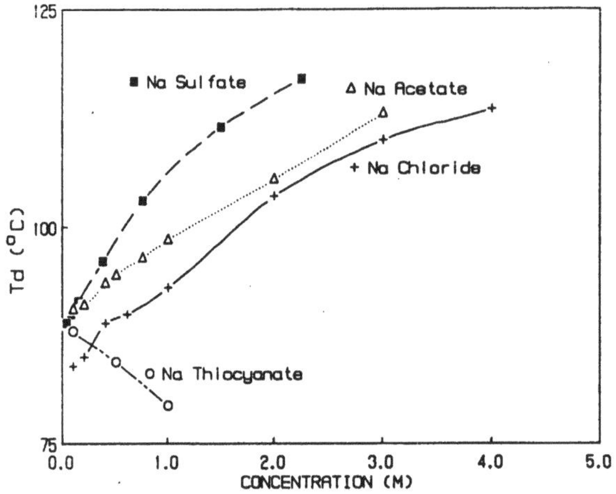


**Figure 9.** Influence of anions of sodium salts on the denaturation temperature (Td) of vicilin in a micelle protein isolate from fababean as a function of concentration. [10]

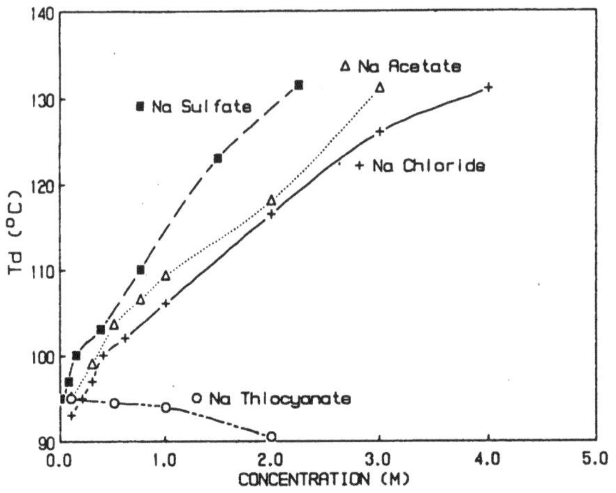


**Figure 10.** Influence of the anions of sodium salts on the denaturation temperature (Td) of legumin in a micelle protein isolate from fababean as a function of concentration. [10]

Furthermore, if the effect of sulfate for both vicilin and legumin is considered in terms of ionic strength rather than concentration (i.e. charge difference eliminated), the resulting Td values are comparable to $NaCH_3COOH$ and NaCl, suggesting that in an isolate, it may be sufficient to distinguish between chaotropic and non-chaotropic effects and the differential effect of these salts on hydrophobic interactions is minimized. However, one should not dismiss the lyotropic effect entirely. Upon examination of the shapes of the stabilizing curves as a function of concentration, there appears to be two distinct phases with a break at a concentration of 0.5 M (Figs 9 and 10). This break is more apparent for the legumin curves (Fig. 10). In fact, the curves have been described as biphasic linear relationships with an inflection point at 0.5 M salt.[10] The first phase corresponds to that region in which electrostatic influences dominate while stabilization in the second phase is primarily associated with the influence of these salts on hydrophobic interactions. It is clear, therefore, that even though the differences due to various anions is minimized in the isolate, the stabilization of these proteins due to the influence of the salts on hydrophobic interactions is in effect.

## Conclusions

Salts can have a major influence on the thermal stability of proteins as evidenced by changes in the Td values when analyzed using differential scanning calorimetry. The extent of this stabilization is dependent on both salt concentration and the type of anion in the salt. For those anions which have a stabilizing effect on the protein, an increase in salt concentration results in increased Td values. This has been observed for both purified proteins (vicilin) and proteins in a commercial protein isolate from fababean (vicilin and legumin). Interestingly, for proteins in the isolate, the relationship between salt concentration and Td could be described as a biphasic one with the two phases corresponding to the regions where electrostatic and lyotropic influences dominate. Furthermore, the extent of stabilization at a given concentration was dependent on the anion type; those with higher molal surface tension increments had a greater influence on hydrophobic interactions resulting in higher Td values. This relationship was more apparent for the purified vicilin. The differential effect is lessened in an environment containing other proteins and non-proteinaceous components.

The destabilization of these proteins by NaSCN is associated with the binding capacity of the thiocyanate anion. This is also a reflection of the lower $\sigma$ and thus the position of NaSCN in the lyotropic series.

The significance of the change in protein stability in terms of structure formation has been shown for both a self associated micelle type network and a network produced by heat denaturation of the protein. Interestingly, stabilization of the protein resulted in decreased protein-protein interactions and overall structure formation for heat induced vicilin networks. At high Td values (i.e. those with 0.5 M $Na_2SO_4$) the nature of the network was also shifted from a crosslinked structure to a viscous mass. The NaSCN also inhibited network formation, possibly due to the increase in charge associated with the binding of thiocyanate which promoted solubility even in the denatured state.

## References


[1] Kinsella, J.E.: Functional properties of proteins in foods: A survey. CRC Crit. Rev. Food Sci. Nutr. 7 (1976) 216-280.

[2] Murray, E.D., C.D. Myers, and L.D. Barker: Protein product and process for preparing same. Can. Patent #1,028,552. 1978.

[3] Murray, E.D., C.D. Myers, L.D. Barker and T.J. Maurice: Functional attributes of proteins - A noncovalent approach to processing and utilizing proteins. In: Utilization of Protein Resources. D.W. Stanley, E.D. Murray and D.H. Lees (Eds.) pp. 158-176. Food and Nutrition Press, Inc., Westport, CT. 1981.

[4] Arntfield, S.D. and E.D. Murray: The influence of processing parameters on food protein functionality. I. Differential scanning calorimetry as an indicator of protein denaturation. Can. Inst. Food Sci. Technol. J. 14 (1981) 289-294.

[5] Privalov, P.L. and N.N. Khechinashvili: a thermodynamic approach to the problem of stabilization of globular protein structure: a calorimetric study. J. Mol. Biol. 86 (1974) 665-684.

[6] von Hippel, P.H. and T. Schleich: The effects of neutral salts on the structure and conformational stability of macromolecules in solution. In: Structure and Stability of Biological Macromolecules. S.N. Timasheff and G.D. Fasman (Eds.) pp. 417-573. Marcel Dekker Inc., New York. 1969.

[7] Arakawa, J. and S.N. Timasheff: Preferential interactions of proteins with salts in concentrated solutions. Biochemistry 24 (1982) 6545-6552.

[8] Melander, W. and C. Horvath: Salt effects on hydrophobic interactions in precipitation and chromatography of proteins: An interpretation of the lyotropic series. Arch. Biochem. Biophys. 183 (1977) 200-215.

[9] Ismond, M.A.H., E.D. Murray and S.D. Arntfield: The role of non-covalent forces in micelle formation by vicilin from Vicia faba. II. The effect of stabilizing and destabilizing anions on protein interactions. Food Chem. 21 (1986) 27-46.

[10] Arntfield, S.D., E.D. Murray and M.A.H. Ismond: Effect of salt on the thermal stability of storage proteins from fababean (Vicia faba). J. Food Sci. 51 (1986) 371-377.

# PHASE EQUILIBRIA IN BROAD BEAN LEGUMIN-NEUTRAL SALT-WATER SYSTEM

V.V.Suchkov, I.A.Popello, V.Ya.Grinberg, V.B.Tolstoguzov[1)]

One of the most clear-cut manifestations of intermolecular interactions in multicomponent protein systems is phase demixing. It may end with a liquid and solid (amorphous or crystalline) phase or with two liquid phases. Particularly, liquid-liquid phase demixing takes place in Protein-Polysaccharide-Water systems or in Protein1-Protein2-Water systems. This type of demixing is characterized by separation of protein and polysaccharide or by separation of proteins when a system is demixed. This phenomenon is known as thermodynamic incompatibility of protein and polysaccharide or of different proteins with each other and it is discussed in some detail in literature [1].

Another significant example of phase demixing in multicomponent protein systems is the behaviour of salt solutions of globulins near the isoelectric point. On cooling these solutions separate into two liquid phases differing very much in protein contents. This process is completely reversible. On heating systems become again homogeneous. The phenomenon of liquid-liquid demixing was first observed by Show and coworkers [2] on ß-Lactoglobulin-Glycin-Water system. Later on this phenomenon was revealed for other proteins as well [3-5]. The few investigations do not furnish an explanation of the nature of interactions causing liquid-liquid demixing in Globulin-Salt-Water systems.

In the present study we tried to estimate the contributions of different types of interaction to demixing in the Broad Bean Legumin-Salt-Water system.

The molecular mass of broad bean legumin (11S globulin) is 300 kD. Its molecule is a compact globule and consists of 12 (6 basic and 6 acidic) polypeptide chains. According to the data published elsewhere, the pH value of the legumin isoelectric point is 4.8 [6]. Legumin does not dissolve in the range of pH 4.6 - 6.0 in the absence of a neutral salt. When 0.3-0.8 moles of salt are added, liquid-liquid demixing is observed in this pH range. In this case the protein concentration in the lower phase runs to 50%. As the temperature rises, the system may go over into a homogeneous state. But once the temperature is lowered, liquid-liquid demixing occurs again.

Figure 1 shows phase diagrams of the Legumin-Sodium Sulphate -Water system at pH 4.8. One can see that the binodal has an upper critical point, which is characterized by the values of critical temperature, Tc, and protein critical concentration, Cc. The binodal is symmetric about the

---

1) A.N.Nesmeyanov Institute of Organoelement Compounds of the USSR Academy of Sciences, V-312, Vavilov Street 28, 117312 Moscow, U.S.S.R.

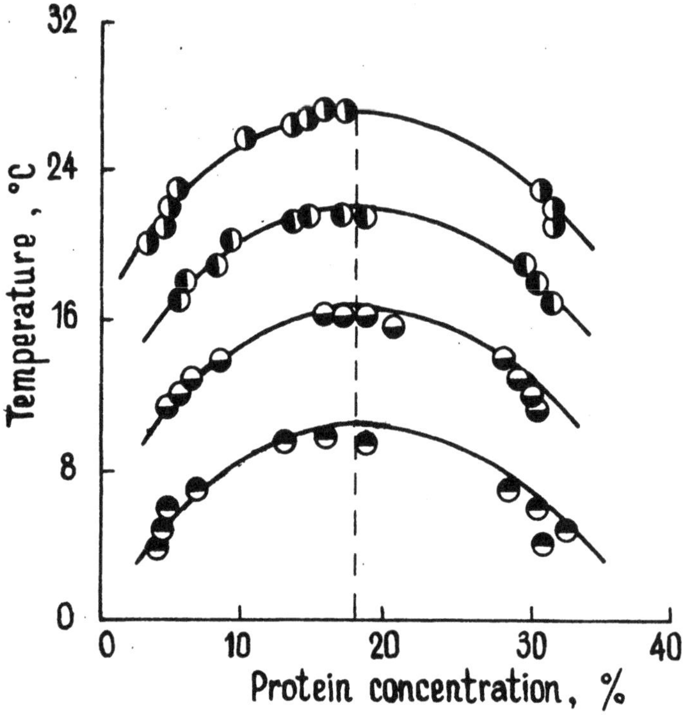


Fig. 1. Phase diagrams of Broad Bean Legumin-Sodium Sulphate-Water system for various sodium sulphate concentrations:
◐ - 0.5 M; ◐ - 0.54 M; ◒ - 0.6 M; ◓ - 0.69 M.
—— - binodal, --- - rectilinear diameter.

rectilinear diameter over a studied temperature range . When the neutral salt concentration is varied only the binodal position relative to the temperature scale is changed, while the shape of the binodal curve and the value of protein critical concentration remain constant. In our system, the latter value was equal to 18% w in the whole studied range of salt concentration. This value is in agreement with that of protein critical concentration established for arachin [4] . The value of critical temperature decreases with an increasing concentration of sodium sulphate.

Figure 2 presents the critical temperature as a function of molar concentration of various salts. For all the salts studied, the critical temperature is lowered with an increasing salt concentration. The plots of critical temperature against salt concentration for 1-2 electrolytes are shifted to the region of lower salt concentrations and are steep, as compared to those for 1-1 electrolytes. If we represent the critical temperature as a function of ionic strength, the nature of salt will not practically affect this relationship.

Such behaviour of the studied system is, probably, a consequence of the polyampholytic nature of protein molecules. In a solution, protein molecules carry both positive and negative charges. It results in rath-

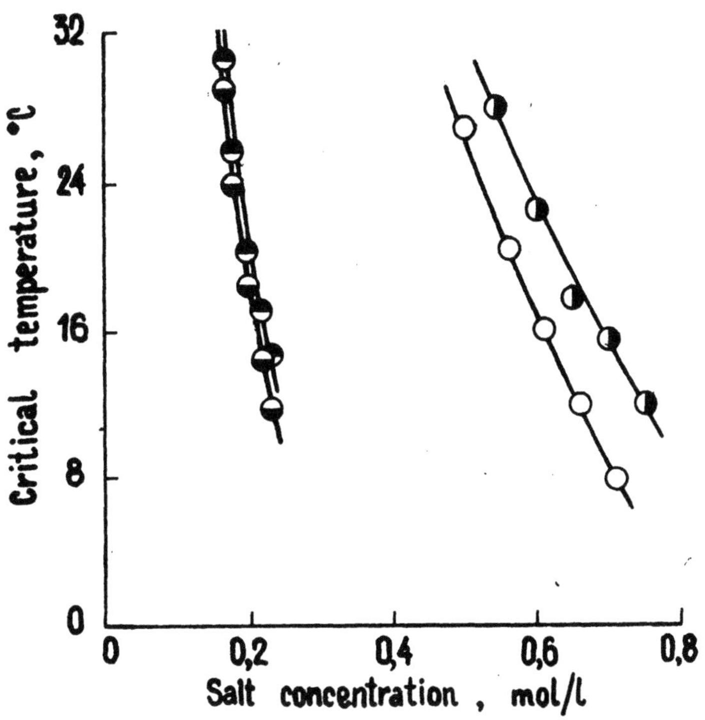


Fig. 2. Plots of critical demixing temperature of Broad Bean Legumin-Salt-Water system versus salt concentration: ○ - NaCl; ◑ - KCl; ◒ - $Na_2SO_4$; ◓ - $(NH_4)_2SO_4$.

er large dipole moments of protein molecules [7] . It is known that the dipole moment of the edestin molecule (11S globulin of hemp) is 1500D. Broad bean belongs to the same class of protein, so its molecules are expected to have the same value of the dipole moment.

Thus, near the isoelectric point in the absence of salt, protein molecules interact as dipoles. In this case, the interaction energy of protein molecules, W, equals the energy of dipole-dipole interaction, $W_{DD}$, and exceeds substantially the energy of thermal motion, kT:

$$W = W_{DD} \gg kT.$$

Therefore globulins are insoluble at their isoelectric point.

On addition of salt, two types of interaction take place: interaction between protein molecules and interaction of protein molecules with the ionic environment. Here the interaction energy of protein molecules will be equal to the difference of energies of the dipole-dipole interaction, $W_{DD}$, and of the ion-dipole interaction, $W_{ID}$. At some salt concentrations, the interaction energy of protein molecules becomes comparable with the energy of thermal motion:

$$W = W_{DD} - W_{ID} \simeq kT,$$

i.e. the energy of thermal motion is sufficient for system transition to a homogeneous state. So, the critical temperature is a measure of relationship between the protein molecule interaction energy and the thermal motion energy.

A salt attenuates the interaction between protein molecules. The energy of interaction between salt ions and protein molecules, i.e. the energy of ion-dipole interaction, is proportional with the ionic strength of a solution [8] . It is evident from Fig.3 that the higher the ionic strength, the lower the critical temperature of demixing.

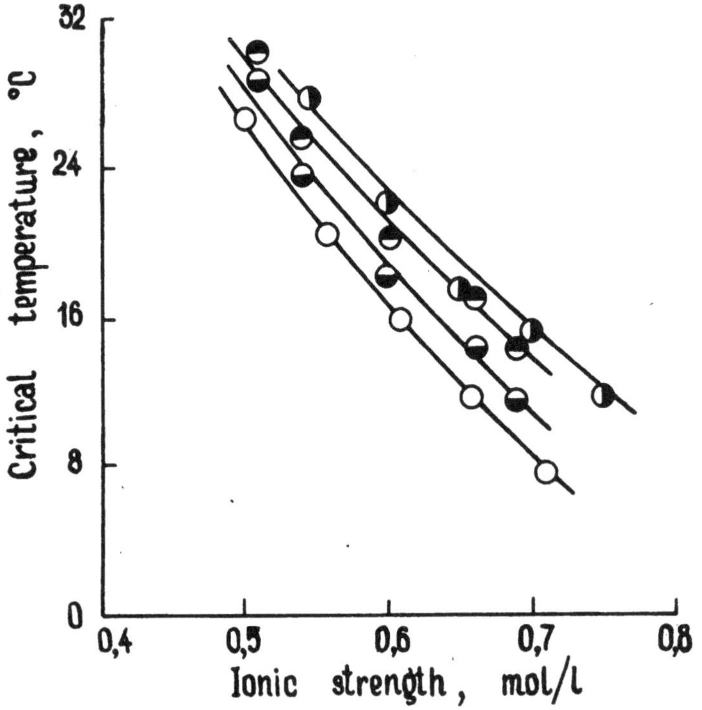


Fig. 3. Plots of demixing critical temperature of Broad Bean Legumin-Salt-Water system versus ionic strength:
○- NaCl; ◐- KCl; ◒- $Na_2SO_4$; ◓- $(NH_4)_2SO_4$.

It is known that the energy of interaction between protein molecules also depends on the dielectric constant of a medium [8,9] . Addition of low molecular weight substances into a system may change markedly the solvent dielectric constant. Water has a fairly high dielectric constant equal to around 80 at 20°C. The dielectric constant of a solution increases on addition of high-polar substances, say, amino acids, and decreases on introduction of low-polar substances, such as alcohols.

Figure 4 shows the effect of glycin and ethanol on the value of the critical temperature of demixing. One can see that on addition of glycin the solution dielectric constant increases, while the demixing critical temperature is lowered. Introduction of ethanol, which decreases the dielectric constant of a solution, causes the demixing critical temperature to rise.

Figure 5 plots demixing critical temperature versus pH value. It is evident that the plotted curves have maxima. The value of critical tem-

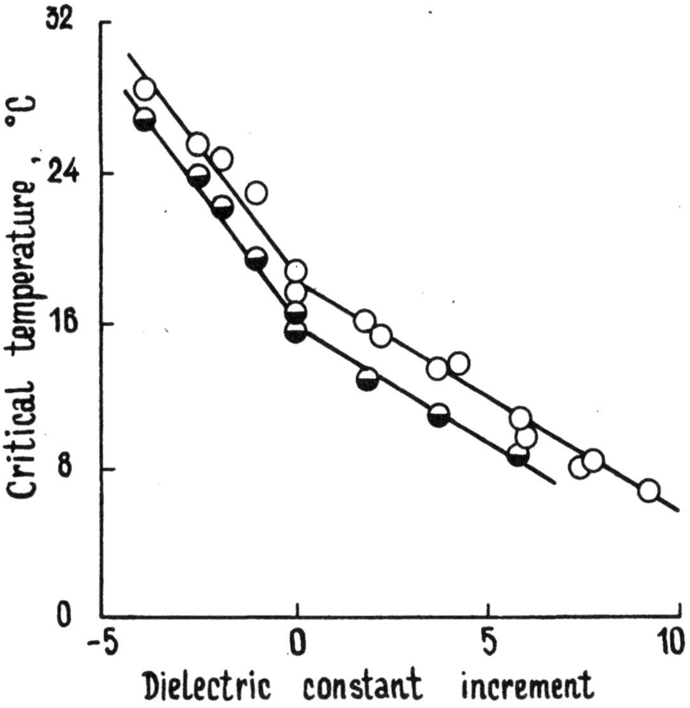


Fig. 4. Plots of demixing critical temperature of Broad Bean Legumin-Salt-Water system versus increase of the dielectric constant for various concentrations of NaCl:
○ - 0.6 M; ◒ 0.63 M.

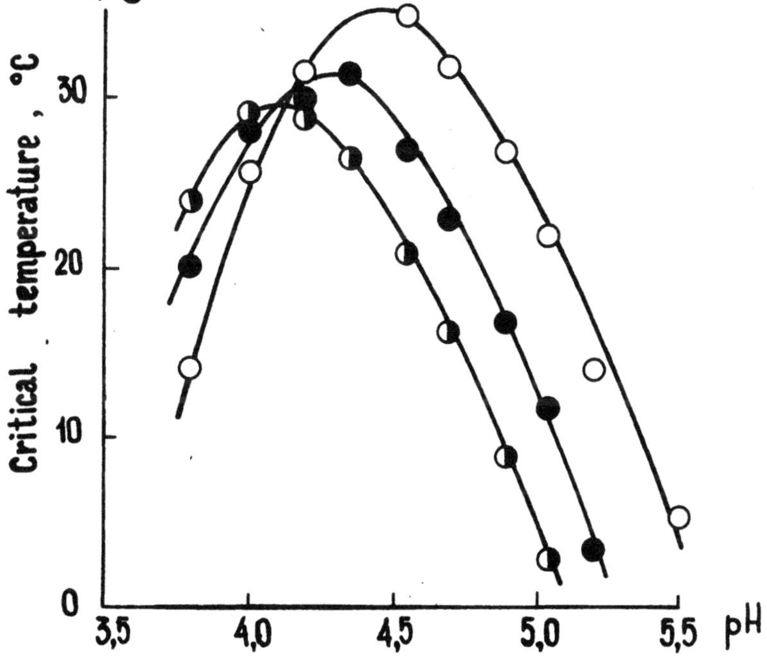


Fig. 5. Plots of demixing critical temperature of Broad Bean Legumin-Salt-Water system versus pH for various concentrations of NaCl:
○ - 0.5 M; ● - 0.6 M; ◑ - 0.7 M.

perature at a maximum goes down monotonically as the ionic strength increases.

When pH of a solution differs from pH of the isoelectric point, the protein molecule has an excess charge. This leads to electrostatic repulsion between protein molecules carrying like charges. Then the energy of interaction between protein molecules at a certain specific pH value different from pH of the isoelectric point consists of three terms:

$$W = W_{DD} - W_{ID} - W_{CC}$$

where $W_{CC}$ is the energy of electrostatic interaction of charged protein molecules (charge-charge interaction energy).

Obviously, an increasing charge of protein molecules, i.e. an increasing energy of electrostatic interaction should lower the demixing critical temperature at a constant ionic strength. At the distance from the isoelectric point, the electrostatic interaction energy is mainly defined by the energy of charge-charge interaction, $W_{CC}$, and the system remains homogeneous up to the freezing point of a solution. At the same time, as a glance at Figure 5 shows, when the salt concentration increases, the position of a maximum shifts to the region of lower pH values. This may be attributed to the shift of the protein isoelectric point due to the specific interaction of protein molecules with low molecular weight ions [10] . The shift of a solubility minimum of legumin with an increasing salt concentration may give information about the shift of the isoelectric point (Figure 6).

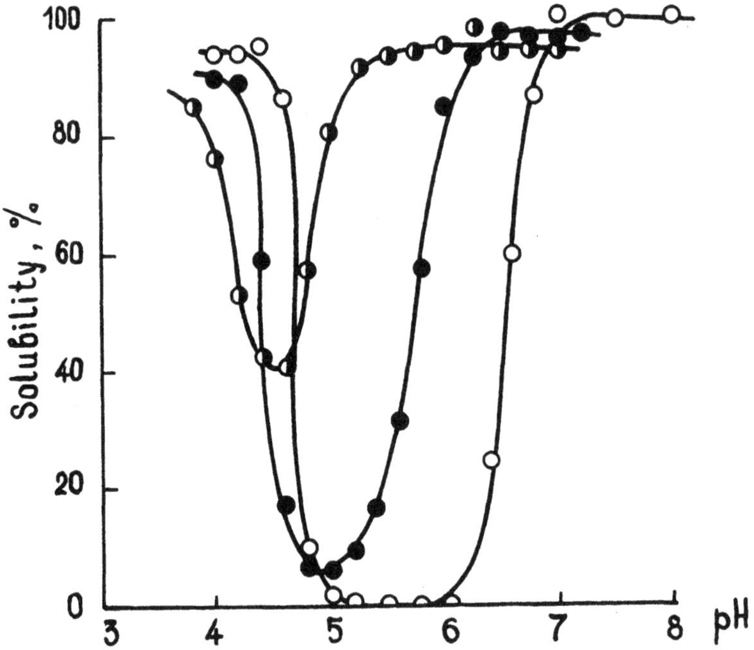


Fig. 6. Plots of solubility of Broad Bean Legumin-Salt-Water system versus pH for various concentrations of NaCl:
◐- 0 M; ●- 0.3 M; ◑- 0.5 M

The shift of a solubility minimum of legumin to the region of more acidic pH values is indicative of the predominant specific interaction of protein molecules with anions - chloride ions.

The reported data permit a conclusion that the phenomenon of liquid-liquid phase demixing in the Broad Bean Legumin- Neutral Salt-Water system relies on a certain relationship between the attractive forces (dipole-dipole interaction) and the forces of repulsion (ion-dipole and charge-charge interactions) between protein molecules. This phenomenon is aggravated by the specific interaction of protein molecules with low molecular weight ions.

Investigation of liquid-liquid phase demixing in Globulin-Salt-Water systems is a matter of interest for protein isolation, concentration, and processing. Tombs [11] proposed a method of processing highly concentrated globulin solutions into food protein fibres with an oriented microstructure. In our laboratory a preparation method has been developed for isolating legumins and vicilins from broad bean and pea seeds [12]. This method enables concentrated protein solutions to be produced. The investigation of liquid-liquid phase demixing made it possible to optimize the isolation conditions. Liquid-liquid phase demixing permits production of two-phase systems based on the globulin fraction of seeds and processing of these systems into food protein fibres of an oriented structure.

REFERENCES


1 Tolstoguzov. V.B., Grinberg,V.Ya., Guruv, A.N. J.Agric.Food Chem. 33 (1985) 151-159.

2 Show, T.M., Janson, E.F., & Lineweaver, H. J.Chem.Phys. (1944) 12, 439-448.

3 Van Megen, W.H.J. Agric. Food Chem. 22 (1974) , 126-129.

4 Tombs, M.P., Newsom, B.G., Wilding, P. Int.J.Peptide Protein Res. 6 (1974) , 253-277.

5 Ishimoto,C., Tanaka, T. Phys.Rev.Letters .39(1977) ,474-477.

6 Derbyshire, E., Wright, D.J., Boulter, D. Phytochem.15(1976) ,3-24.

7 Stuart, H.A.,Julfs, J. In: Die Physik der Hochpolymeren.Bd.2/Ed.H.A. Stuart.Springer-Verlag,Berlin 1953,618-638.

8.Kirkwood, J.G.In: Proteins, AminoAcids and Peptides as Ions and Dipolar Ions/Eds. Cohn,E.J. & Edsall, J.T. Reinhold Publishing Corporation, New York 1943,276-306.

9 Fuoss,R.M. J.Am.Chem.Soc. 58 (1936) ,982-984.

10 Longsworth,L.G., Jacobson,C.F. J.Phys.Coll.Chem 53(1949) ,126-134.

11 Tombs, M.P. Brit.Pat. 1265661, 1972.

12 Popello, I.A., Suchkov, V.V., Grinberg, V.Ya., Tolstoguzov, V.B. Prikladn. biokhim. mikrobiologhiya, 24 (1988) 1, 50-55.(in Russian).

# SOME PHYSICO-CHEMICAL AND TECHNOLOGICAL ASPECTS OF INTERACTIONS IN PROTEIN MULTICOMPONENT SYSTEMS

V.Tolstoguzov[1)]

## INTRODUCTION

Foodstuffs are practically always multicomponent systems. They usually contain proteins or protein-polysaccharide mixtures. Proteins and polysaccharides are the most important types of emulsifiers, stabilizers, foaming and gelling agents used by food industry. Their interactions determine the feature of the structure, rheological and other physico-chemical properties of many processed food systems and foods. That is why the interactions of these main kinds of food macromolecules are of great value to the understanding of the relationships between the composition, structure, and physico-chemical properties of real food systems. But until recently no information about the interactions in biopolymer mixtures, the most important for food modelling, has been available at all. I mean sufficiently high-concentrated systems containing globular proteins and their mixtures with polysaccharides. Systematic investigations in this field were started 20 years ago in our laboratory. What I am going to do today is to talk about some recent findings, namely about the phenomenon of incompatibility of proteins and polysaccharides. After that we will take up some general questions: What are the applications of these findings ? What is the significance of the phenomenon of biopolymer incompatibility to food science and technology ?

## 1. THERMODYNAMIC INCOMPATIBILITY OF PROTEINS AND POLYSACCHARIDES

The phenomenon of thermodynamic incompatibility of biopolymers has been so far studied using more than 150 systems containing the main types of food proteins and polysaccharides [1-5]. This phenomenon is that solution mixtures of biopolymers may undergo liquid-phase separation, with the macromolecular components concentrated mainly in different phases. If we mix, for example, aqueous solutions of a protein and a polysaccharide, providing their rather high bulk concentration, this mixture may break down spontaneously into two phases, one of which is relatively rich in protein and the other is relatively rich in polysaccharide. This phenomenon is essentially opposite to the phenomenon of formation of intermacromolecular complexes. It takes place under the conditions where complex formation is inhibited. This means that mixtures of biopolymer solutions can undergo phase separation only under certain specific conditions, namely at pH va-

1) A.N.Nesmeyanov Institute of Organoelement Compounds of the USSR Academy of Sciences, V-312, Vavilov Street 28, 117312 Moscow, U.S.S.R.

lues and salt concentrations which inhibit interactions between the different macromolecular species and encourage their self-association, i.e. under the conditions promoting interactions between macromolecules of the same type. As a result, every macromolecule in solution mixtures should be preferentially surrounded by macromolecules of the same type. If the difference between biopolymers in hydrophilicity increases, their incompatibility increases, too. Phase separation occurs only where the mixing of biopolymer solutions is an endothermic process.

Thermodynamic incompatibility of biopolymers is a rather general phenomenon. It takes place, first, in solution mixtures of all classes of proteins and polysaccharides; second, in solution mixtures of proteins belonging to different classes, according to the Osborn classification and of proteins having different conformations, including the solution mixtures of the native and denatured forms of the same protein; and third, in solution mixtures of structurally unlike polysaccharides. Among all studied systems containing globular proteins, only two were found to remain single-phase over a wide range of pH values, ionic strength and biopolymer concentrations. These are mixtures of serum albumin with ovalbumin as well as with pectin. A small difference between biopolymers in hydrophilicity making for their compatibility is apparently characteristic of mixtures of proteins belonging to the same class within the Osborn classification or of the same mixtures of proteins and polysaccharides.

It is noteworthy that incompatibility of proteins and polysaccharides is usually typical of food systems. It shows up at pH values above the protein isoelectric point and at sufficiently high ionic strength. This means that the biopolymer incompatibility phenomenon is characteristic of real foods owing to the features of their composition. That is why this phenomenon is of importance to the formation of structure and properties of foods. It is also worth noting that the Osborn classification of proteins according to their solubility in different aqueous media reflects the difference between proteins in their interaction with solvent. This classification is essentially thermodynamic and convenient for use in this field of investigation.

Phase equilibrium in biopolymer mixtures has been studied by means of chemical analysis of coexisting phase compositions and by the phase volume ratio method. The latter permits us to determine phase diagrams without chemical analysis [5, 6] . Figure 1 shows a series of phase diagrams for protein-polysaccharide-water, polysaccharide-polysaccharide-water, and protein-protein-water systems [3-5,7] . As a rule, phase diagrams of three components are presented in the form of triangular coordinates, as can be seen from Figure 1A. In the case of food systems, however, the concentration of the water component is considerably higher compared to those of biopolymers. That is why it is easier to make use of the rectangular coordinates, as is shown in Figures 1B, C, and D. It is important to check experimentally that the conditions of mixing of biopolymer solutions and the conditions of centrifugal separation of the coexisting phases are

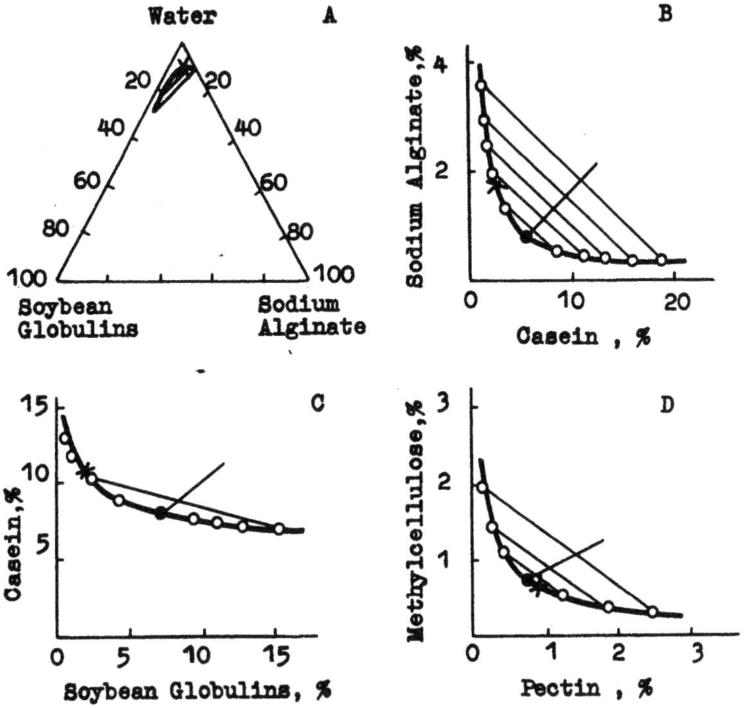


Fig. 1. Phase diagrams for biopolymer I-biopolymer II-water systems at 20°C: A- soybean globulins-sodium alginate (pH 9.0); B- casein-sodium alginate (pH 7.0); C- soybean globulins-casein (pH 6.9); D- pectin-methylcellulose (pH 5.0, 0.5 M NaCl).

sufficient to determine an equilibrium phase diagram.

In phase diagrams, the concentrations of biopolymers are plotted in per cent. The positions of the binodal curve, the critical points, the tie-lines, the phase separation threshold, and the rectilinear diameter are indicated. The composition area of single-phase biopolymer mixtures is separated by the binodal curve from mixtures which are two-phase systems. At a critical point the two coexisting phases are equal to one another in volume and composition. The phase separation threshold is a minimum total concentration of biopolymers required for phase separation to occur. The thin lines are tie-lines . The tie-line connects the points representing the compositions of the coexisting phases. The compositions of mixtures separating into phases of the same volume are represented by a rectilinear diameter. This is the curve passing through the center of the tie-lines.

The obtained results show that the phase state of biopolymer mixtures and the compositions of the coexisting phases depend on the following factors: pH values, concentrations of salts and biopolymers as well as the difference between biopolymers in hydrophilicity, molecular masses and conformational state of their molecules.

The first feature of biopolymer mixtures is rather high values of

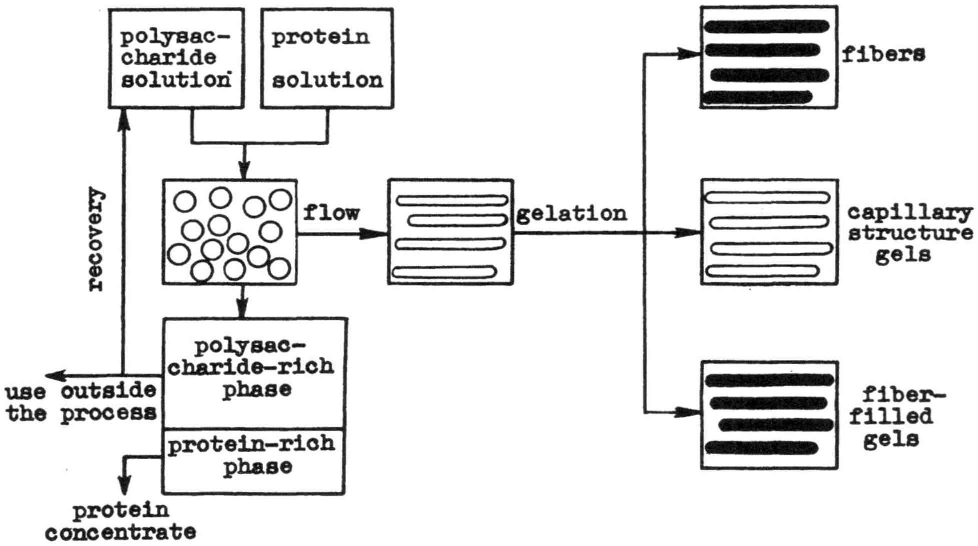


Fig.2 General scheme for the membraneless osmosis and the spinneretless spinning processes.

their phase separation thresholds. This means that biopolymers are better compatible than synthetic polymers. The relatively high values of phase separation threshold may be attributed to the compactness of globular protein molecules. The phase separation threshold decreases on transition to proteins with unfolded conformation and then to polysaccharides of a linear structure.

For instance, the value of phase separation threshold usually exceeds 15% for mixtures of globular proteins. It is about 2 to 4% or higher for globular protein-polysaccharide mixtures and about 2% for gelatin-polysaccharide mixtures as well as for mixtures of structurally unlike polysaccharides [3-7] . The phase separation threshold for biopolymer mixtures is in a concentration area corresponding to transition from dilute to moderately concentrated solutions or within the concentration range corresponding to the molecular volume overlapping. This transition from dilute to moderately concentrated solutions of compact globular proteins can obviously take place at markedly higher concentrations, as compared to other polymers.

The second feature of biopolymer mixtures is a high degree of asymmetry of their phase diagrams. There are two types of asymmetry. The first is related to the effect of molecular mass and the second reflects the effect of relative hydrophilicity on biopolymer compatibility. Accordingly, firstly the binodal curve usually lies closer to the axis of the component with a lower molecular mass. Secondly, the critical point does not coincide with the phase separation threshold but instead it is shifted towards the concentration axis of the biopolymer of a lower hydrophilicity value.

It is obvious that in mixtures of various biopolymer species the difference of macromolecules in hydrophilicity and conformational state may be greater than in mixtures of globular proteins. Therefore, protein-polysaccharide mixtures are characterized, as a rule, by a lower phase separation threshold and by a higher asymmetry of phase diagrams, compared to solution mixtures of proteins. Now we will briefly consider the applied significance of this phenomenon. We will start with the membraneless osmosis process.

## 2.THE MEMBRANELESS OSMOSIS PROCESS

This is a new method for concentrating protein solutions. Behind this process are the phenomena of thermodynamic incompatibility of proteins and polysaccharides as well as of high asymmetry of phase diagrams of these biopolymers. The phase diagram asymmetry implies that there is a great difference between the concentrations of macromolecules in the two coexisting equilibrium phases (Figure 2). This difference in the concentrations may be 10- to 25-fold or even more. As a result, one phase of a two-phase system is a relatively high-concentrated protein solution, while the other is a rather dilute polysaccharide solution. The membraneless osmosis process (Figure 2) is notable for the transfer of the solvent between the solutions of two incompatible biopolymers, namely, water transfer from the protein solution to the polysaccharide solution. The function of a membrane in this process is performed by the interface between the two phases [4,7]. This process was first successfully employed to concentrate milk proteins from skimmed milk by means of apple pectin. On addition of 1% pectin to skimmed milk the system breaks down into two liquid phases one of which contains about 85-91% of milk proteins with concentrations around 20-30%. The degree of the milk protein concentration depends on the quantity of added pectin, its molecular mass and esterification degree, as well as on the temperature of a system. Phase equilibrium establishes itself one minute after the pectin solution and skimmed milk were mixed up. This is provided by a very small diameter of dispersed particles and, accordingly, by the highly developed interface between the two phases of water-in-water emulsions. This type of emulsions is characterized by a very low interfacial tension and by similar phase viscosities. The emulsion phases are then separated by means of a separator. Pectin can be precipitated from the dilute polysaccharide-rich phase in the form of complexes with milk proteins at pH below the protein isoelectric point and re-used in the process [7].

The membraneless osmosis process is also useful for food protein fractionation and purification. In this case it is of importance that phase separation thresholds of various protein solution mixtures with the same polysaccharide may be significantly different. The partition coefficient of a dissolved (thermodynamically compatible) biopolymer in the two coexisting phases seems to be also of great value for successful application of the membraneless osmosis method. For instance, in the concentration of skimmed milk proteins the obtained pectin-rich phase did not prove to contain bovin serum albumin. It has been found out, however, that bovin serum albumin is compatible with pectin under a wide range of conditions. This means that it can be concentrated in the protein-rich phase owing to its better co-solubility with proteins, as compared to polysaccharides. An important consideration for this process is distribution of metal ions between the phases of a system. This opens up new ways for controlling the composition and functional properties of food protein isolates. Now we will also briefly consider the spinneretless spinning process. Here the biopolymer incompatibility phenomenon is used to prepare processed two-phase systems.

## 3.THE SPINNERETLESS SPINNING PROCESS

The basic idea of the spinneretless spinning process is clarified in Figure 2. The initial systems, namely water-in-water emulsions, can be obtained, for instance, by mixing solutions of various proteins or of proteins and polysaccharides. Spinneretless spinning is a process of shaping heterophase liquid systems. This process makes use of nozzles just as the spinneret spinning technique does. The difference between these two processes lies in the fact that in the spinneret process each nozzle produces only a single fibre, whereas in spinneretless spinning each nozzle provides simultaneously many fine fibres. Thus, spinneretless spinning (or maybe better to say spinneretless fibre shaping) is the process of shaping an anisotropic fibrous structure of heterophase liquid systems in flow and fixing the shape of deformed dispersed particles through rapid gelation of one or both phases of a system. Using various compositions of two-phase liquid systems as well as different procedures for generating flow and gelling the jet we are able to produce a wide range of food protein products with a fibrous structure, as shown in Figure 2.

If the dispersed phase is gelled in flow, fibres are formed, namely fibres of protein or polysaccharide. It depends on the composition of emulsion phases and on the gelation conditions. It is important that both short and very long fibres can be produced. The latter are possible due to the orientation and coalescence of the deformed dispersed particles in flow by sufficiently high volume fraction of a dispersed phase. If the dispersion medium of a system is converted into the gelled state we obtain gels filled with oriented liquid filaments. These gels are called gels of a capillary structure. And finally, gelation of the two phases of a liquid system in flow may give rise to gels filled with oriented fibres [2,4,7,8] . In the latter case two-phase liquid systems containing two gelling agents which are concentrated in different phases of a system are used. The food gelling agents can be various proteins or proteins and polysaccharides which are incompatible with each other. The two system phases can be converted into the gelled state consequently or simultaneously. This means that the initially obtained gels of a capillary structure can be converted into gels filled with fibres. Various coagulating baths, say, heated salt solutions, as well as heating in a gas medium or other gelation procedures can be used to gel a dope jet [8] .

Textured food products produced by spinneretless shaping can be regarded as composite solids. They are notable for an anisotropy of structure and strength and, hence, can closely simulate traditional meat products. What is the significance of the studied physico-chemical phenomena lying behind spinneretless spinning to food science and technology? I mean the phenomena of thermodynamic incompatibility of biopolymers in solution mixtures, membraneless osmosis and deformation of dispersed particles of water-in-water emulsions in flow. Their significance is obviously based on the heterophase nature of foods. Moreover, it is noteworthy that the manufacture of foodstuffs usually involves shaping of liquid heterogeneous systems which are subsequently converted into the gel- or the glass-state. That is why the spinneretless spinning process is so important to the formation of structure and a set of properties of many foodstuffs. Just for this reason a wide range of traditional and novel food technologies can be regarded as particular versions of spinneretless spinning. For many of them the membraneless osmosis process is important, too [8] . Now let us briefly discuss some other promising applications for the phenomenon of incompatibility of biopolymers [7-10] .

## 4. FUNCTIONAL PROPERTIES OF FOOD PROTEINS

The problems of successful use of food protein additives and of protein processing into foods make it necessary to estimate and control the structural functions of proteins in food systems. Our knowledge of the area of protein functional properties is still rudimentary. This depends to a large degree on the multicomponent nature of real food systems in which the behaviour of protein may be exceedingly various and more complicated than that in model systems of a lower concentration and a less complex composition that are usually the object of study. It is quite obvious that moderately concentrated mixtures of interacting macromolecules, containing colloidal particles at the same time, are far richer in properties than dilute binary solutions of biopolymers. What is the role of studying biopolymer incompatibility in the understanding of food protein functional properties? The logical starting point is to discuss some volume properties of multicomponent protein systems. A protein added to a food system may be incompatible with the macromolecular components of this system. As a result, the functional properties of an added protein may show up within the volume of one of the system phases in a different manner and to a larger measure than they will in the whole volume of the system. Phase separation of biopolymer solution mixtures in flow may invite the membraneless osmosis and spinneretless spinning processes to take place. This means that the composition, structure, and properties of the two phases and of the whole system may be altered considerably. In view of the fact that biopolymers are limited compatible, i.e. limited co-soluble in aqueous media some system phases may be mixed, filled , or complex gels whose properties differ strongly from those of gels of particular macromolecular components of the system taken separately [7,9,10] . For instance, on gelation of biopolymer solution mixtures three interesting effects manifest themselves. First, critical concentrations for gelation of each of the components in solution mixtures are low compared to their binary solutions. Second, the gelation rate of biopolymer mixtures is accelerated and the elastic moduli of single phase mixtures increase. And finally, if one of the three-dimensional networks of a mixed gel is thermoreversible over its melting temperature range, such a mixed gel is notable for an anomalously high deformability. Studies of mixed gels are still in the development phase. Nevertheless, the obtained results indicate substantial effects of protein interactions with other proteins and polysaccharides on the gelling behaviour of food systems [7,9,10] .

Now I should like to call your attention to the problem of protein surface activity in multicomponent systems. Two key factors determine the effect of any protein on the surface properties of food systems. They are (1) the relative hydrophilicity of a protein compared to the other ones of the same system and (2) the relative conformational stability and ability of proteins for intermolecular interactions at the interface. We will only discuss the former, because it is related to the biopolymer incompatibility phenomenon. It is essential that addition to a protein solution of some other biopolymer incompatible with this protein will degrade the quality of the solvent, as compared to a pure solvent. This promotes protein concentration at the interface. The least hydrophilic protein of any system, i.e. the protein for which an aqueous solvent is a worse one than for other proteins of the system, usually concentrates at the interface. Therefore, evaluation of the relative hydrophilicity of proteins in sufficiently concentrated systems is of great importance. This value can be obtained by two techniques. First, the asymmetry of phase diagrams for protein-protein-water systems is useful as a measure of relative hydrophilicity of proteins. The water concentration is always higher in the phase containing protein of higher hydrophilicity. The phase diagram asymmetry can be evaluated by several methods : first, by the ratio of the critical point coordinates, second, by the length of the segment of a binodal curve between the critical point and the phase separation threshold, as well as by the angle made by the tie-lines with the concentration axis of one of system components. Once an increasing protein concentration in one of the system phases results in intensification of intermolecular interactions, association of protein molecules, and reduction of hydrophilicity of protein particles and finally in gel formation, the tie-lines become nonparallel, thereby changing the angle made by the tie-lines with the concentration axis. Thus, phase diagrams of systems containing proteins and protein-polysaccharide mixtures can yield valuable information not only about the phase state, composition and volume properties of system phases but also about relative hydrophilicity of proteins in moderately concentrated food systems, i.e. the information which is of great importance to the understanding of a wide range of food protein functional properties.

The second approach to evaluation of relative hydrophilicity of proteins relies on their ability to alter surface properties of gelatin gels. For this purpose, a studied protein is dissolved in a gelatin solution; then the obtained solution is gelled by cooling and, finally, the contact angle of a water drop at the gel surface is measured. Here gelatin is used as a standard protein to estimate relative hydrophilicity of any other proteins. The choice of gelatin permits us to obtain gels containing various proteins. The surface of gelatin gels obtained in contact with air is extremely high-hydrophilic. For instance, the value of the contact angle of water at the surface of 15% gelatin gel is about 116 to 129°, depending on the gelatin sample used [11-13] . The contact angle of water at the gel surface is not altered on introduction of up to 40% (relative to gelatin concentration) of serum albumin or ovalbumin into these gels. However, the value of this angle drops rapidly as a result of introduction of several per cent of casein into the gelatin gel [10, 14] . This method is very convenient in terms of simplicity of manipulation and reproducibility of results. It is remarkable that the two methods have been employed in our laboratory, i.e. the method of phase diagram determination for protein-protein mixtures, including gelatin-containing ones, and the method of measurement of the contact angle of water on gelatin gels containing food proteins.

Another important functional property of proteins is their ability to stabilize food dispersed systems. Phase separation of biopolymer solution mixtures may proceed, as mentioned in the above discussion, through two different mechanisms: first, incompatibility of these biopolymers and, second, formation of insoluble complexes by these biopolymers. What will happen if one of the system components is made of colloidal particles, say, dispersed particles consisting of protein or stabilized by adsorbing protein? In this case the same phenomena may take place as do in solution mixtures but they can be strongly expressed in view of the colloidal particle dimensions of one of the system components. This means that interactions in such systems containing both colloidal particles and free molecules of biopolymers or adsorbed and dissolved polymer molecules of different species, may result in aggregation of dispersed particles and in destabilization of the dispersed system at very low concentrations of a dissolved biopolymer acting as a flocculent. Flocculation, i.e. the reversible process of formation of aggregates of colloidal particles, can occur by two different mechanisms: first, owing to macromolecules dissolved in the dispersion medium (depletion flocculation) and second, by means of linkages of colloidal particles by an adsorbed biopolymer (bridging flocculation). The mechanism of depletion flocculation was systematically discussed by D.H.Napper. This phenomenon comes about as follows. If two colloidal particles under the Brownian motion happen to approach one another at a distance shorter than the dimensions of biopolymer molecules dissolved in the dispersion medium, between these particles there is a gap containing a pure solvent and surrounded by the solution of another biopolymer. As a result, the solvent flows out from this gap (microvolume) between two approaching particles by action of the osmotic pressure, the dispersion medium is diluted and the dispersed particles become aggregated. Depletion flocculation seems to be favoured by the lower concentration of the dissolved, nonadsorbing biopolymer near the surface of colloidal particles, i.e. by its negative adsorption by these particles. It is usually the case under thermodynamic incompatibility between the nonadsorbing biopolymer dissolved in the dispersion medium and another biopolymer adsorbing at the surface of colloidal particles or a biopolymer making up colloidal particles.

Apparently, one of the earliest studied instances of depletion flocculation is the process of milk casein concentration from skimmed milk by means of pectin. The mixture of skimmed milk and pectin solution separates into a micelles-rich and a solvent-rich phases. It is also noteworthy that addition of phosphate or citrate ions giving rise to dissociation of casein micelles is responsible for a much higher phase separation threshold and a lower degree of protein concentration. This latter example is to emphasize that interactions in multicomponent protein systems resulting in flocculation are of importance to both protein isolation and control of protein functional properties.

In conclusion, I should like to note that by today only the first steps have been taken in understanding the interactions in multicomponent protein systems. This field of investigation is of key importance to getting insight into the formation of structure and properties of many foods, to improving traditional and developing some new processes of food technology.

REFERENCES


1 Tolstoguzov, V.:Physikochemische Aspekte der Herstellung künstlicher Nahrungsmittel. Nahrung. 18(1974) 5, 523-531.

2 Tolstoguzov, V.:New Protein Foods.Agropromizdat, Moscow 1987,302 (in Russian).

3 Tolstoguzov, V.:Artificial Foodstuffs.Nauka,Moscow 1978,231 ( in Russ.)

4 Tolstoguzov, V., Grinberg, V., and Gurov,A.:Some physico-chemical approaches to the problem of protein texturization.J.Agric.Food Chem. 33(1985) 2, 151-159.

5 Antonov, Yu., Pletenko, M., and Tolstoguzov, V.:Phase state of water-polysaccharide-1 - polysaccharide-2 systems. Thermodynamic compatibility of polysaccharides in aqueous media.Visokomol.soed. 29 (1987), 2477-2481, 2482-2486.

6 Polyakov, V., Grinberg, V., and Tolstoguzov, V.:Application of phase-volume ratio method for determining the phase diagram of water-casein-soybean globulins system. Polymer Bul. 2 (1980) 757-760.

7 **Tolstogusov**, V.: Functional properties of protein-polysaccharide mixtures. In: Functional Properties of Food Macromolecules /Eds. Mitchell, J. and Ledward, D. Elsevier Applied Science, London and New York 1986, 385-415.

8 Tolstoguzov, V.: Creation of fibrous structures by spinneretless spinning. In: Food Structure - Its Creation and Evaluation /Eds. Mitchell, J. and Blanshard, J. Butterworths, London 1988, Chapter 10.

9 Tolstoguzov, V. and Braudo, E.: Fabricated foodstuffs as multicomponent gels. J. of Texture Studies.14 (1983) 183-212.

10 Braudo, E., A.Gotlieb, I.Plashina, and V.Tolstoguzov: Protein-containing multicomponent gels. Nahrung.30 (1986) 3-4,355-364.

11 Braudo, E., V.Tolstoguzov, and E.Nikitina:Investigation of the wettability of gelatin gels. Kolloid.Zh. 35 (1974) 2,208-213 (in Russian).

12 Braudo, E., E.Nikitina, and V.Tolstoguzov:Benetzbarkeit von Gelatingelen durch wässrige Elekrolyt- und Harnstofflösungen.253(1973) 5-6,300-310.Z.phys.Chem.

13 Braudo,E., E.Mikhailov, and V.Tolstoguzov:Zur Frage des Kontaktwinkels des Flüssigkeitstropfens auf der Oberfläche deformierbarer Festkörper.Z.phys.Chem.253 (1973) 5-6.369-378.

14 Braudo, E., V. Tolstoguzov, V. Ershova, and G.Slonimsky: Wetting by water of jellies containing gelatin and globular proteins. Kolloid. Zh. 33 (1971) 5, 653-656 ( in Russian).

15 Napper, D.H.:Polymeric Stabilization of Colloidal Dispersions. Academic Press, London 1983.

Stephen E. Harding & Michael P. Tombs[1)]

## I. Introduction

The way in which proteins diffuse in solutions of polymers has attracted much interest recently, giving insight into the way in which non-ideal interactions can affect diffusion. There has however been very little work on the events at the water-water interface in incompatible two phase systems [1]. This is surprising since it would appear to offer excellent opportunities to model systems of biological and biotechnological importance - such as the enzymatic modification of lipids in the food industry and the mobilisation of seed protein bodies [2]. We have therefore attempted to extend some of the ideas of non-ideal diffusion behaviour to polyethylene glycol (PEG) - Dextran two phase systems, to study the way in which proteins move through solutions of macromolecules to the water-water interface and penetrate it in terms of 1. diffusion kinetics, 2. potential density inversion & fingering phenomena [3,4,5] and 3. interfacial accumulation phenomena [6].

## II. Theoretical considerations

1. Diffusion in concentrated systems. In both phases the protein must diffuse through solutions of other polymers. By analogy with dilute solution behaviour [7], these can affect the flux or (translational) apparent diffusion coefficient D, in two ways [5] (i) a hydrodynamic effect, which tends to decrease D largely as a result of an increase in viscous drag, related to the translational frictional property; (ii) a thermodynamic affect related to exclusion volumes and Donnan effects, which tends to increase D. Depending on the relative effects of (i) or (ii) diffusion can be retarded or enhanced.

In ´classical´ diffusion

$$d\,(Q/C_0)^2/dt = D\,(A^2/\pi) \tag{1}$$

where Q is the quantity crossing the boundary in time t with initial concentration $C_0$. A is the cross sectional area. In concentrated ternary solutions, according to [6] this is replaced by

$$d\,(Q/C_0)/dt = k \tag{2}$$

where k is a transport rate. For intermediate concentrations diffusion can commence according to (1) and change to (2) as concentrations shift.

2. Two phase systems. These, with added protein, are quarternary systems, but the same considerations apply. In the PEG-Dextran systems we have used, the polymer concentrations are probably high enough to produce linear kinetics (eqn. 2) for the polymer diffusion behaviour. However as Ogston has shown [8] for some typical globular proteins $D/D_0$, where $D_0$ is the ´ideal´ or ´infinite dilution´ value for D, falls steadily up to concentrations of 20% for the matrix polymer, and it is doubtful if polymer protein interactions would ever cause an enhanced diffusion rate for this class of proteins.

3. Approach to equilibrium. The flux equations (including cases where diffusion must occur up the concentration gradient to achieve equilibrium) can be written

---

1) University of Nottingham, Department of Applied Biochemistry & Food Science, Sutton Bonington, LE12 5RD, UK.

$$\text{Flux } A \rightarrow B,\ J_{AB} = D_0 \cdot d\,(C'_P + A^*_{P.DEX} \cdot C'_P C_{DEX} + \ldots)/dx \qquad (3)$$

$$\text{Flux } B \rightarrow A,\ J_{BA} = D_0 \cdot d\,(C''_P + A^*_{P.PEG} \cdot C''_P C_{PEG} + \ldots)/dx \qquad (4)$$

where $C_P'$, $C_P''$ are the protein concentrations (m/v) in phases A (dextran rich) & B (PEG rich) respectively and $C_{DEX}$, $C_{PEG}$ the concentrations of dextran (dextran rich phase) and polyethylene glycol (PEG rich phase). The ability to diffuse up a concentration gradient depends on the magnitude of the cross interaction terms, $A^*_{P.DEX}$, $A^*_{P.PEG}$. Within the two phases, diffusion will be mainly viscosity dependent, and slow. There will be a large viscosity gradient in the interface, which might be the major factor in determing the concentration profile, and will be markedly asymmetric depending on the direction of diffusion.

4. Transient water fluxes: ´density inversions´ & ´fingering´. Wells [9] has recently proposed a theory to describe disequilibria due to diffusion in moderately concentrated polymer solutions. Although this was originally intended for layered solutions, as shown in Fig. 1a, where A is described as the matrix solute and P the cosolute (in our case, protein), it can also be applied to the quarternary two phase systems shown in Fig 1b, 1c. The question is what happens to the transient water flows, because it is a matter of experimental observation that these systems behave initially as if there were a semi-permeable membrane between the layers. This would of course restrict the movement to that of solvent only, an effect no doubt due to the much greater mobility of water.

The local density, ρ, (for a given phase) in the quarternary 2-phase system is given by

$$\rho = \rho_0\,(1 + \alpha\, C_A + \beta\, C_P) \qquad (5)$$

where $\rho_0$ is the density of pure solvent and α, β are the density increments of A and P (whose partial specific volumes are $\bar{v}_A$ and $\bar{v}_P$) respectively:

$$\alpha = (1/\rho_0) - \bar{v}_A \quad ; \quad \beta = (1/\rho_0) - \bar{v}_P \qquad (6)$$

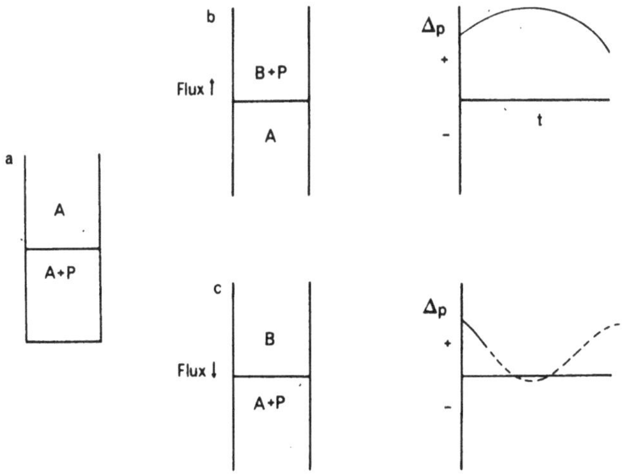


Fig. 1. "a" represents layered solutions containing a matrix polymer A together with protein P. "b" and "c" represent the two possibilities where two polymers A and B are used to produce phase separation, followed by the addition of protein to one or other of them (although both phases contain both A and B the dominant component only is indicated). Also given are the water fluxes and likely transient density changes for situations b and c.

Suppose a lamina of solvent is transferred, of volume $\Delta V$ as a result of osmotic flux effects. If $\rho'$ and $\rho''$ are the local densities in the lower & upper phases respectively, the condition for instability or 'fingering' of protein passing through the interface [5] is that $\Delta\rho = (\rho' - \rho'')$ must become negative. Wells [9] has shown that for Fig 1a, and after making the rather unrealistic assumption of thermodynamic ideality, this condition for instability leads to

$$\alpha/\beta > M_P/M_A \tag{7}$$

(where $M_P$, $M_A$ are the molecular weights of cosolute P & matrix solute A respectively), although the same concepts apply to quarternary systems (Figs 1b, 1c).

It is clear that since the density increment for the two phases is different, shifting a solvent lamina will have different effects in b. and c. However the protein is the source of the osmotic flux, and adapting the arguments we can write

$$\alpha_{PEG}/\alpha_{DEX} > M_P/M_{PEG} \qquad \alpha_{DEX}/\alpha_{PEG} > M_P/M_{DEX} \tag{8}$$

as instability criteria for 1c & 1b respectively. Taking PEG as $M_r \sim 6000$ by this test case '1c' fails to give fingers whereas for dextran ($M_r \sim 500000$) the situation '1b' could. Thus by this test we might expect density inversion & fingering for protein initially in the denser dextran rich phase ("B") but not in the PEG rich phase ("A"), based on the expected osmotic fluxes involved.

By using more general arguments, in '1c' with protein in the upper phase, addition of protein will reduce the initial density difference: in addition, there will be water flux which reduces the density downwards faster than it will increase the density of the lower phase. Thus the interface will be stabilised since the density difference between the phases will tend to increase. By contrast, in '1b' addition of protein will cause an increase of the density of the upper phase more rapidly than the lower phase loses density, so the density difference could reach zero.

The nearer to the critical point composition, the more nearly alike the composition of the phases, and the more nearly alike the rate of change of density, but also the lower the initial density difference. There will be an optimum composition for density inversion, if it occurs.

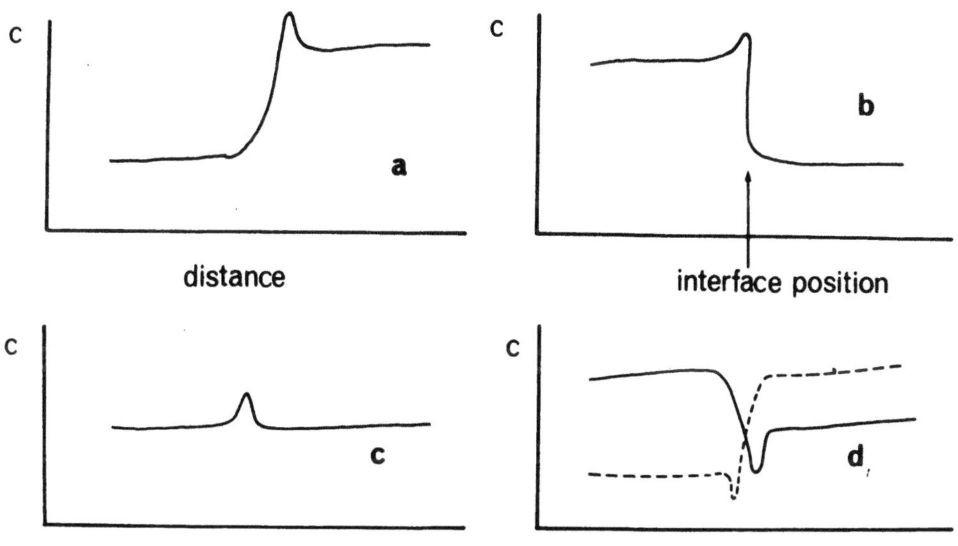


Fig. 2. Predicted concentration profiles across the interface for various combinations of interfacial tension between particles and phases.

5. Interfacial accumulation. Some possible profiles can be predicted from theoretical considerations, and Albertsson [6] has analysed the possibilities in terms of surface energies. By considering the energy associated with a spherical particle at various positions in and near an interface, Albertsson was able to predict accumulations depending on the relative values of the interfacial energies $\gamma_1$, $\gamma_2$ & $\gamma_{12}$ between the particle and the two phases, where $\gamma_1$, $\gamma_2$ & $\gamma_{12}$ are the interfacial energies betwen phase 1 and the particle, phase 2 and the particle and between the two phases respectively. Two possibilities arise: Condition "1" ($\gamma_1 - \gamma_2 < \gamma_{12}$): energy minimum criteria are satisfied when particle totally contained within one of the phases; Condition "2" ($\gamma_1 - \gamma_2 > \gamma_{12}$): energy minimum when particle either totally in one of the phases or in the interface. The interfacial tension between PEG and dextran is low, ( < 0.02 dyne/cm), but $\gamma_1 - \gamma_2$ is also likely to be very low (cf partition coefficients near one) so that the latter condition allowing a build up at the interface is by no means unlikely. Fig. 2 gives some possible profiles. Since in general terms the partition coefficient

$$K = (C_1/C_2) = \exp\,[-\Delta E/kT] = \exp\,[-4\pi R^2(\gamma_1-\gamma_2)/kT] \tag{9}$$

(where $\Delta E$ is the energy difference between the phases) we can write for condition "1" and more interestingly, for the partition between the interfacial region and the phase, with condition "2"

$$C_i/C_1 = \exp[\pi R^2(\gamma_2-\gamma_1-\gamma_{12})^2/\gamma_{12}kT] \tag{10}$$

where $C_i$ is the concentration (g/ml) in the interface and $C_1$ the concentration in phase 1. We have to choose a value for $\gamma_1 - \gamma_2$. This is likely to be small, and for example 0.001 yields $C_i/C_1 = 1.009$. If we assume that $\gamma_1 - \gamma_2$ will be negligible compared with $\gamma_{12}$ (which will not always be the case, but in suitable examples is justified) then

$$C_i/C_1 = \exp\,[6.8\gamma_{12}] \tag{11}$$

Values for the interfacial energy in the PEG-Dextran system are quoted as variable between 0.00046 and 0.066 dyne/cm (or erg/cm$^2$) [6] depending on the precise composition: the further from the critical point, the higher the value. These results suggest that excess concentrations of the order of 60% of the bulk concentration are not impossible. In the dynamic system approaching equilibrium there are other factors which may tend to make this build up greater. A sharp change in viscosity or density in one phase may slow down migrating molecules. Such effects should be revealed by comparing migration in opposite directions.

## III. Experimental

We examined the concentration profiles by using the scanning absorption optical system of an MSE Centriscan analytical ultracentrifuge equipped with a monochromator. We loaded 0.22 ml of lower phase followed by the same volume of top phase into 10mm cells. At the position of the interface the cross sectional area was 25.9 mm$^2$. The rotor was run at 4000rpm at 20$^\circ$C or 25$^\circ$C which should produce no significant sedimentation. Appropriate blanks were included, mainly the two phases with no added protein. Most experiments were done in the two phases produced by mixing 5g of PEG 6000 (BDH Biochemical grade, with low 280nm absorbance), 5.3g of Dextran T-500 (Pharmacia) with 100ml of 50mM sodium phosphate, pH 7.0. After equilibration phases were separated and protein added to the appropriate phase. Four protein systems were analysed: FITC labelled bovine serum albumin, FITC labelled ovalbumin, chromobacter lipase and cytochrome c. Protein concentrations of $\sim$1 mg/ml ($\equiv \sim 1.5 \times 10^5$ M) were added to either phase.

Measurement of interfacial surface tension (by our colleague, Dr. J. Mead, Unilever Research, Bedford, U.K.) by the spinning drop method gave a value of (0.09 $\pm$

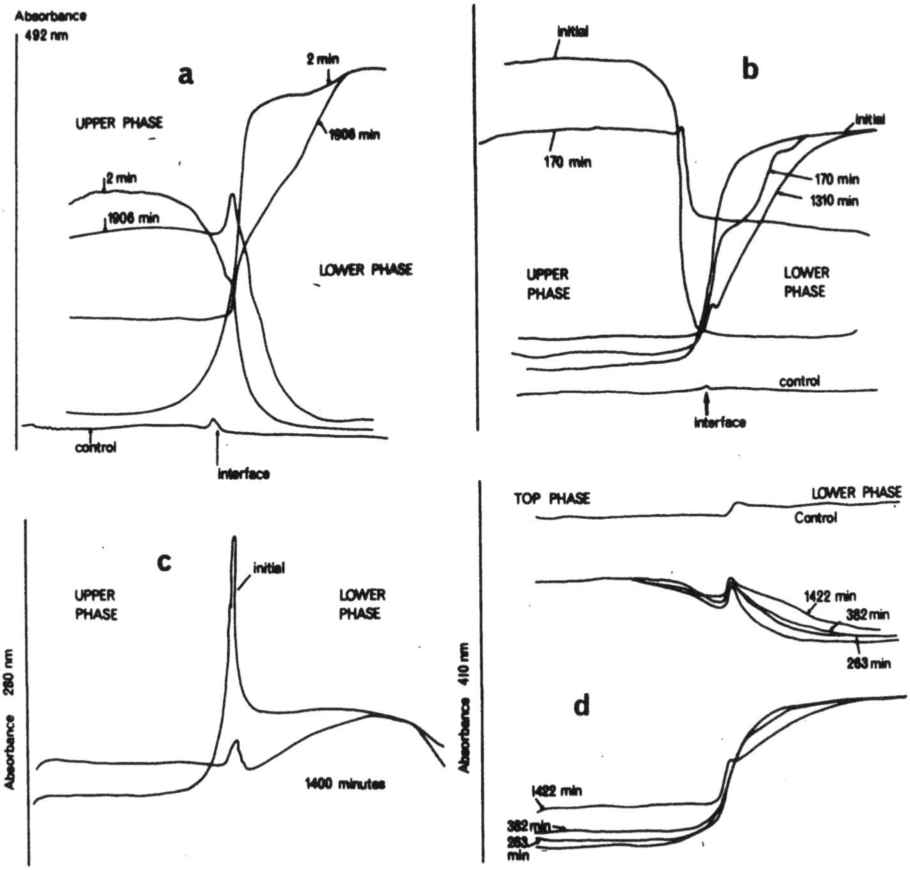


Fig. 3. Protein concentration profiles
a. FITC bovine serum albumin, added at ~1 mg/ml to either the upper or lower phases. Behaviour is different depending on which phase the protein is added to. At the bottom, a control containing no protein. The concentration profiles were measured in three cells run simultaneously.
b. FITC ovalbumin, at 0.2 mg/ml. The complex step pattern was only seen when protein was initially added to the lower phase. Diffusion was apparently much more rapid when protein was added to the upper phase.
c. Lipase, at 0.2 mg/ml, scanned at 280 nm. The initial contact produced a large increase in interfacial accumulation. After ~1400 minutes (near equilibrium) a large excess concentration still persisted.
d. Cytochrome c (after predialysis). At the top, a control trace, in the middle, patterns with protein initially in the upper phase and at the bottom the comparable patterns for the lower phase.

0.03) mN $m^{-1}$ml. $g^{-1}$. The density drop across the interface was ~.03 g/ ml so that the interfacial energy was 0.0027-0.0036 erg. $cm^{-2}$.

## IV. Results

The profiles observed for each of the four proteins are shown in Fig 3. Two regimes are evident:

1. Initial disturbances. Considerable initial turbulence was observed caused by the disequilibrium effects of adding protein to either phase. Considerable transient water flux would be expected and, as shown in Fig. 3 complex steps in the concentration gradients formed. The initial transient fluxes were asymmetric, and were greater when protein was initially in the lower phase than when it was in the upper phase. Pre-dialysis almost completely eliminated them: in this, both phases containing protein were outside the sac. After dialysis to equilibrium, which would result in a small hydrostatic pressure difference, the protein containing phases from inside the sac were placed in contact with the corresponding phase from outside.

2. The overall diffusion process. Classical diffusion theory (cf. eqn. 1) predicts that $Q \propto t^{1/2}$. We have used the areas under the concentration profiles to estimate Q. As is shown by some typical examples in Fig. 4, eqn. 1 does appear to hold, and the overall process regardless of initial turbulence, is one of simple diffusion. The profiles in Fig. 5 were chosen to illustrate the case where diffusion must have occurred against the concentration gradient. Even in this instance, ´classical´ diffusion behaviour can account for the final equilibrium.

## V. Discussion

Diffusion to equilibrium. For most of the proteins used in this work the partition coefficient K (= conc. in upper phase/ conc. in lower phase) is less than 1. For albumin and ovalbumin values of ~0.5 have been reported [6] and this is consistent with the ratios shown in for example Fig. 5 for times of the order of 2000 minutes. Starting with the protein in the less dense phase seems to take longer to reach the equilibrium position by pure diffusion. However as Fig. 5 illustrates, equilibrium can be reached, even if during the process of getting there protein must diffuse up its own concentration gradient [6]. This means the term $d(C'_P + A^*_{P.DEX} . C'_P C_{DEX})/dx$ in eqn. 3 must still be positive even though $dC'_p/dx$ is negative. This is due to the large value for $A^*_{P.DEX}$ and $C_{DEX}$. Because this term changes very rapidly in the interface the concentration gradient is very sharp, at equilibrium. It is not necessary to involve effects caused by agitation to achieve this result. Diffusion alone is sufficient to account for it, providing the effect of interactions is properly taken into account. Shanbag´s observation [10] that the rate of diffusion between phases was dependent on K for proteins of comparable frictional coefficient is also a reflection of the same underlying phenomenon.

Initial disequilibria. What were probably osmotic effects due to the initial disequilibrium proved to be quite easily detectable. Since buffer ions were present some of these effects were probably due to Donnan equilibria. Pre-dialysis eliminated the effects, although it did not in fact pre-equilibrate the samples since the osmotic pressure would have led to a small hydrostatic pressure difference. It might nevertheless have removed the reasons for the transient osmotic flux effects: The Donnan equilibria would already be in existence and the activity of the water in the two phases commences by being equal, and only slowly moves to a new equilibrium as a result of diffusion of the protein. Thus the initial events were different in pre-dialysed and non-predialysed samples. It is interesting to note that the semi-quantitative theory proposed by Wells [9] which we considered above correctly predicts the asymmetry of these effects, and that they would be greater with protein in the lower phase, when adapted to these two phase systems.

Interfacial accumulation. Accumulation in the interface region was consistently observed with all samples. Some of the initial transient effects could produce spikes at the interface but after relatively long periods, at or approaching equilibrium there was always excess concentrations in that region. Blank runs, with no added protein also showed apparent peaks at the interface. These were comparatively small, and probably due to the accumulation of dust. They were more

Fig. 4. Plots of flux through the interface, expressed in arbitrary area units derived from concentration profiles, against $t^{1/2}$.
2 plots for FITC bovine serum albumin, upper to lower phase ( ● , ▲ ); 1 plot for lower to upper phase ( ■ ). The linear fits in each case are consistent with a 'classical' diffusion process.

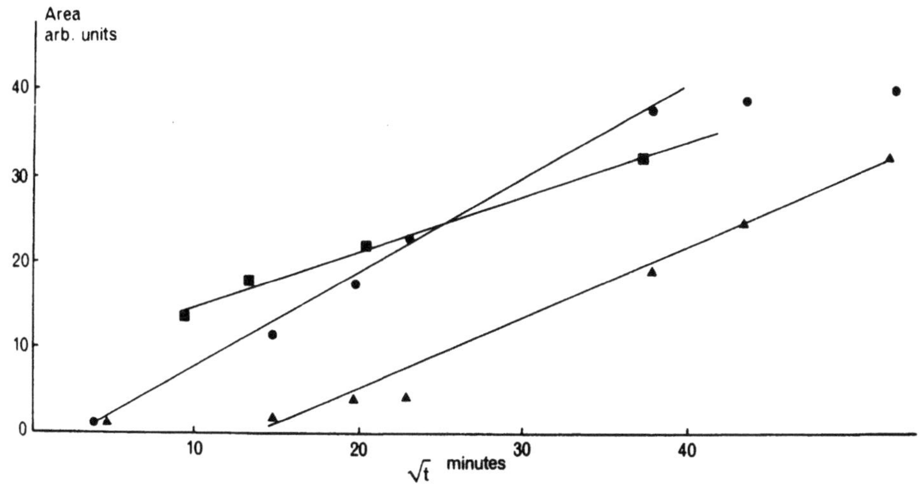


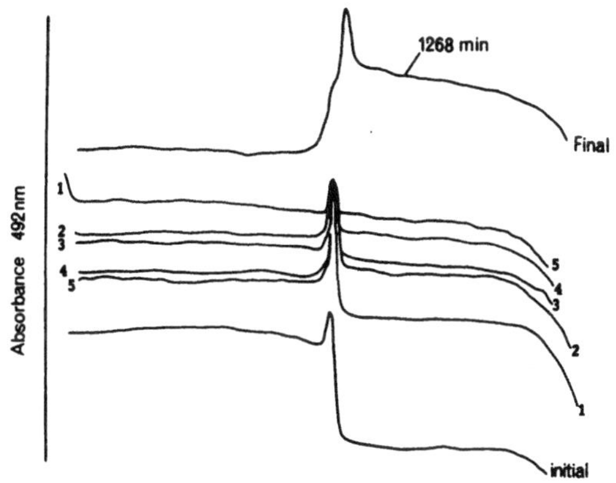


Fig. 5. Profiles for FITC bovine serum albumin, commencing in the upper phase and diffusing to equilibrium, with partition coefficients giving a higher concentration in the lower phase. The initial and final profiles have been shifted for clarity. As the intermediate traces show, diffusion occurred up the concentration gradient.

prominent when scanning at 280 nm than 492 nm as would be expected for scattering. Application of eqn. (11) and estimates of the interfacial tension leads to predictions of an excess of the order of 2-3%. Values found for cytochrome c and chromobacter lipase were far larger than this prediction (Fig. 3), varying up to 50% excess concentrations. FITC-ovalbumin, at ~5% and albumin at ~10% were nearer predicted levels.

All proteins have, on their surface a mosaic of hydrophilic and hydrophobic regions, and if these are distributed so that one side of the molecule has relatively more than the other, then this could produce large excess concentrations, as could the presence of a large heme group. Although lipases are relatively hydrophilic molecules containing carbohydrate, they are also because of their activity, likely to have hydrophobic areas and might well be expected to have considerable asymmetry in the hydrophobic-hydrophilic balance. It is distinctly possible that at the interface the protein concentration rises to a degree which makes it necessary to regard the protein at the interface as a '3rd phase': The possibility also of some self-association behaviour at the meniscus cannot be ignored: we are currently attempting to model this behaviour using advanced sedimentation velocity & low speed sedimentation equilibrium procedures.

## VI. References


1. Tombs, M.P. & Harding, S.E. (1988) in Advances in Seperations using Aqueous Phase Systems in Cell Biology & Biotechnology (Fisher, D. & Sutherland, I.A. eds.) Plenum, NY
2. Tombs, M.P., Newsom, B. & Wilding, P. (1974) Int. J. Prot. Pept. Res. 6, 253-277
3. Laurent, T.C., Preston, B.N. & Sundelof, L-O. (1979) Nature 279, 60-62
4. Preston, B.N., Laurent, T.C., Comper, W.D. & Checkley, G.J. (1980) Nature, 287, 499-503
5. Laurent, T.C., Preston, B.N., Comper, W.D., Checkley, G.J., Edsman, K, & Sundelof, L-O. (1983) J. Phys. Chem., 87, 648-654
6. Albertsson, P-A (1985) Partition of cell particles and macromolecules (3rd edn.) Wiley, New York
7. Harding, S.E. & Johnson, P. (1985) Biochem. J. 231, 543-547
8. Ogston, A.G. (1970) J. Phys. Chem. 74 668-669
9. Wells, J.D. (1986) J. Phys. Chem. 90, 2433-2440
10. Shanbag, V.P. (1973) Biochim. Biophys. Acta. 320, 517-522

# EFFECT OF SUCCINYLATION ON SURFACE BEHAVIOURS OF 12S RAPESEED STORAGE PROTEIN

S. Bollecker[1] , J. Gueguen[1] , K.D. Schwenke[2]

## Introduction

Succinylation is one of the most efficient chemical modification for improving functional properties of proteins [1]. Using succinylation, the change of functional properties of protein isolates from soybean [2], peanut [3], sunflower seed [4,5], cottonseed [6] and faba bean [7-9] has been studied.

In a previously published paper, a first investigation of functional properties of the succinylated rapeseed 12S globulin was described [10]. A certain dependence of functional properties on the kind and level of modification was found but the structure-functionality relationships derived remained mostly phenomenological. This was caused mainly by the methods applied for the determination of the functional properties: they were adapted from a more practical point of view of food protein application. New aspects were opened by the investigations of GRAHAM and PHILLIPS [11 - 17] and TORNBERG [18 - 20] and more recently by DAGORN-SCAVINER et al. [21 - 23], who studied the surface behaviours of the 12S (legumin) and 7S (vicilin) globulins of pea (Pisum sativum L.).

It was the aim of the present work to investigate the surface functional properties, that means the adsorption kinetics at air/water interface, as well as the kinetics of foam destabilisation, of the 12S rapeseed globulin, in dependence on the level of succinylation of this protein.

## Material and methods

The protein was isolated from dehulled, and diethylether extracted rapeseed flour (prepared from Brassica napus, var. Sollux, harvested 1984) as described previously [24].

The succinylation was carried out as previously described [25].

---

[1] Ministère de l'Agriculture, Institut National de la Recherche Agronomique, Laboratoire de Biochimie et de Technologie des Protéines, La Géraudière, 44072 NANTES Cedex, France

[2] Central Institute of Nutrition, Potsdam-Rehbrücke, Academy of Science of GDR

The kinentics of surface tension "gamma" were established at 20°C in sodium phosphate / sodium chloride solution (0.05 M $Na_2HPO_4$, pH 9.2, 0.05 M NaCl) by the Wilhelmy plate technique using a Prolabo tensiometer. The final protein concentration was comprised between $5\cdot10^{-7}$ and $1.04\cdot10^{-4}$ g/ml and the gamma-t curves were recorded till a constant value of gamma.

In order to determine the various parameters which control the successive rate steps of the interfacial pressure ($\pi$) kinetics, the commonly used plots
$\pi = f(t^{1/2})$, $\log(d\pi/dt) = f(\pi)$, $\log(1 - \pi / \pi_E) = f(t)$
[25, 26, 11, 18, 19] were established on a computer.

Foaming properties

Foaming capacity and stability were determined using the conductivity method described by KATO et al. [27] and modified by DAGORN-SCAVINER [21]. The foaming was performed by passing a nitrogen stream through a fritted glass at the bottom of a column containing the protein solution (1 mg protein/ml in 0.05 M $Na_2HPO_4$/0.05 M NaCl, pH 9.2).

Two parameters were chosen for the determination of the foam stability. The first corresponded to the time ($t_{1/2}$) at which the initial conductivity reached half of its value ($C_i/2$). The second was the foam stability index (FSI) according to KATO et al. [27].

To evaluate the rate constants of foam breaking, the method of DRAGORN-SCAVINER [21] adapted by GUEGUEN et al. [28] was used.

## Results

### Adsorption at the air/water interface

The adsorption of the protein samples at the air/water interface was studied both by the pressure isotherms (Fig. 1) the kinetics of adsorption (Fig. 2) and comparing the pressure isotherm for the native and highly succinylated (83 %) sample, it was observed that the same plateau value was reached (about 25 mN/m) and that at lower concentrations the succinylated sample was more efficient to increase the surface pressure. The general profile of the isotherm is not, however, drastically modified by succinylation. The slope of the increasing part is not very affected, neither is the lower concentration value for the $\pi_e$ plateau ($11\cdot10^{-6}$ g/ml).

In order to discuss more generally the effect of the succinylation degree on the $\pi_e$ values, the various succinylated samples were compared at three concentrations. One of them was chosen in the increasing linear part of the isotherm ($4\cdot10^{-6}$ g/ml), and the other two in the plateau region (20 and $40\cdot10^{-6}$ g/ml).

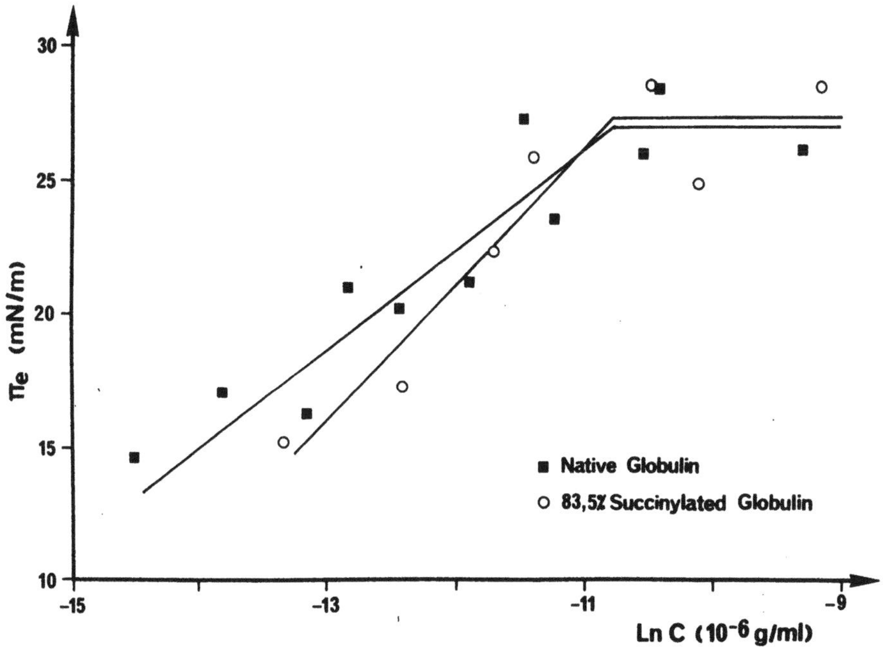


Figure 1: Pressure isotherms of the native and succinylated (83 %) globulin

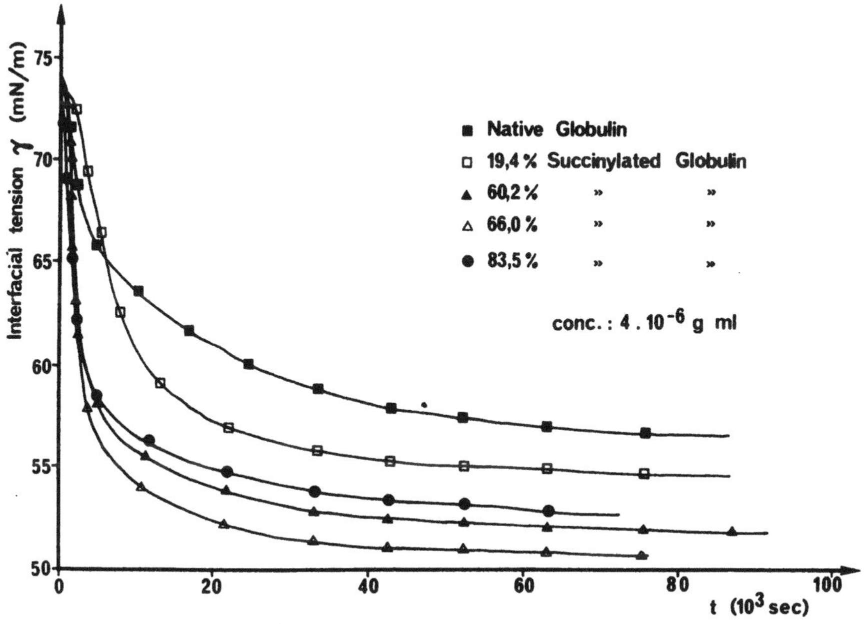


Figure 2: Kinetics of adsorption of native and succinylated globulin at the air/water interface

Whatever the succinylation degree was, the same plateau value was reached (about 25 mN/m). On the other hand, for the lowest concentration, succinylation induced higher pressure values. The increase of $\pi_e$ proceeds parallely with the increase of the level of modification until a degree of about 66 %. A further increase of the level of succinylation (to 83 %) decreases $\pi_e$ (Fig. 2). it might be related to the high degree of dissociation which could inhibit an efficient rearrangement of the dissociated subunits at the interface.

The kinetics of surface adsorption were studied for the three previous concentrations. Succinylation results, moreover, in a decrease of the time necessary for reaching the equilibrium ($t_e$). This effect is more pronounced at higher concentrations where $t_e$ of the native protein drops from 28 to 18 h already after a weak modification, without further significant changes at higher degrees of modification. At the lowest concentration, this effect comes into beeing, however, not early than at 66 % modification, where $t_e$ amounts to 21 h.

The analysis of the kinetics brought about four phases for the interface adsorption of each sample, corresponding to a short latent ("zero") phase, a diffusion phase (n°1), a phase of penetration (n°2), and a phase of rearrangement (n°3). The characteristics of each phase are summarised in figure 3a, b, c.

The very short latent phase did not exceed 1 % of the total time of the kinetics for each sample. During this time, the native protein causes a change of surface pressure of 4.6 %, whereas the modified proteins show a higher effect increasing with the degree of modification from 7 % at 19 % succinylation to 15 % at 83 % succinylation.

The diffusion phase is also relatively short (1.6 - 2.0 %). The time for diffusion does not show a dependence on the level of modification (the 19 % succinylated sample represents an exception with 10 %). The relative changes of interfacial tension in this phase amounts to 25 % for the native protein. It is significantly higher (31 - 60 %) for the modified samples (Fig. 3 a).

The rate constant of this step "1" became higher with the degree of modification (Fig. 3 b). Assuming that this step is mainly ruled by diffusion, it is linked to the fact that highly succinylated proteins are components with lower molecular weight. The native globulin, as well as ~ 90 % of the 19 % modified protein sedimented around 12S, and have rate constants of $1.2 \cdot 10^{-4}$ s. But when the degree of succinylation was over 60 %, high amounts of 3S components appeared, leading to a rate constant of about $4.5 \cdot 10^{-4}$ s.

As generally observed, the energy barriers ($\Delta A$) are low for all samples in this phase and do not show differences between the native and the modified proteins (Fig. 3 c).

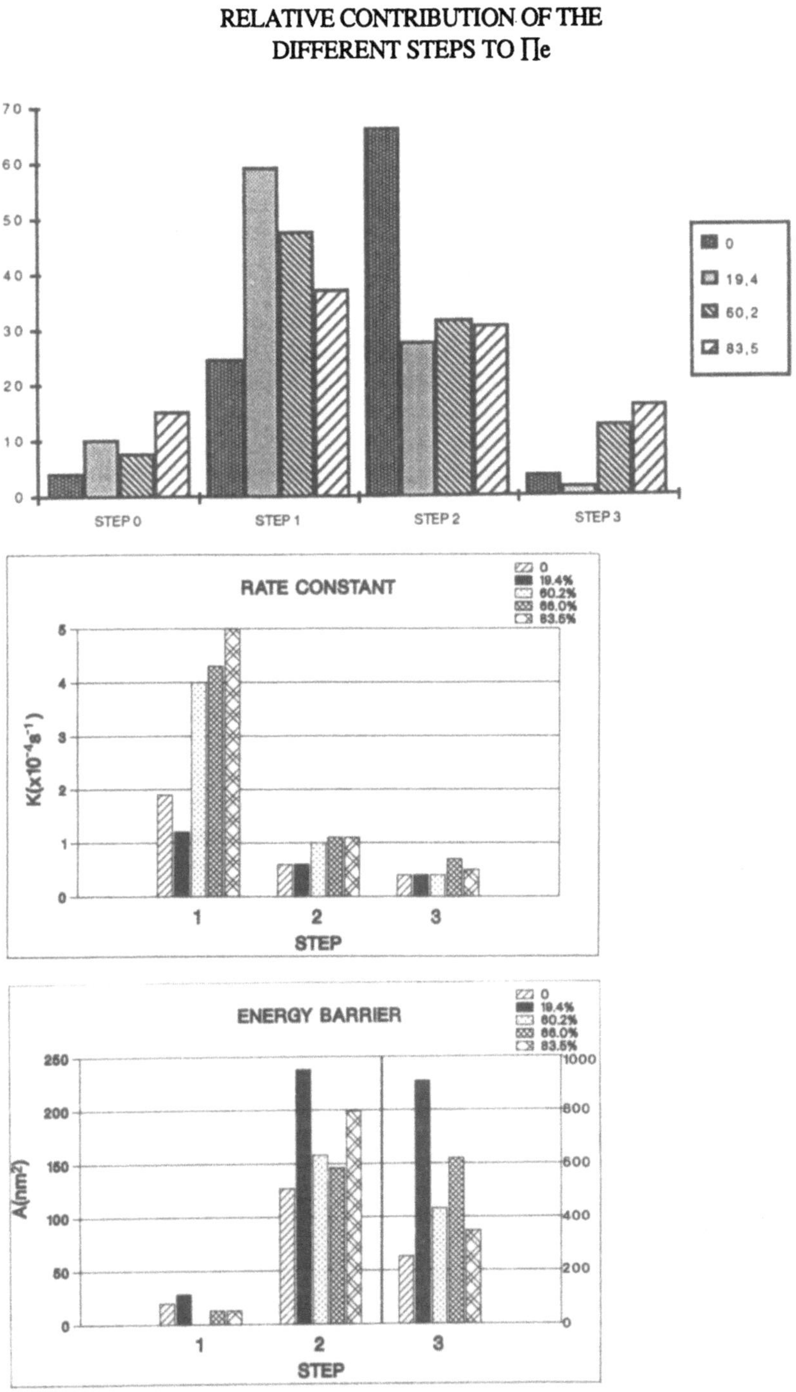


Figure 3: Characteristics of the adsorption kinetics of the rapeseed globulin (native and succinylated) at air/water interface.
(Buffer: phosphate, pH 9.2; Concentration: $4 \cdot 10^{-6}$ g/ml)
(3 a-c downward)
3 a: Relative contribution of the different steps to $\pi_e$
3 b: Rate constants for the different steps
3 c: Energy barriers for the different steps

The penetration phase is characterised by a long duration for the native and weakly (19 %) succinylated protein, amounting to 50 - 60 % of the total time, and a significant shorter duration for the highly modified ( > 60 % succinylation) samples. The change of $\pi_e$ induced by the native protein is the highest one during the total adsorption process, amounting to 66 % of the change. The modified proteins cause a change of $\pi_e$ of 30 - 40 % without a clear dependence on the level of succinylation (Fig. 3a). The energy barriers ($\Delta A$) and the rate constants (k) are increased for the highly ( > 60 %) modified proteins in this phase (Fig. 3b, c).

The phase of rearrangement (n=3) is significantly shorter (33 - 36 % of the total time) for the native or weakly modified proteins than for the highly ( > to 60 %) succinylated ones (about 80 % of the total time). The latter causes a pressure variation of 8 - 16 %, the former ones a change of only 2 - 4 % (Fig. 3 a). Figure 3 c shows also an increase of the energy barrier for all succinylated proteins without a clear dependence on the degree of modification. Nevertheless, the change of k is less significant in this phase (Fig. 3 b).

Foaming properties

Figure 4 shows the kinetics of collapse of the foam of the native and succinylated rapeseed globulin in comparison with BSA. Taking into account the initial conductivity $C_i$ as a measure of the foam capacity, one can notice an improving of the latter at high degrees of modifiction (Fig. 5 a). $C_i$ of highly modified proteins reaches a value of 1, 100 S/cm. The native and weakly modified samples have $C_i$s in the range of 860 - 910 µS/cm.

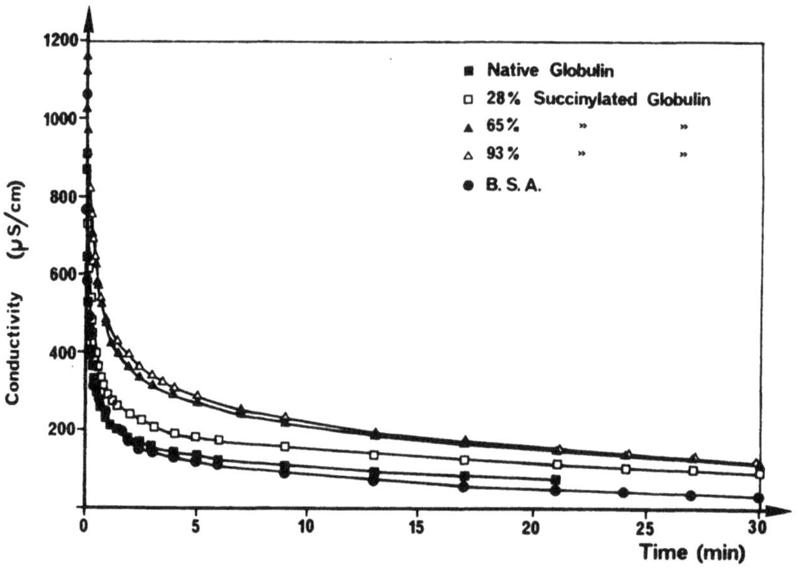


Figure 4: Kinetics of foam breaking for native and succinylated rapeseed globulin

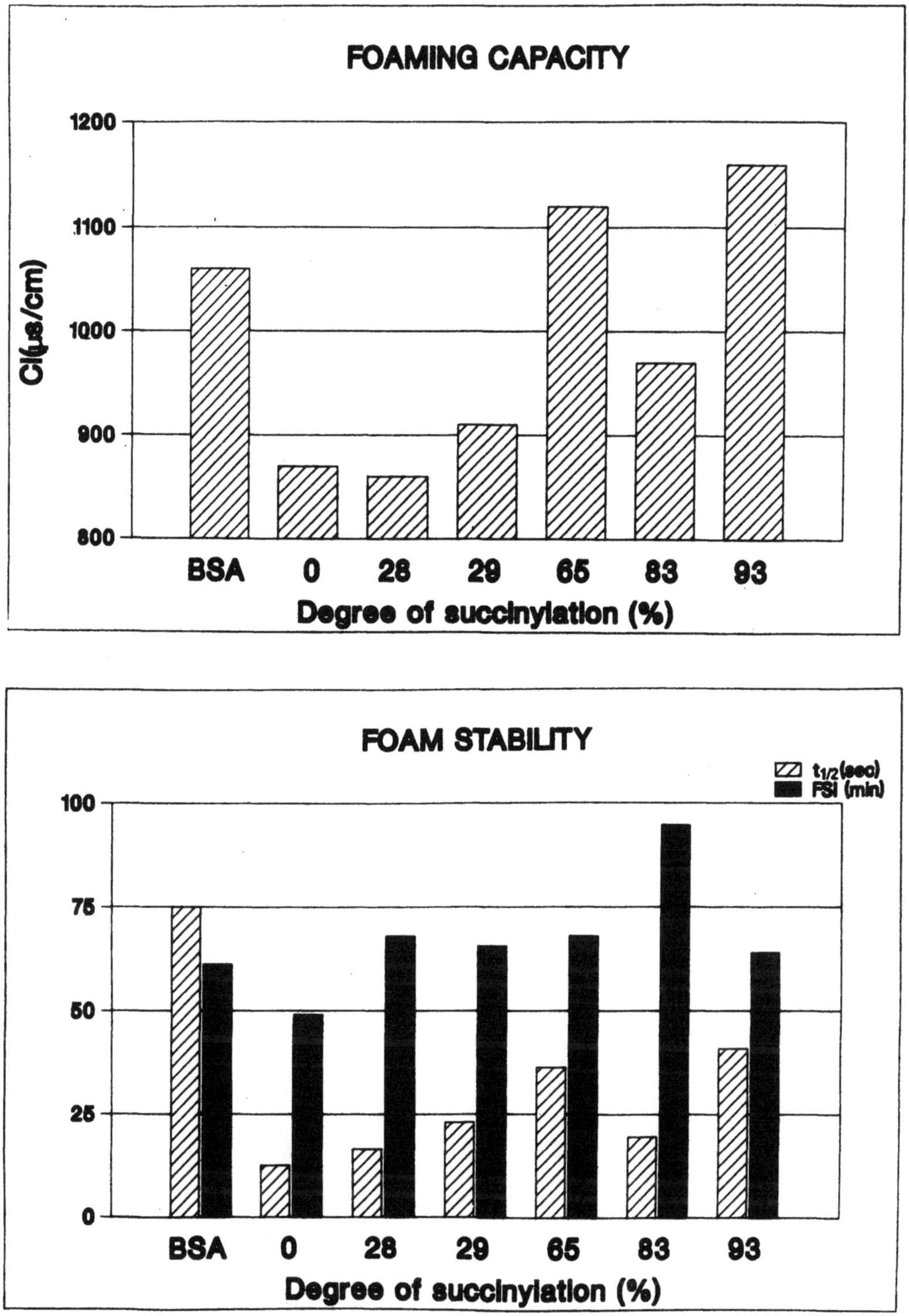


Figure 5: Influence of the succinylation on the foaming properties of the 12S rapeseed globulin (5 a, b downward).
5 a: Foaming capacity
5 b: Foam stability

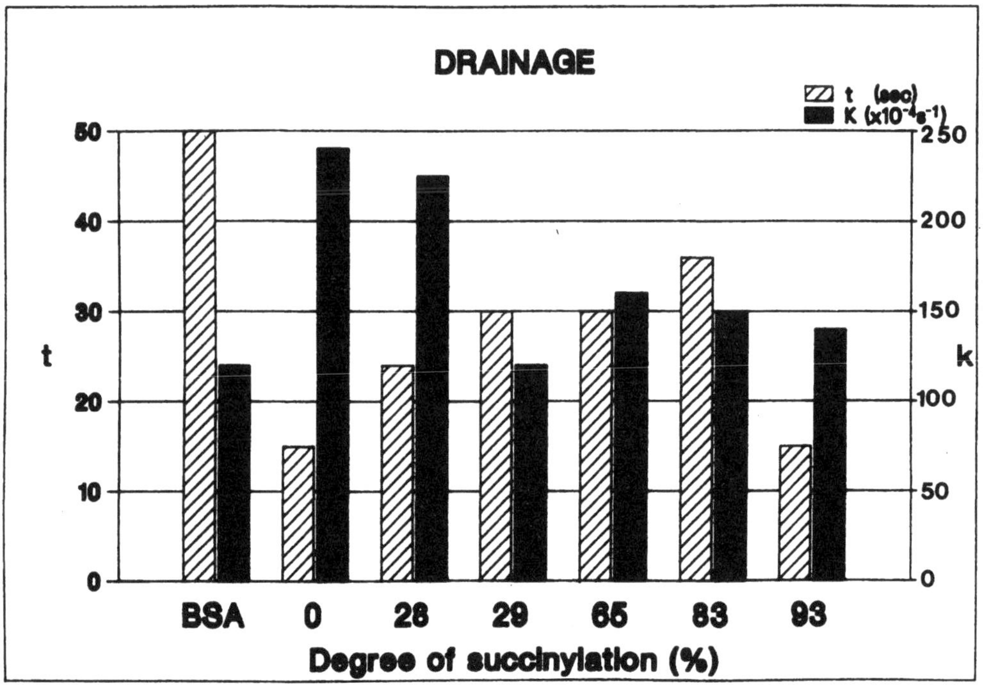


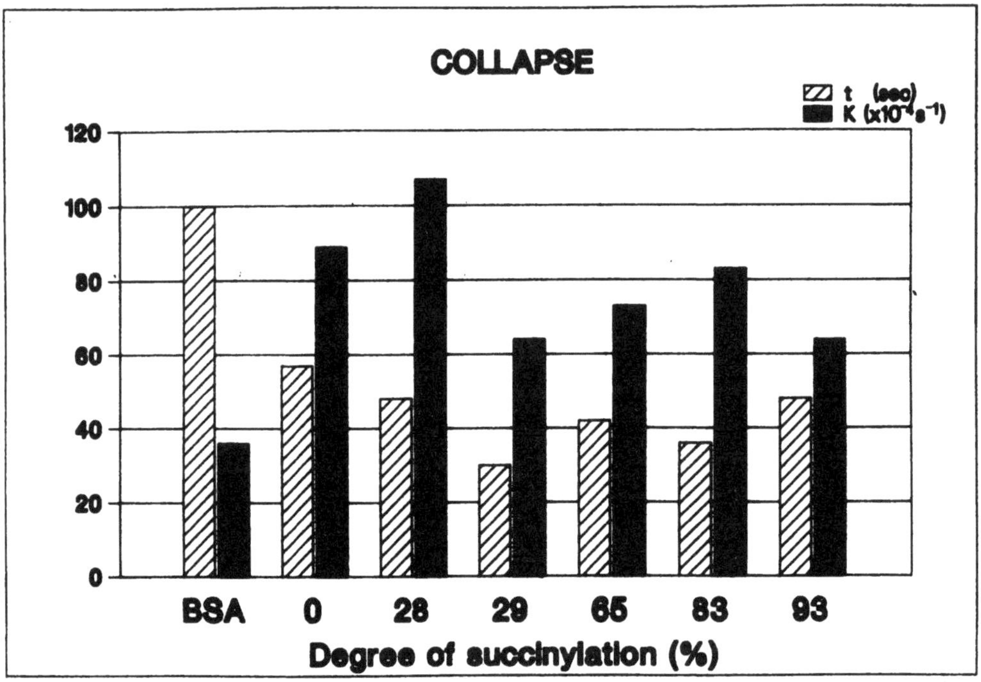


Figure 6: Influence of the succinylation on the foaming properties of the 12S rapeseed globulin (6 a, b downward).

6 a: drainage: duration and rate constant for the first step of the foam breaking kinetic.

6 b: collapse: duration and rate constant for the second step of the foam breaking kinetic.

The two measures of foam stability ($t_{1/2}$ and FSI) represent different stages of foam destabilisation. Whereas $t_{1/2}$ reflects an early stage of foam destabilisation, FSI gives informations about the state of the foam just before its collapse. $t_{1/2}$ describes therefore the capability of the protein to diffuse at the interface and to be adsorbed, stabilising the air bubbles just after formation. Contrary to that, FSI, as a measure of coalescence phenomena, is more related to the protein film characteristics. The native protein showed a $t_{1/2}$ of 12.6 S which increased to 36 - 41 S in the case of highly modified proteins (Fig. 5 b). The high value of BSA (75 S) was not reached, however. Contrary to that, the FSI of the native globulin, amounting to 49 min increased just after a moderate level of succinylation of 26 % and reached values of 64 - 68 min which were higher than that of BSA (62 min).

In general, the rate constant of drainage decreased with time. Drainage is more important just after foam formation for step "1", it is related to the ability of the protein to adsorb quickly at the interface and to stabilise the air bubbles. The last step ("3") mainly reflects the drainage due to collapse of the air bubbles and the behaviour of the adsorbed film. From the data obtained, it was clearly observed that an increasing degree of succinylation make easier adsorption of the protein and stabilisation of bubbles (Fig. 6 a, b). Moreover, the results corresponding to step "3" showed that collapse is more drastic for native and weakly modified proteins (Fig. 6 b). It was clearly observed that the rate constants were generally higher for the native and weakly modified proteins. It indicates that the electrostatic repulsions between bubbles are more important for highly modified proteins because of a higher charge of the adsorbed film.

**Discussion**

The change in the functional properties of the 12S globulin depending on the degree of succinylation can be explained by the structural alterations of the proteins, taking into account the change in molecular mass (dissociation) and shape (unfolding) as well as the increase of negative charge resulting in an increase of hydratation of the protein molecules [5, 29]. Generally, these alterations improve the surface activity at the air/water interface as well as the foaming properties of the native protein under the conditions applied in this paper.

The differences in the adsorption kinetics of the native and the succinylated samples reflect the structural changes and the charge increase. Indeed the comparison of the behaviour of the native and weakly (19 %) modified samples in the various phases of kinetics points to a significant influence of small changes in charge and size of the proteins molcules. Increasing the degree of modification does not modify very much the duration of the preliminary phase "0". On the other hand, it increases significantly the contribution of this phase to decrease the surface tension (Fig. 3 a).

According to BLANK et al. [30], this preliminary phase mainly results from an electrostatic barrier to adsorption, due to orientated water molecules at the interface. Adsorption of the first protein molecules disorganizes this water interface layer and induces positive surface pressure. Therefore, this last phenomenon seems to be more efficient for succinylated protein, probably because of their charge. Modifications of size and charge also induced a remarkable change of surface tension in the diffusion and penetration phases ($\pi$ / $\pi_o$ amounts to 60 and 26 %, resp., of the total) and a significant increase of the energy barrier $\Delta A$ in the phases of penetration and rearrangement. The latter ones ought to be caused by electrostatic repulsion. In the case of higher succinylated samples, the energy barrier are smaller in these phases than for the weakly modified ones, though the negative charges are much more increased. Apparantly, the inhibiting repulsive effect of the charge is compensated by the decay of the big oligomeric 12S molecule into dissociated 3S molecules [26]. Furthermore, protein-protein interaction between hydrophobic regions exposed after the unfolding of the protein might be taken into account.

The more obvious phenomenon is the existence of small dissociation products which leads to an increase of the rate constant in the first phase of kinetics corresponding to the diffusion. Moreover, the high charge density of the strongly succinylated proteins are obviously responsible for the prolongation of the third phase consisting in the rearrangement of the molecules at the interface. Additionaly, some relaxation effects induced by the more stretched unfolded molecules may be discussed for the 83 % modified sample, too [5, 29].

The first oligomeric proteins studied by measuring the interface adsorption kinetics were the legumin (12S protein) and the vicilin (7S protein) of pea [22]. The different adsorption kinetics of both proteins were discussed by the authors in relation with the molecular properties. It was concluded for the concentration dependence of the energy barrier in the penetration phase that vicilin, lacking in disulfide bridges, possesses a higher molecular flexibility than legumin. Moreover it was observed that the constant rate for the first step of adsorption was increasing when the molecular weight of the protein was decreasing, indication that this step was mainly ruled by diffusion.

On the basis of the isotherms, it seems that the equilibrium state of adsorption was not so much different between the native and the 83 % succinylated proteins. The interface area per molecule in the adsorbed monolayer, calculated from the slope of the adsorption isotherm were 0.61 $nm^2$ and 1.25 $nm^2$ respectively. These values are close to the corresponding one obtained by DAGORN-SCAVINER et al. [22] for pea legumin (1.04 $nm^2$). From these results on adsorption, we may conclude that succinylation affects more the kinetic parameters (rate constant of diffusion, energy barriers) of the adsorption, due to the size and charge of the modified proteins, than the equilibrium characteristics.

According to the differentiated effect of a variation of the degree of succinylation on the different phases of kinetics of adsorption, one can expect a similar influence of the succinylation on the foaming properties, too.

It is interesting to note that the succinylation exerts various effects on the foaming capacity and the foam stability. It needs an explanation considering a simultaneous influence of particle size and shape as well as charge effects. The foaming capacity increased with higher degree of succinylation; it is related to the higher rate constant for the diffusion of the dissociated components to the interfacial layers. This kinetic parameter could explain the higher ability of these samples in stabilizing the air bubbles just after formation. The stability of the foam was also improved by increasing levels of modification. It has to be related to the electrostatic repulsive effects between the air bubbles which are due to the increasing charge of the adsorbed proteins. That is probably reinforced by the rheological properties of the interfacial layers owing to the increased viscosity of the succinylated proteins. However the degree of succinylation has to be above 60 - 65 % to improve significantly the foaming properties. This degree has been defined as a critical one ot which the dissociation to 3S subunits is finished and the unfolding of the protein begins [5, 29].

The peculiar behaviour of the 83 % succinylated samples needs an explanation considering a simultaneous influence of particle size and shape as well as charge effects. Its low stabilisation ability in the first phases (decrease of $t_{1/2}$) compared to its high stabilisation effect in the last phase (highest value of FSI) has to be discussed with regard both to the continuous increase of negative charge and the unfolding process which takes place at this level of modification. These effects are probably compensated by the higher flexibility of the most unfolded, highly hydrated 93 % modified protein sample.

The kinetic approach applied in this paper opens new possibilities of derivation of structure-functionality relationships for the foaming properties. In conclusion, the succinylated proteins appeared to be more efficient foaming agents, mainly due to their charge and size. Whereas the effect of modification on the equilibrium interfacial pressure is fairly weak, the kinetics aspects of adsorption seems to be very important in explaining these functional properties, this fact beeing very consistant with our previous results on pea globulins [23]. Moreover, the charge and the increased viscosity of the modified proteins induced positive effects on the stability of foams.

## References


[1] Kinsella, J.E.; Crit. Rev. Food Sci. Nutr. 7, 219 (1976)

[2] Franzen, K.L. and J.E. Kinsella;
J. Agric. Food Chem. 24, 788 (1976)

[3] Beuchat, L.R.; J. Agric. Food Chem. **25**, 258 (1977)

[4] Canella, M., G. Castriotta and A. Bernardi; Lebensm. Wiss. U. Tech. **12**, 95 (1979)

[5] Schwenke, K.D., E.J. Rauschal, D. Zirwer and K.J. Linow; Int. J. Pept. Prot. Res. **25**, 347 (1985)

[6] Choi, Y.R., E.W. Lusas and K.C. Rhee; J. Food Sci. **46**, 954 (1981)

[7] Rauschal, E.J., K.J. Linow, W. Pähtz and K.D. Schwenke; Nahrung **25**, 241 (1981)

[8] Schwenke, K.D., B. Raab, P. Plietz and G. Damaschun; Nahrung **27**, 165 (1983)

[9] Prahl, L. and K.D. Schwenke; Nahrung **30**, 311 (1986)

[10] Nitecka, E. and K.D. Schwenke; Nahrung **30**, 969 (1986)

[11] Graham, D.E.; Thesis Ph. D. C.N.A.A., London (1976)

[12] Graham, D.E. and M.C. Phillips; Theory and practice of emulsion technology, Ed. Smith, A.L., Academic Press, London (1976)

[13] Graham, D.E. and M.C. Phillips; J. Coll. Interf. Sci. **70**, 403 (1979)

[14] Graham, D.E. and M.C. Phillips; J. Coll. Interf. Sci. **70**, 415 (1979)

[15] Graham, D.E. and M.C. Phillips; J. Coll. Interf. Sci. **70**, 427 (1979)

[16] Phillips, M.C.; Chem. Ind. **5**, 170 (1977)

[17] Phillips, M.C.; Food Technol. **35**, 50 (1981)

[18] Tornberg, E.; J. Coll. Interf. Sci. **64**, 391 (1978)

[19] Tornberg, E.; J. Sci. Food Agric. **29**, 762 (1978)

[20] Tornberg, E., Y. Granfeld and C. Hakansson; J. Sci. Food Agric. **33**, 904 (1982)

[21] Dagorn-Scaviner, C; Thesis, Universite de Nantes, France (1986)

[22] Dagorn-Scaviner, C., F. Gueguen and J. Lefebvre; Nahrung, **30**, 337 (1986)

[23] Dagorn-Scaviner, C., J. Gueguen and J. Lefebvre; J. Food Sci. **52** 335 (1987)

[24] Raab, B. and K.D. Schwenke; Nahrung, **28**, 863 (1984)

[25] Ward, A.F.H. and L. Tordai; J. Chem. Phys., **14**, 453 (1946)

[26] Ward, A.F.H. and L. Tordai; Rec. Trav. Chim. **71**, 572 (1952)

[27] Kato, A., A. Takashashi, N. Matsudomi and K. Kobayashi; J. Food Sci., **48**, 62 (1983)

[28] Gueguen, J., S. Bollecker, K.D. Schwenke and B. Raab; J. Sci. Food Agric. Submitted

[29] Schwenke, K.D., K.J. Linow and D. Zirwer; Nahrung, **30**, 263 (1986)

[30] Blank, M., B.B. Lee and J.S. Britten; J. Coll. Interf. Sci. **50**, 215 (1975)

# THE EFFECT OF SELF-ASSOCIATION OF PROTEINS ON THEIR ELECTROSTATIC COMPLEXATION

Vainerman, E.S., Kurskaya, E.A., Rogozhin, S.V. [1]

The process of electrostatic complexation in view of its employment for the isolation, purfication and transformation of the proteins into food forms arouses cosiderable interest. The regulation of electrostatic interactions between the proteins and their subunits makes it possible to vary the composition of protein complexes and the structure of such oligomeric proteins as 11S globulins of oilseeds. The electrostatic complex formation is observed within the pH range, limited by the isoelectric points of interacting protein compounds. The macromolecules have an opposite net charge within this range. The process of electostatic interaction between polyelectrolytes can be well described by the multiple equilibrium scheme presented on Fig.1 [1]. In this case the protein component with an excess net charge density is an acceptor, the less charged one is a ligand of the complexes. As it is shown on the scheme, the charge of the complexes formed in the initial stages of the process, decreases as the ligands are attached. Electroneutral complexes associate with each other when affected by nonelectrostatic forces and precipitated from the solution in the "complex coacervate" form. The composition of residue corresponds to the equivalence requirement: the mole ratio of the electroneutral complex components is inversely proportional to their net charges ratio [2]. However, when the proteins with highly ordered globular structure form complexes, steric hindrance can cause the incomplete mutual neutralization of macromolecule charges in insoluble complexes. The composition of the formed insoluble complexes cannot be stoichiometric. Moreover, the multiple equilibrium scheme of electrostatic protein complexation does not take into account the possibility of macromolecules to self-association processes affected by hydrogen and Van der Waals bonds as well as hydrophobic interactions. The regulation of the composition and the pysico-chemical properties of protein complexes are hindered by protein self-association.

In the present work we have investigated the self-association effect on the electrostatic complexation of acid-process and alkali-process gelatins. Acid-process gelatin (A) is known to be a collagen acid-hydrolysis product with isoionic point 9, while alkali-process gelatin (B) has an isoionic point of 5. Within the range of pH 5 - 9 protein macromolecules have opposite net charges and form electrostatic complexes [3]. The conformation of gelatin macromolecules is random coil, when they are heated up to 40°C. This causes the decrease of steric hindrance in the formation of intermolecular electrostatic complexes.

---

[1] Institute of organoelement compounds of Academy of sciences of the USSR. 117813 Moscow, Vavilova, 28, USSR

$$A^{Z_a} + B^{Z_b} \overset{k_1}{\rightleftharpoons} AB^{Z_a+Z_b}$$

$$AB^{Z_a+Z_b} + B^{Z_b} \overset{k_2}{\rightleftharpoons} AB_2^{Z_a+2Z_b}$$

..........................................

$$AB_{n-1}^{Z_a+(n-1)Z_b} + B^{Z_b} \overset{k_n}{\rightleftharpoons} AB^{Z_a+nZ_b}$$

---

$$A^{Z_a} + nB^{Z_b} \overset{K}{\rightleftharpoons} AB_n^{Z_a+nZ_b}$$

$$K = k_1\, k_2\, \dots\, k_n = \frac{|A| \cdot |B|^n}{|AB_n|}$$

Figure 1: Multiple equilibrium scheme of electrostatic interactions of oppositely charged molecules.

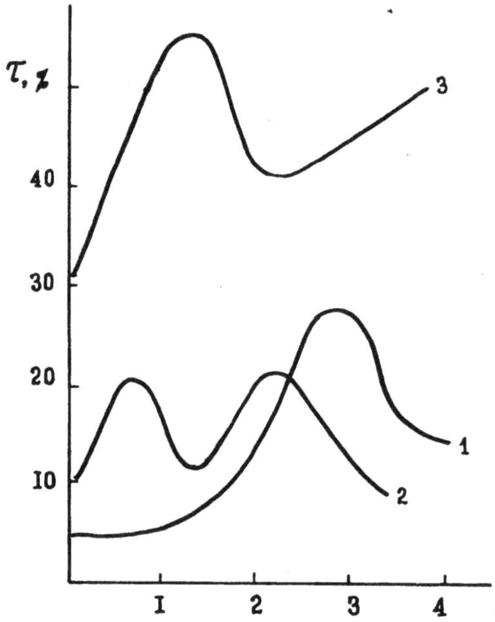


Figure 2: Turbidity value versus the mole ratios P = ligand: acceptor at different conditions:
1 pH = 6.8 T = 40°C, P = A:B;
2 pH = 5.5 T = 40°C, P = B:A;
3 pH = 5.5 T = 23°C, P = B:A.

Due to the abnormally high content of apolare amino acid residues and the significant amount of functional groups capable to form H-bonds, A, B-macromolecules incline to indefinite self-association caused by non-Coulomb forces. The self-association is favoured by approaching the isoionic point of one component because of the weakening of the repulsion between similarly charged macromolecules. It is also favoured by increasing the protein concentration due to the stengthening of Van der Waals interactions. In favourable cases the gelatin aggregates were established to attain the size of colloid particles [4]. The indicated features make the A-B system as a convenient model for the investigation of self-association effects in the formation of electrostatic complexes between two polyampholytes with low charge density, i.e. proteins.

The original samples A and B obtained by hydrolysis of collagen had a high polydispersity and were fractionated by alcohol precipitation [5]. A and B fractions with molecular mass of 100 kD were employed in the experiments.

Interactions between protein molecules were studied under conditions of favouring and inhibiting the protein self-association. Under conditions avoiding self-association (40°C, concentration is not more than 0.01%, pH value 6.8 is far from the isoionic points of both proteins) the mixing of the solutions with various A and B mole ratios led to the formation of soluble and insoluble complexes. The fact that the complexation did not occur in the presence of neutral salts pointed out the electrostatic nature of the process. The formation of insoluble complexes resulted in an augmentation of the turbidity of the system. The determination of the composition of insoluble complexes was based upon the investigation of turbidity versus the mole ratios of A and B according to Job's method of continuous variation [6]. This method allowes to determine the stoichiometry of protein complexes. Fig. 2 (curve 1) illustrates the turbidity values as a function of mole ratios p = ligand : acceptor. The position of the turbidity maximum on pH 6.8 curve proved to be in accordance with the $AB_3$ complex composition. The determination of net charges of A and B macromolecules based on potentiometric titration data indicated that the insoluble complex is electrically neutral. The mole ratio of A and B in the complex is inversely proportional to the net charge of protein macromolecules at the experimental pH value [7]. The existence of soluble electrostatic complexes of A and B was determined by ultracentrifugation, gel-permeation chromatography and by turbidimetric titration with ethanol [7]. The abrupt increase of turbidity with adding the precipitant to the A and B initial solutions was observed when the excess ethanol volume was approximately three times of that of water solution. In this case the turbidimetric curves are S-shaped ones which is characteristic for monodisperse polymers (Fig. 3, curve 1). At the same time the turbidimetric titration curve of an equimolar mixture of A and B was more complicated and has an additional extremum at approximately 1.5 volume excess of the ethanol in the system (Fig. 3, curve 2). This shows that the solution contains components of heavier molecular weights, i.e. soluble complexes of A and B. The equimolar composition of this complex was ascertained by sedimentation equilibrium studies. The excess of negative charge hinders the coagulation of the complex from the solution.

It has to be emphasised that physico-chemical properties of the soluble A - B complexes deviate notably from these of A and B. For example the helix-coil transition temperature range for the A - B gelatin mixture was 3 - 5°C higher than that for A or B. Higher thermal stability of the helix conformation may arise from weaker repulsion between equally charged protein groups on account of their mutual neutralization during complex formation. The value of the intrinsic viscosity of soluble complex was two times decreased, and the value of second virial coefficient $A_2$ was four times decreased. (Table 1).

Table 1: Some physico-chemical parameters of the solutions of individual A and B and their equimolar mixture in 5 mM phosphate buffer and 0.5 M urea pH 6.8 at 40 °C

| | [ν] dl/g | $k' = tg\ \alpha/[\nu]^2$ | $A_2 \cdot 10^{-4}$ | $\bar{M}w$ |
|---|---|---|---|---|
| B | 0.23 | 2.8 | 12.0 | 80,000 |
| A | 0.26 | 4.9 | - | - |
| A:B = 1:1 | 0.13 | 32.0 | 2.9 | 156,000 |

The decrease of intrinsic viscosity of soluble complexes and increase of their molecular weight suggest that their structure becomes more compact. The increase of the Huggins constant (k') and decrease of the second virial coefficient ($A_2$) indicate that hydrophilicity of complex structure is reduced.

In order to study the effect of self-association of A and B on electrostatic complex formation, the conditions of experiments were varied. Protein solutions with concentrations more than 0.01 % were mixed at room temperature and pH 5.5 which is near isoionic point of B. The decrease of the temperature favoured the formation of H-bonds between protein molecules. The variation of pH value decreased electrostatic repulsion of B macromolecules, promoting their assembling. The polydispersity of solution B in such conditions was evidenced by, for instance, turbidimetric titration with precipitant. The composition of insoluble complexes formed by A and B, mixed at pH 5.5 was affected by the self-association process. This can be seen from the complicated profile of turbidimetric curve. The curve possesses two turbidity maxima (Fig. 2, curve 2). The first one corresponds to the complex, the composition of which differed from the electroneutrality. This complex appeared to be formed by the interaction between A and associated form of B. The aggregation stability of the system decreased with the increase of protein concentration up to 0.05 - 0.10 %. The composition of insoluble complexes differed progressively from an equivalent one (Fig. 2, curve 3). Perhaps within the range of high protein concentrations, when the size of aggregates attains the size of colloid species, the process of phase separation resembles that of colloid heterocoagulation. In these conditions the composition of the precipitation can be significantly differed from the electroneutral one.

The electrostatic complexation and self-association process are competing. The mechanism of interaction between the protein molecules is affected not only by pH values, temperature and concentration but also by the sequence of mixing of the components and by the presence of some ions and urea in the solution, which prevent the self-association of the gelatin as well. The influence self-association upon the electrostatic complex formation was lowered with the growth of macromolecules charges, for example after succinylation and phoshorylation. As a result of chemical modification a decrease of protein self-association was observed. As a consequence the insoluble complexes of acid-process gelatin with modified samples of alkali-process gelatin possessed an equivalent composition regardless of mixing order of the components and of temperature value. The characteristic feature of these complexes was their higher resistance to dissociation under the effect of ionic strength.

Thus, the interaction between oppositely charged polyampholytes of low charge density is determined by Coulomb forces forming soluble and insoluble complexes in the case of suppressing the self-association process. This can be achieved by reducing protein concentration, working at pH values far enough from their isoionic points, adding urea, increasing net charge density through chemical modification.

When low charge protein macromolecules are interacting the simultaneously occurring processes of eletrostatic complexation and self-association turned out to be competing. The preferred interaction mechanism is that one determined by the ratio the binding constants of macromolecules affected by electrostatic or non-Coulomb forces. The quantitative investigation of the electrostatic complex formation between A and B was performed using the ion-exchange resins method. This method allows to determine the association constants under equilibrium conditions in the process of interaction between molecules corresponding to the multiple equilibrium scheme [8]. The method consists in the comparision of the ion-exchange resin solution distribution coefficients of acceptor in the absence ($K_{d_o}$) and in the presence of the ligand ($K_d$) from which the apparent association constants of acceptor-ligand electrostatic complexes can be calculated.

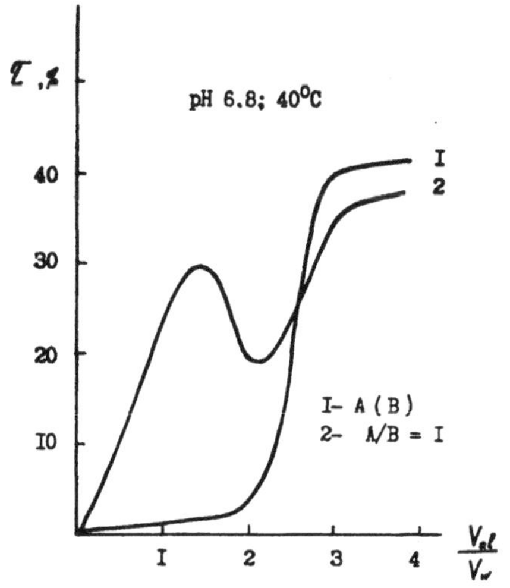


Figure 3: Turbidity of protein solutions (C = 0.01 %) versus alcohol concentration at pH 6.8 and T = 40°C: 1- A or B;
2- A:B = 1:1.

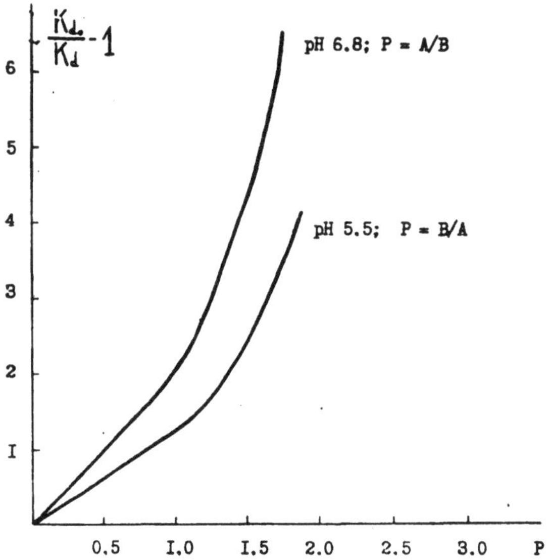


Figure 4: $K_{d_o}/K_d-1$ versus mole ratios P = ligand:acceptor curves at different conditions (5 mM phosphate buffer, T = 40°C)

Studying the interaction of A and B under various experimental conditions promoting the suppression of proteins self-association the following has been estimated. At the first stage of the process, that means under the conditions of ligand shortage complexes with an equimolar A/B composition only were formed. Fig. 4 illustrates the experimental curves of $K_{d_o}/K_d-1$ as a function of mole ratios p = ligand:acceptor. These curves characterize the process desorption of the acceptor from the ion-exchange resin under conditions of electrostatic complexation of proteins in the solution. In all the cases at $p < 1$ the curves had a linear character. For these conditions of equal concentrations of A and B associated in the complex, the values of free concentrations of ligand [B] were calculated. The values of apparent association constants $k_1$ were determined according to the following equation:

$$K_{d_o}/K_d-1 = k_1\cdot[B] + k_1k_2\cdot[B]^2 + \ldots + k_1k_2 \ldots k_n\cdot[B]^n$$

The $k_1$ values have been established to be dependent on A and B net charges and determined by the pH of the medium. The variation of temperature from 20 to 40°C didn't affect the association constant when self-association processes were suppressed. This fact indicated the electrostatic nature of A - B complexes.

With further increase of the ligand mole fraction, electrostatic protein complexes of other composition were formed and acumulated in the solution. As it is shown on Fig. 4 the plots are rather curvilinear in the range of ligand concentrations higher than those of the acceptor. The production of electroneutral complexes led to their coagulation. The process of phase separation limited the application of the ion-exchange resins method for the investigation of proteins interaction in the case of high mole fractions in the system.

**References**


[1] Vainerman E.S., W.Ya. Grinberg, W.B. Tolstoguov: Untersuchung der Wechselwirkung von Eiweissen mit Polysaccariden im Wassermedium. Kolloid Z.u.Z. Polymere. **250** (1972) 10, 945-949.

[2] Tolstoguzov, W.B., E.S. Vainerman: Untersuchung der Wechelwirkung einiger Eiweissstoffe mit sauren Polysaccariden in wässrigem Medium. Nahrung. **19** (1975) 1, 45-60.

[3] Kurskaya, E.A., E.S. Vainerman, S.V. Rogozhin: On complex formation of acid-process and alkaline-process gelatins. Nahrung. **26** (1979) 6, 581-588.

[4] Boedtker H., P. Doty: Study of gelatin molecules, aggregates and gels. J. Phys. Chem., **58** (1945) 11, 968-983.

[5] Steinsby G.: The fractionation of gelatin by coacervation. Disc. Farad. Soc. **18** (1954) 2, 288-294.

[6] Rossotti, F.J.C., H. Rossotti: The determination of stability constants and other equilibrium constants in solutions. McGraw-Hill, New York 1961.

[7] Kurskaya, E.A., E.S. Vainerman, S.V. Rogozhin, G.I. Timofeeva: A study of soluble complexes of alkaline-process gelatins by turbidimetric titration. Colloid Polym. Sci. **258** (1980) 9, 1086-1091.

[8] Nakai, C., W. Glinsmann: Interactions between polyamines and nucleotides. Biochemistry, **16** (1977) 25, 5636-5641.

# METHODIC ASPECTS IN STUDYING POLYELECTROLYTE COMPLEX FORMATION

Dautzenberg, Herbert und Linow, Karl-Joachim [1)]

## 1. Introduction

Polyanion-polycation complexes (symplexes) are known for a long time on an empirical basis from the mutual precipitation of proteins. Already at the end of the previous century Kossel /1/ recognized the electrostatic interaction between the oppositely charged polyions as the driving force for precipitation. Up to now complex formation between proteins as well as proteins and synthetic polymers plays an important part in preparation and purification of proteins.

In the recent years we dealt with complex formation between synthetic polyions /2/. However the basic effects and the methods of investigation are the same for the different types of polyelectrolyte complexes. Therefore some methodic experiences and results obtained on synthetic polymers may be of general interest.

Mixing of solutions of oppositely charged polyions leads to complex formation due to Coulombic interaction. This complex formation is accomponied by a change of different physical parameters of the system, e. g. conductivity, pH-value (free acid-base pairs), conformation of the molecules, degree of aggregation. All methods, which are sensitive about these parameters, are suitable to observe complex formation. In sufficiently diluted solutions a macroscopic flocculation may be avoided and the complex formation can be stopped at a colloidal level. In this case the physico-chemical methods, employed for polymer solutions, can be used to study polyelectrolyte complex formation.
More infomation may be obtained by a combination of different methods.

## 2. Methods of investigation

Table 1 shows the methods used in our work. The first three methods usually are employed to study the stoichiometry of the symplexes. Observation of dye binding and liberation by fluorescence measurements allow to judge the symplex stability. In principle density measurements should give similar information, but only in the case of components with very different densities reliable results may be obtained. The last three

-------

1)
Institut für Polymerenchemie der AdW der DDR, 1530 Teltow,"Erich Correns"

methods cannot only be applied to determine the stoichiometry, but also to characterize size and structure of the generated symplex particles. In this report we will demonstrate the meaningfulness of the mentioned methods by some representative results and discuss more general features of complex formation.

Table 1: Methods of investigation

- conductometry
- potentiometry
- turbidity
- UV/VIS spectroscopy (fluorescence of dyes)
- density measurements
- viscometry
- sedimentation measurements
- light scattering (quasielastic)

## 3. Materials

Complex formation was studied between a great number of polyions, this report is however restricted to the polymers given in Table 2. In the series A0 - A8 and C0 - C8 of anionically and cationically modified poly (acrylamide) the charge density was varied systematically. Poly(acrylic-acid) and Cellulosesulphate differ in the strength of the ionic groups.

Table 2: Selected samples employed in symplex formation

| Polyanion Name | Abbr. | Polycation Name | Abbr. |
|---|---|---|---|
| Poly(sodiumacrylate) | A0 | Poly(N-methyl-N,N-diethyl-aminoethylacrylate) | C0 |
| Copolymer of A0-units and acrylamide | | Copolymer of C0-units and acrylamide | |
| 1 : 4 | A4 | 1 : 4 | C4 |
| 1 : 8 | A8 | 1 : 8 | C8 |
| Cellulose sulphate | | Poly(dimethyldiallyl-) ammoniumchloride | PDMDAAC |
| salt | NaCS | | |
| free acid | HCS | | |
| Sodium lignosulphonate | NaLS | Poly(ethyleneimine) | |
| | | linear | $PEI_{lin}$ |
| | | branched | $PEI_{br}$ |

Also branched polymers (lignosulphonate and branched PEI) were included in the investigations.

### 4. Stoichiometry of symplexes - titration methods

To observe the macroscopic course of symplex formation a titration cell was constructed, which allows a simultaneous registration of the pH-value, conductivity and turbidity. Results obtained for the system acid form of cellulosesulphate/PEI $_{br}$ are represented in Fig. 1.

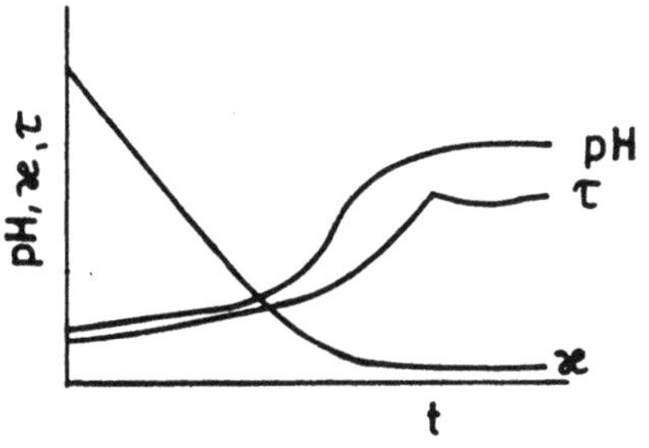


Fig. 1: pH-value, conductivity and turbidity of cellulose sulphate (acid form) titrated with PEI $_{br}$ in $H_2O$

During the addition of the PEI $_{br}$ solution the conductivity decreases, due to the neutralization of the excess of $H^+$ ions, reaching a constant level in the neutral range. The breakpoint in the conductivity agrees with the steepest slope of the pH-curve. The molar ratio of the cationic sites to the anionic ones at this point was determined to $N_C/N_A$ = 1.3. The turbidimetric endpoint yields 1.6, indicating that the flocculation point must not be identical with the balance of charges of the polyions. The pH-measurement is limited to the case of free acid/base pairs. In the case of polysalts also another behavior of the conductivity should be expected. In the solution of polyions the low molecular counterions are concentrated in the enviroment of the polyions, yielding a low conductivity. Complex formation leads to a liberation of the counterions and therefore to a stronger increase of the conductivity. After finishing of complex formation the conductivity enhances only slightly. The endpoint of titration is again expressed as a breakpoint in the conductivity. Fig. 2 shows the titration curves of AO with CO, C4 and C8. While for all systems the flocculation point is clearly expressed, the determination of the breakpoint in conductivity for the systems AO/C4 and AO/C8 is no more reliable. This result is caused by the misfit of the charge density of the symplex components. Table 3 gives the stoichiometry of the symplexes CO/AO, C4/A4, C8/A8 with comparable charge densities.

Table 3: Molar ratio $N_C/N_A$ at the turbidimetric and conductometric endpoint for symplexes of components with equal charge density

| PEL-combination | $N_C/N_A$ |
|---|---|
| CO/AO | 0.6 |
| C4/A4 | 1.8 |
| C8/A8 | 3.1 |

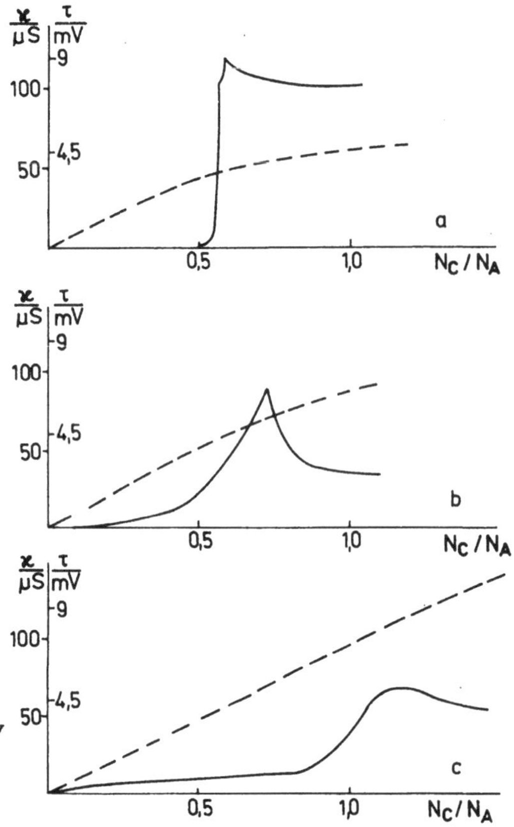


Fig. 2: Conductivity and turbidity of AO titrated with CO, C4, and C8 in $H_2O$

The data suggest a strong deviation from the 1 : 1 stoichiometry, depending on the charge density of the components. Generally our investigations showed that in highly diluted systems the 1 : 1 stoichiometry is more an exception than the rule. This result is in contradiction to the 1 : 1 stoichiometry of washed and dried polyelectrolyte complexes. It must be stated here that the titration studies are no direct methods for the determination of the symplex stoichiometry. More explicit information may be obtained by sedimentation measurements.
We will return to this topic, but before that, some remarks about a special titration technique. Fluorescence measurements of dyes can be used to observe the formation of dye-polyion complexes and the liberation of the dye due to polyanion-polycation complex formation. Such investigations allow the estimation of symplex stability and preferential binding. Fig. 3 gives the fluorescence intensity of acridine orange during addition of AO, A4 and A8. With decreasing charge density an increasing amount of anionic sites is necessary to quench the dye, see also Table 4.

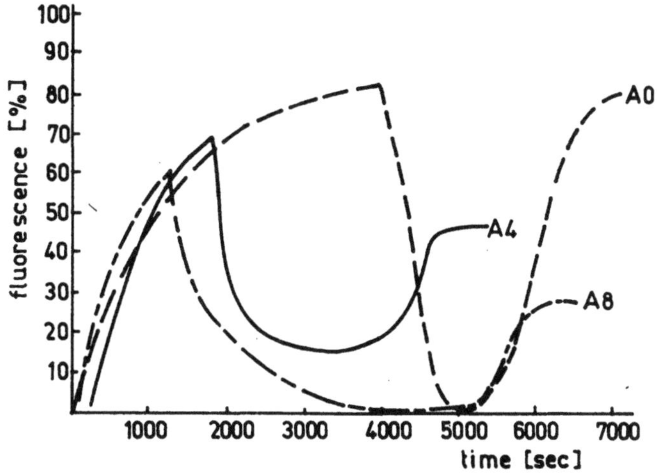


Fig. 3: Change in fluorescence intensity of acridine orange due to binding of AO, A4, A8 and liberation by subsequent addition of CO

Table 4: Binding and liberation of acridine orange in symplex systems of AX and CO

| Polyanion | anionic sites required per quenched dye molecule | % fluorescence recovered after addition of CO |
|---|---|---|
| AO | 4 | 90 - 95 |
| A4 | 40 | 71 |
| A8 | 60 | 42 |

The dispelling of the dye by addition of CO depends also strongly on the charge density of the polyion. For AO a nearly complete liberation of acridine orange was found, while for A8 more than 50 % of the dye remained bound. This result suggest a preferential binding between polyelectrolyte components with appropriate charge density.

## 5. Characterization of symplex particles

The methods covered hitherto, give no information about the structural parameters of the symplex particles in diluted systems. Sedimentation measurements, viscometry and light scattering offer a better access to this problem.

Sedimentation in a medium with a density gradient or zonal sedimentation allow a separation of the PEL-complex and the single components. A quantitative analysis yields the mass fractions of all components and

above that a characterization of their size distribution. Due to a lot of trouble with our instruments we could not carry out such investigations up to now, but the work is in progress.
Viscometry is one of the simplest method to observe structural changes of the solvated polymer coils in solution. Complex formation is accompanied by an aggregation to more compact particles, resulting in a decrease of the viscosity. In Table 5 the intrinsic viscosities of the single components A4 and C4 and of the symplex system at different degrees of conversion are given.

Table 5: Viscometric data of the system A4/C4 in 0.1 n NaCl

| sample | $[\eta]$ $cm^3/g$ |
|---|---|
| A4 | 863 |
| C4 | 1054 |
| A4 + C4 ( 50 %) | 459 |
| A4 + C4 (200 %) | 220 |
| C4 + A4 ( 50 %) | 221 |
| C4 + A4 (200 %) | 461 |

As expected, PEL-formation led to a significant decrease in viscosity, which is stronger in the case of cation excess. This result corresponds to the deviation from the 1 : 1 stoichiometry, found by the titration studies. The viscosities obtained for the same composition of the systems, but different sequence of mixing, agrees quite well, indicating the same stoichiometry of the symplex. But without additional information quantitative results about the stoichiometry cannot **be derived from** the viscometric data.

In our work light scattering proved to be one of the most informative methods in the study of PEL-complex formation in diluted systems. While in viscometric measurements the contribution of the polyelectrolyte components dominates, in light scattering the formed complex yields the main part of the measured intensity and the influence of the single polyelectrolytes may be neglected. Therefore light scattering allows directly the characterization of the mass and size of the symplex particles.

In our investigation we used a wide-angle-light scattering photometer (Sofica 42000, Wippler and Scheibling, Strasbourg, France), which was equiped with a He-Ne-laser as light source. Thereby the accuracy of measurements could be improved to be better than 1 %, which is a necessary condition for a reliable interpretation of the scattering curves.

To study the process of complex formation, the polyelectrolyte solutions were mixed directly in the scattering cell and the scattered intensity at the scattering angle of 30° was recorded continuously. The solutions were purified by filtration through membrane filters of pore size 0.45 μm. To obtain complete scattering curves we interrupted the titrant dosage at different degrees of conversion and measured the scattering intensity at 31 angular positions.

The analysis of the scattering curves by a Zimm or a Guinier plot /3/ yields the mass average value of the particle mass and the z-average value of the square of the radius of gyration.
For that an extrapolation of the scattering curves to the scattering angle 0 must be carried out, which may be connected with great errors (up to an order of magnitude), due to the strong curvature in the small angle region for polydisperse systems of large particles. Therefore we derived an algorithm of data evalution, basing on an assignment of the experimental curves to a section of an appropriate theoretical curve. This allows a reliable extrapolation, taking advantage from the known course of the theoretical scattering curve. The main problem consists in the fact that even assuming a monomodal system of particles with known structure, a two-dimensional variety of scattering curves exists in dependence on the size and polydispersity parameter ($a_m$, $\sigma$) of the distribution function. To solve this task, we used a special logarithmic distribution function /4/, which separates the influence of size and polydispersity and yields the intensity at the scattering angle 0 independent of $\sigma$. Fig. 4 shows the distribution function for different polydispersities.

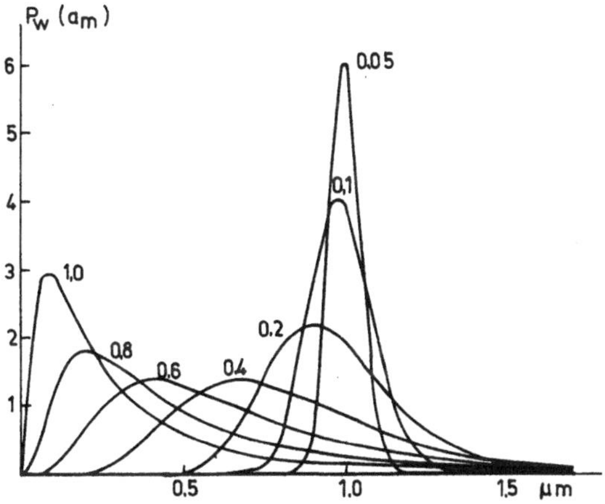


Fig. 4: Logarithmic distribution functions used in light scattering calculations

In the framework of the Rayleigh-Debye-approximation the size parameter $a_m$ generally occurs in the scattering function as a product with the scattering parameter h. Therefore the $a_m$-dependence of the scattering curves may be represented by a single curve. In a double logarithmic plot log I versus log($a_m$ . h) a variation of $a_m$ corresponds only to parallel shifts along the axis. Consequently the two-dimensional dependence on $a_m$ and $\sigma$ is reduced to a set of scattering curves with different values of $\sigma$. Such Master curves were calculated for spheres of homogeneous density and Gaussian coils /5/, see Fig. 5.

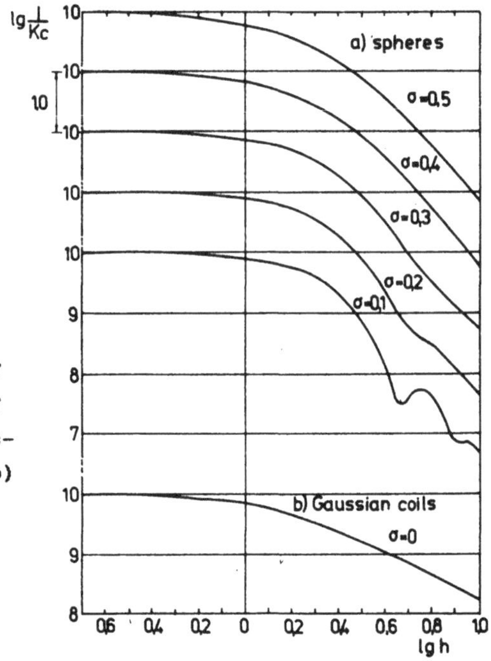


Fig. 5: Master curves for light scattering of polydisperse systems of spheres (a) and monodisperse Gaussian coils (b)

In the abscissa range 0.25 to 1.0, the scattering curves are so different that a corresponding experimental curve can be unambiguously assigned to a particle typ and for spheres also to a certain polydispersity. This range of the scattering curves corresponds to particle sizes between 200 nm and 1 µm. From the position of the experimental curve on a theoretical one we obtain the mass and size of the particles. Alltogether we get the following information :
typ of particles, polydispersity of the system, weight average value of the particle mass $M_w$, size parameter $a_m$ and from $M_w$ and $a_m$ the polymer packing density in the particles

$$\rho = M_w / \frac{4\pi}{3} a_m^3$$

The detailed information allows a deeper understanding of the processes, occurring during symplex formation or addition of salt to a symplex system. This should be demonstrated by some examples. In Fig. 6 the dependence of $M_w$ on the degreee of conversion is represented for different PEL-complexes.
With exception of the system A8/C8 only a slight variation of $M_w$ was observed up to a degree of conversion of 80 %, suggesting that the buil-

ding of new particles and not particle growing is the dominating process with increasing conversion. The particle size is already fixed from the very beginning of the reaction. The absolute value of M ist not a relevant parameter, because it can be changed to a great extent by a variation of the polymer concentration (compare $M_w$ of the symplexes NaCS/PDMDAAC).

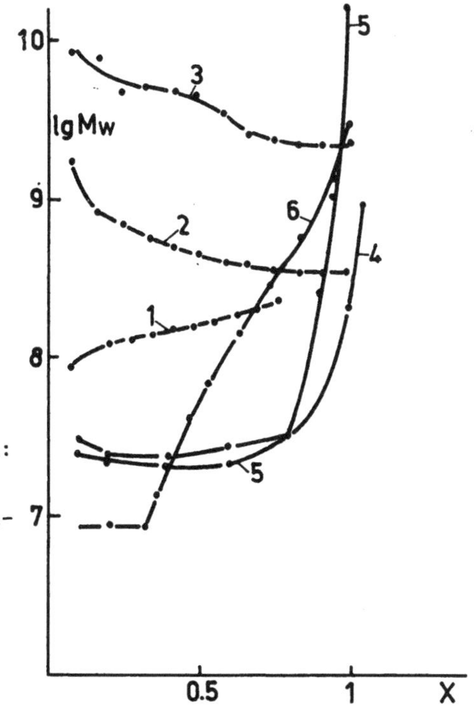


Fig. 6: Dependence of $M_w$ (g/mole) on the degree of conversion: 1-CO/AO, 2,3-NaCS/PDMDAAC, at different polymer concentrations (factor 5), 4-NaLS/PDMDAAC, 5-$PEI_{lin}$/A4, 6-A8/C8

In the system A8/C8 a strong dependence of all particle parameters on the conversion occurred. The scattering curves are represented as Guinier plot in Fig. 7 and as Master plot in Fig. 8. While the Guinier plot doesn't allow a reliable determination of the particle parameters, we obtain from the Master plot a lot of information. At the beginning of the symplex formation highly swollen particles were formed and the scattering curves correspond to Gaussian coils. With increasing conversion the particles become more compact and the structure typ changes to homogeneous spheres. The polydispersity of the systems decreases. The particle parameters determined from the Master curves, are given in Fig. 9 (for more details see /5/). The quantitative results show that up to a conversion of about 50 % the particles mass increases slightly, but the polymer packing density rises drastically. Afterwards a progressive aggregation without change of the internal particle structure occurs.

The last example demonstrates the effect of the addition of salt to a symplex formed in pure water; Fig. 10.

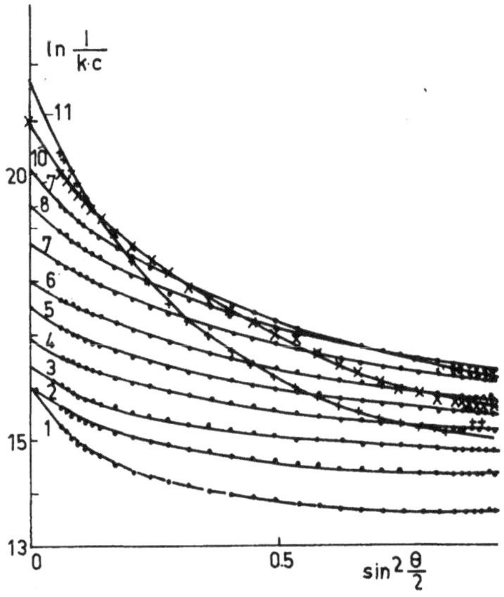


Fig. 7: Scattering curves of the system A8/C8 in dependence on the degree of conversion as Guinier plot

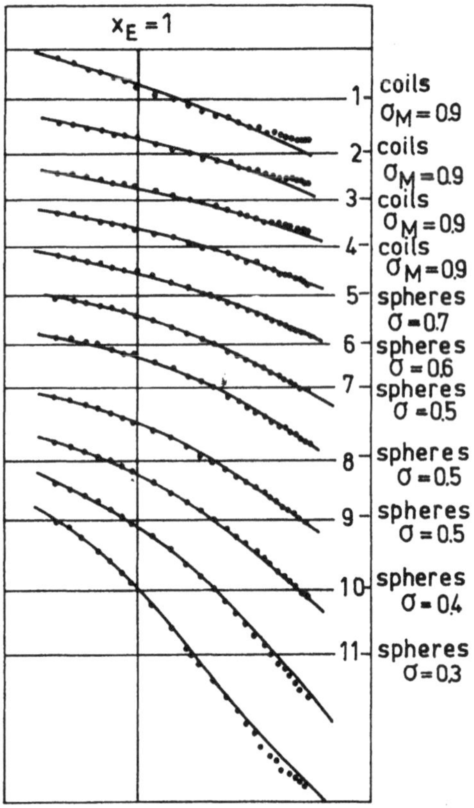


Fig. 8.: Scattering curves of the system A8/C8 as Master plot

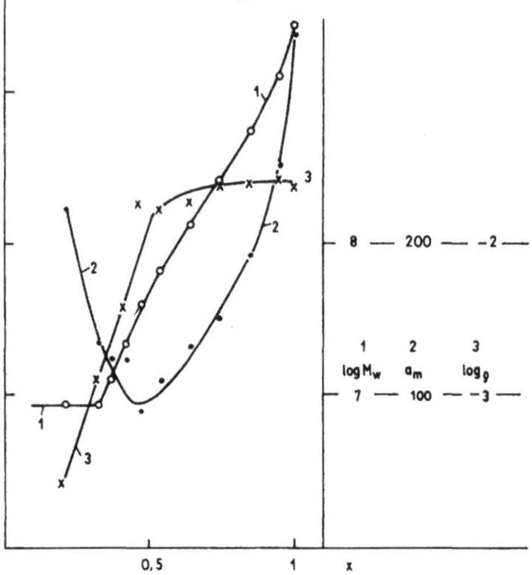


Fig. 9: Conversion dependence of the parameters $M_w$, $a_m$ and $\rho$ for A8/C8 in $H_2O$

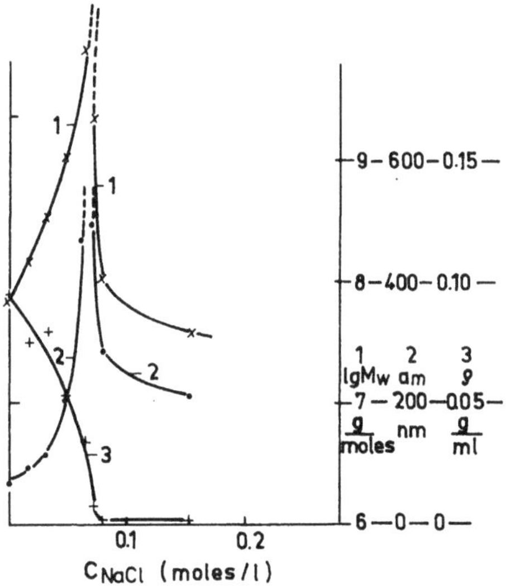


Fig. 10: Dependence of the particle parameters of a symplex C4/A4 on NaCl content at subsequent addition of salt

The addition of salt leads to two effects: aggregation and swelling. At a certain critical salt concentration a dissolution up to the molecular level was observed. In this range the scattering curves indicate a transition from compact spheres to Gaussian coils. The critical salt concentration depends on the charge density of the components, as Table 6 illustrates. In this Table the values of the polymer packing density are given too, which also correlate with the charge density.

Table 6: Polymer packing density and critical NaCl concentration in dependence on charge density

| PEL-combination | $\rho$ g/ml | $c_{NaCl}$ mole/l |
|---|---|---|
| CO/AO | 0.13 - 0.17 | 0.45 |
| C4/A4 | 0.07 - 0.13 | 0.065 - 0.09 |
| C8/A8 | 0.02 - 0.08 | 0 - 0.02 |

The response of a symplex to addition of salt may be very different. For the symplex NaCS/PDMDAAC with strong ionic groups a macroscopic flocculation occurs at a certain salt concentration.
It should be mentioned here that no significant influence of branching on symples formation was observed for poly(ehtyleneimine). On the other hand NaLS/PDMDAAC yields symplex particles with extremely high polymer packing density of about 1.

## 6. Conclusions

The examples reported demonstrate that the application of methods, usually employed in characterization of polymer solutions, yields detailed information about the process of PEL-complex formation and moreover about the mass, size and internal structure of the generated particles.
Especially an improved interpretation of light scattering data allows to analyse different processes as aggregation, swelling, dissolution, change of the particle structure and the polydispersity of the systems.
The combination of different methods increases the reliability of the results obtained.

We are grateful to Mrs. Dr. G. Rother for her involvement in the calculations of the theoretical light scattering curves and Dr. J. Kötz (Institut für Polymerenchemie) for his work in the titration experiments.

Literature:

/1/ Kossel, A.: J. Physiol. Chem. 22 (1896)

/2/ Dautzenberg, H., Linow, K.-J., Kötz, J. and Philipp, B.
Acta Polymerica 32 (1981), 225; 33 (1982), 619, 37 (1986), 108,
39 (1988), 157
and Plaste und Kautschuk 29 (1982), 631

/3/ Kerker, M. "The scattering of light and other electromagnetic radiations"
Chapter 8, p. 414, New York/San Francisco/London, Academic Press (1969)

/4/ Hartmann, M. and Dautzenberg, H.: Acta Polymerica 34 (1983), 52

/5/ Dautzenberg, H. and Rother, G.: J. Polym. Sci. Part B, Polymer Physics, 26 (1988), 353

# RAPESEED PROTEIN-POLYANION INTERACTIONS

K.D. Schwenke[1], R. Mothes[1], K. Gast[2] and D. Zirwer[2]

**Abstract**

The binding of pectic acid (PA), polyphosphate, phytic acid and two cellulose sulfates (CS) to the main storage proteins from rapeseed, the high molecular mass neutral 12S globulin and the low molecular mass basic 2S protein (napin), in insoluble complexes has been studied at pH < pI by means of turbidimetry and chemical analysis of the supernatant after coprecipitation. In most cases the precipitation of the proteins took place at a substoichiometric polyanion-protein ratio. An excess binding of polyanion was observed in the systems globulin-phytic acid, globulin-PA and napin-PA at pH-values where the acidic groups of the polyanion were partially neutralized.

In PA-containing systems an intensive polyanion binding took place beween pH 5 and 3 which corresponds to the region of carboxyl groups titration both in the proteins and in the polyanion.

The napin precipitation by CS at pH 2.5 - 3.0 resembles the interaction between strong polyelectrolytes: the CS-protein ratio in the coprecipitates is nearly independent on the CS concentration. This behaviour was only approached by the globulin at pH 2.5.

The formation of soluble complexes was investigated in the system napin-phytic acid by means of gel chromatography, dynamic light scattering, circular dichroism spectroscopy, potentiometric titration and turbidimetry. Depending on the napin-phytic acid ratio and the salt concentration dimeric and oligomeric complexes were formed. This complexation did not influence the protein secondary structure but resulted in a total inhibition of heat induced coagulation. The dynamic light scattering study revealed the presence of high-molecular mass soluble aggregates which were stable at 60°C.

## Introduction

The study of the interactions between rapeseed proteins and polyanions is motivated by two facts: The first one is the low recovery of rapeseed protein due to the high percentage of a water soluble isoelectrically non-precipitable protein fraction which can be pre-

---

[1] Central Institute of Nutrition, Potsdam-Rehbrücke, Academy of Sciences of the GDR,
1505 Bergholz-Rehbrücke, Arthur-Scheunert-Allee 114 - 116
[2] Central Institute of Molecular Biology, Academy of Sciences of the GDR,
1115 Berlin-Buch, Robert-Rössle-Str. 10

cipitated by complexing with polyanions [1]. The second one is the presence of a low molecular mass polyanion in rapeseed, phytic acid or myo-inositol hexaphosphate, which forms electrostatic complexes with the rapeseed proteins [2, 3]. This interaction is favoured owing to the basic nature of the main rapeseed protein fractions. These are proteins with a quite different structure: the oligomeric 12S globulin with a molecular mass of 300 000 g/mol and an isoelectric point of 7.2 [4, 5] and the 1.7S protein fraction ("albumin" or "napin") with a molecular mass of 12 000 - 14 000 g/mol and isoelectric points higher than 10 [6, 7]. From a practical point of view it is necessary to know the conditions of maximum protein precipitation with a minimum use of the polyanion as flocculating agent. The complexes obtained must possess a definite composition (polyanion - protein ratio). From a more theoretical point of view such problems as the stoichiometry of complex formation, the equilibrium between insoluble and soluble complexes, if it exists, and last not least the structure of the electrostatic complexes - if there are definite ones - are of interest.

A number of papers were published on the problem of protein precipitation by polyanions (vide for example [8, 10]), some of which are concerned with the use of polyanions for rapeseed protein recovery [1, 11]. There is however, a lack of knowledge on the interaction between isolated definite rapeseed proteins and polyanions.

The present paper deals with the complexation of the two main protein fractions from rapeseed by various polyanions and characterization of soluble rapeseed protein - phytic acid complexes.

**Insoluble complexes between rapeseed proteins and high molecular mass polyanions**

The formation of insoluble electrostatic complexes between a protein and a polyanion takes places generally in the pH-range below the isoelectric point of the protein. This can be followed quickly by turbidity measurements [9, 10]. Figure 1 shows the pH-dependence of complex formation in the system 12S rapeseed globulin - cellulose sulfate (CS). A distinct maximum of precipitation appears for each polyanion - protein ratio, the position of which shifts to lower values of pH with increasing percentage of the polyanion [12].

There are three different steps of complexation of special interest:

- The maximum precipitation taking place mostly at a substoichiometric polyanion-protein ratio
- the (1 : 1)-stoichiometric composition, at which the turbidity curves approach sigmoid shape corresponding to a mass part of 0.33 for the polyanion in Fig. 1
- the polyanion-protein ratio, at which the solubilization of the complexes is complete.

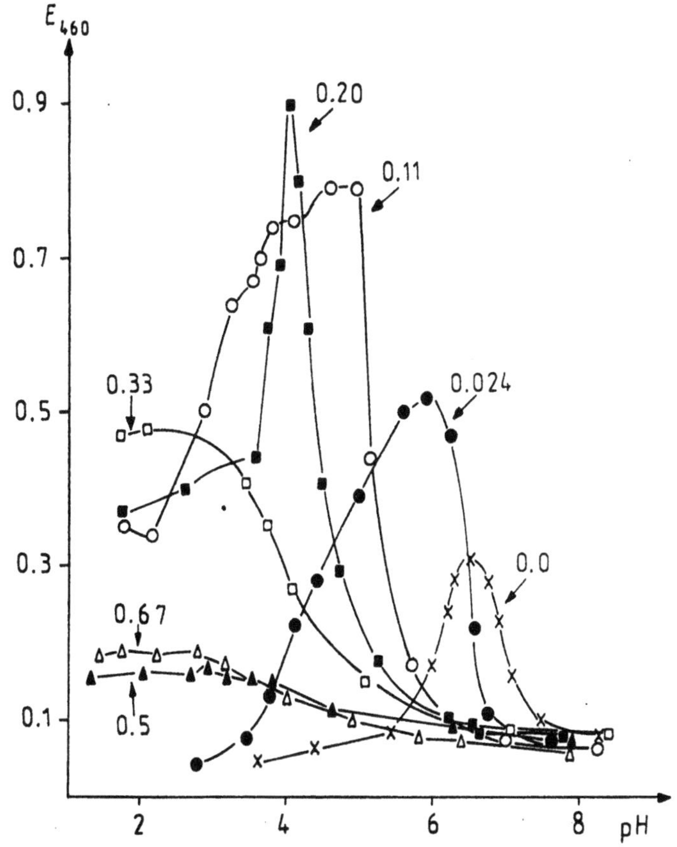


Fig 1: Estimation of pH-dependence of globulin precipitation by different amounts of a cellulose sulfate (DS 0.6) using turbidimetric titration with hydrochloric acid, according to [12]. The numbers on the curves designate the mass part of the polyanion.

A (1 : 1)-stoichiometric composition means the equivalence both of the total of basic groups of the protein and the negative charges of the polyanion. This important composition can be estimated quickly by plotting the maximum position of the turbidity curve versus the polyanion-protein mass ratio [13]. Fig. 2 shows this plot for the systems pectic acid (PA)-rapeseed proteins. The resulting curves contain an inflection or breaking point which corresponds fairly well to the (1 : 1) stoichiometric ratio of both components.

The turbidimetric titration of the protein with the polyanion was used for the determination of polyanion binding. The bound amount of polyanion can be determined from the precipitation point which is seen as a sudden increase of turbidity in most cases and which coresponds to the midpoint of sigmoid turbidity curves. Figure 3 shows the turbidimetric titration curves of the rapeseed globulin with PA at pH 4.0 using various protein concentrations.

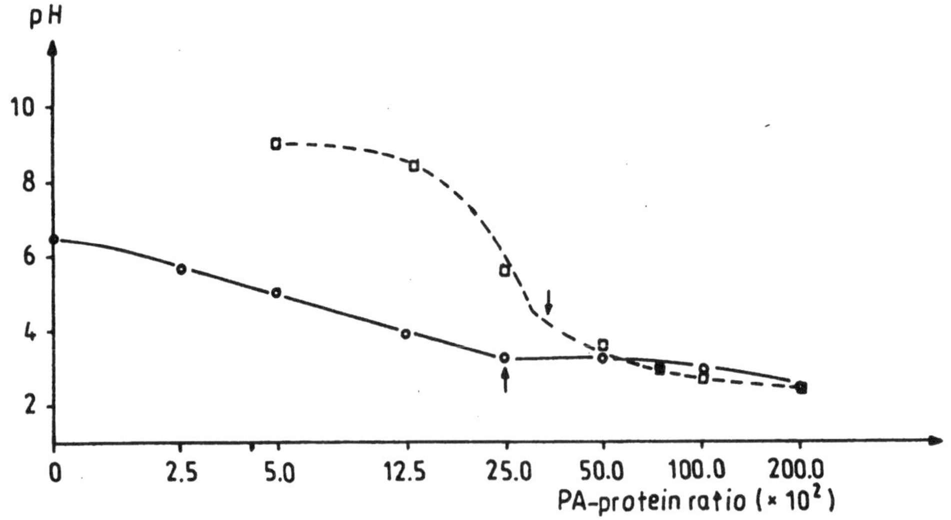


Fig. 2: Dependence of the maximum position of the turbidity curves of rapeseed protein-PA mixtures on the PA-protein ratio, according to [13].
The arrows designate the (1 : 1)-stoichiometric composition.
o globulin □ albumin

Corresponding to the increase of positive net charge of the proteins, the amount of bound PA increases with decreasing pH (Fig. 4). The prolongation of the curves of pH-dependence of PA binding gives pH-values for the "zero"-binding which correspond to the isoelectric regions of both proteins. A (1 : 1)-stoichiometric ratio is observed for the PA-globulin complex at pH 3.3 - 3.4 and for the PA-albumin complex at pH 4.2 - 4.3. Both proteins bind a molar excess of PA at lower pH. The highest amount of bound PA was determined to be 1.9 (mol COOH per mol positively charged groups of the protein) for the globulin and 1.4 for the albumin at pH 3.0. The PA-albumin binding curve is characterized by an inflection point at pH 5 which clearly separates a region of high PA binding at low pH from that of low PA binding at higher pH. The first one corresponds to the titration of carboxyl groups both of proteins and pectic acid. This titration has an opposite effect in proteins and pectic acid. It favours the interaction of positively charged groups in the protein by neutralizing the carboxyl groups. It reduced, on the other hand the reactive carboxyl groups in the polyanion.

At pH below the pK amounting 3.3 - 3.5 for galacturonic acid the carboxyl groups are partially neutralized and only the charged ones are able to interact with basic groups of the proteins. Therefore, the "excess" binding as to the total amount of carboxyl residues at pH lower the pK is plausible.

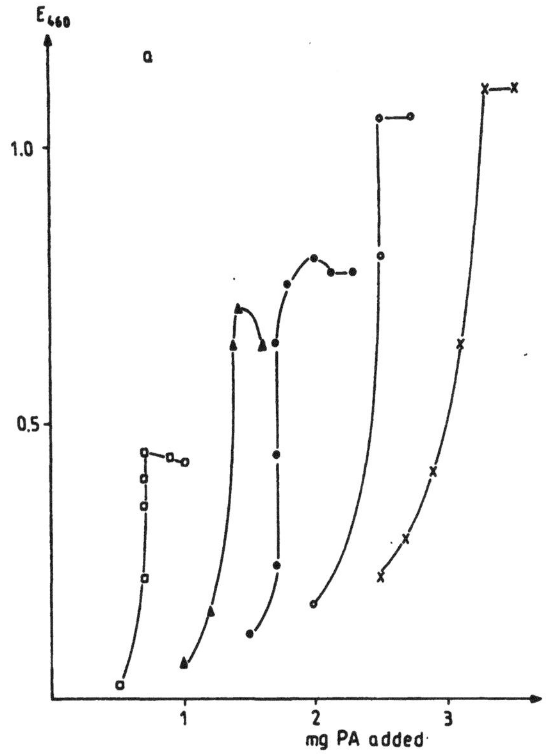


Fig. 3: Turbidimetric titration of the globulin with PA at pH 4.0 using various amounts of protein, according to [13].
□2.0 mg ▲4.3 mg •6.1 mg o8.0 mg x10.4 mg

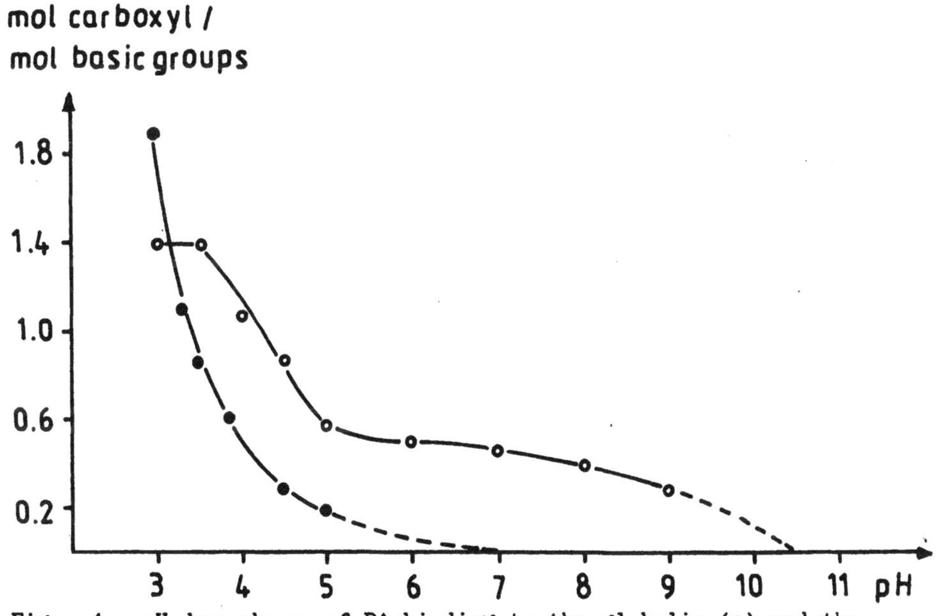


Fig. 4: pH-dependence of PA-binding to the globulin (•) and the albumin (O) according to [13]

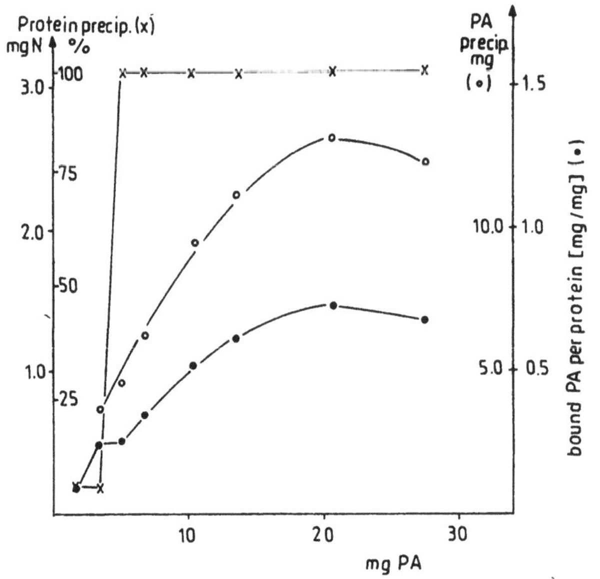


Fig. 5: Coprecipitation of globulin and PA at pH 3.0 in dependence on the amount of PA used, according to [13] (Protein = 0.07 %)

The PA binding to both proteins has also been studied by means of chemical analysis of the supernatant after PA-protein coprecipitation. A complete globulin precipitation takes place at pH 3.0 - 4.5 in a broad range of PA concentrations, This was attained by a (1 : 1)-stoichiometric ratio at pH 3.0 (mass ratio 0.25) (Fig. 5) and a lower ratio at higher pH. Increasing the amount of PA results in a rising excess binding of PA until a 1.4 fold mass ratio corresponding to a nearly 6 fold molar ratio. Contrary to that, the complete albumin recovery is obtained only at discrete pH values and PA-protein ratios [13]. An excess of PA results in an increasing solubilization. The binding of a surplus of PA was found, too.

There are differences in the interaction of polyanions with proteins depending on the nature of the anionic group (acid strength) and their charge density. Mixtures of highly or moderately substituted cellulose sulfates and rapeseed albumins are strong polyions with a high charge density. Practically all of the charged groups of the protein are available. As Figure 6 shows, the polyanion precipitates the protein in such a way that a nearly constant composition - corresponding to a (1 : 1)-stoichiometric one of the coprecipiate results notwithstanding the amount of precipitating agent. Contrary to that, the composition of the coprecipitate of the globulin and the same polyanion, obtained under comparable conditions (pH 3.0) depends remarkably on the amount of the polyanion. At lower pH (pH 2.5), where the globulin is more unfolded and the positively charged groups are more available, a constant composition of the coprecipitate is approached, too [12].

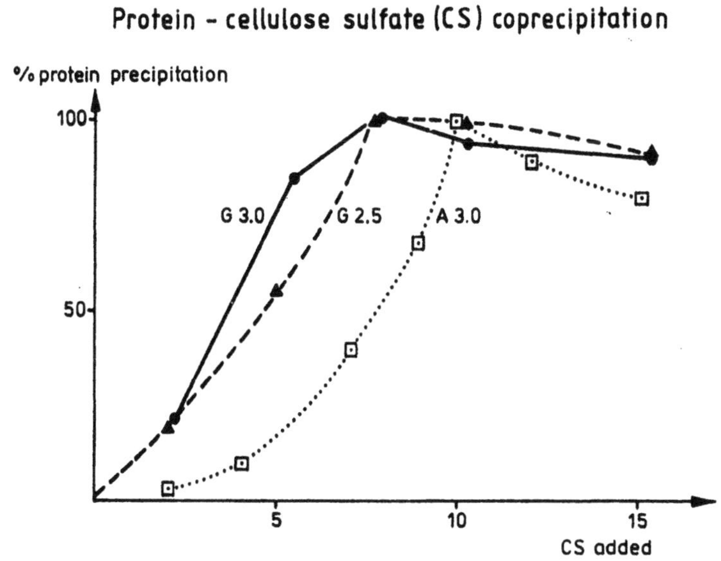


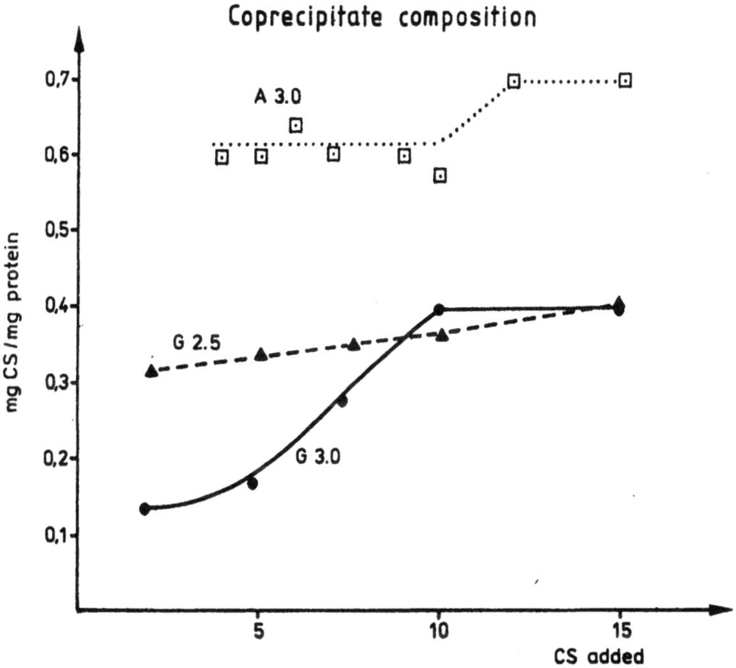


Fig. 6: Precipitation of globulin and albumin by a cellulose sulfate (DS 0.6) depending on the amount of the polyanion.
upper part: percentage of protein precipitation,
lower part: coprecipitate composition
A 3.0: albumin pH 3.0,
G 2.5 and G 3.0: globulin pH 2.5 and pH 3.0

**Phytic acid - rapeseed protein complexes**

As other polyanions, too, phytic acid forms insoluble complexes at pH values below the isoelectric points both with the globulin and the albumin [12, 13]. Though the isoelectric points of the proteins are in the neutral and strong basic region, their phytic acid complexes can be precipitated in the acidic region as the native globulins of most other oilseeds and legumes [14, 15]. Therefore, the commonly prepared rapeseed protein isolates are mostly phytic acid complexes. Owing to the incomplete dissociation of the phytic acid phosphorus at low values of pH, an excess binding is observed at the globulin at pH $< 3$ [15]. An increasing amount of phytic acid exerts a strong solubilizing effect on the albumin resulting in the coexistence of soluble and insoluble complexes. The comparison of the results of turbidimetric titration, reflecting the formation of insoluble complexes, and those of potentiometric titration, reflecting the total amount of charges occupied by the binding of phytic acid, revealed a constant percentage of insoluble complexes amounting to 74 - 78 independently on the pH.

Three discrete steps of complexation can be distinguished:

Insoluble complexes at a substoichiometric phytic acid-protein ratio, neutral complexes existing in a mixture between soluble and insoluble complexes, negatively charged soluble complexes with a definite phytic acid content amounting to about 2 mol per mol protein at pH 6 - 8.

Table 1 summarized the data obtained at pH 6 and 8. As a result of potentiometric titration it was found that the neutralization of the positively charged groups in the protein was attained by 8 - 9 negative charges per mol of phytic acid. This is in accordance with the degree of dissociation of the phosphate ester groups in the phytic acid in this pH-range as determined by Evans et al. [16].

Table 1: Binding of phytic acid to the basic low-molecular mass albumin fraction from rapeseed at pH 6 and 8*)

| pH | method | bound phytic acid mg/g protein | mol/mol protein |
|---|---|---|---|
| 6 | turbidimetry | 39 | 0.80 |
| | potentiometry | 55 | 1.20 |
| | gel chromatogr. | 84 | 1.80 |
| 8 | turbidimetry | 29 | 0.60 |
| | potentiometry | 40 | 0.85 |
| | gel chromatogr. | 80 | 1.70 |

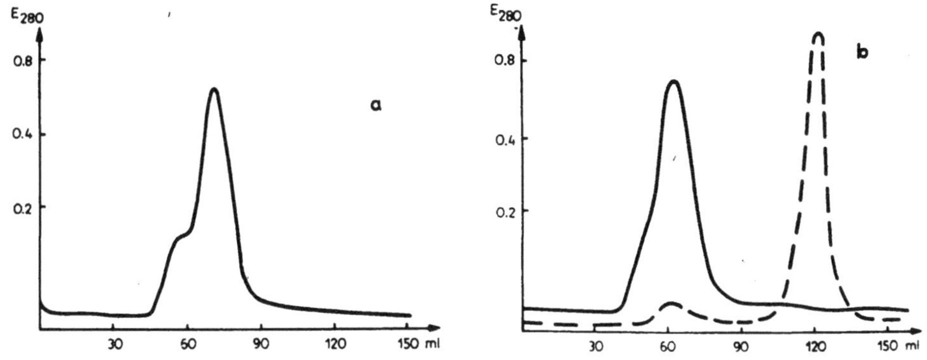


Fig. 7: Gelchromatographic separation of the albumin-phytic acid complex from free phytic acid (b) and gelchromatography of the albumin alone (a) on Sephadex G-75 (buffer: Tris-HCl, pH 7.2, ν = 0.05)
- absorbance at 280 nm
- phytic acid determined by means of the FeSCN-decoloration method

It was found by means of gel chromatography (Fig. 7) that this complex formation results in an oligomerization of the protein. The predominant product is a dimer. Its molecular mass was determined to be 30 000 ± 2 000 in good agreement with the composition mentioned above. The presence of small amounts of oligomers beside the dimer was ascertained by means of dynamic light scattering. After heating, high-molecular mass soluble aggregates appeared which did not precipitate. While the native protein undergoes a heat-induced aggregation at 40 - 50°C, the soluble phytic acid complexes are stable against heating until 100°C. The albumin phytic acid interaction does not influence, however, the secondary structure of the protein.

**Literatur**


[1] Gillberg, L. and B. Törnell, J. Food Sci. **41**, 1070 (1976)

[2] Maga, I.A., J. Agric. Food Chem. **30**, 1 (1982)

[3] Gillberg, L. and B. Törnell, J. Food Sci. **41**, 1063 (1976)

[4] Schwenke, K.D., M. Schultz, K.-J. Linow, K. Gast and D. Zirwer, Int. J. Peptide Protein Res. **16**, 12 (1980)

[5] Schwenke, K.D., B. Raab, K.-J. Linow, W. Pähtz and J. Uhlig, Nahrung **25**, 271 (1981)

[6] Lönnerdal, B. and J.-Ch. Janson, Biochim. biophys. Acta **278**, 175 (1972)

[7] Schwenke, K.D., B. Raab, J. Uhlig, H. Tkocz, J. Behlke, M., Bötger and U. Freimuth, Nahrung **17**, 791 (1973)

[8] Vainerman, E.S., W.J. Grinberg and W.B. Tolstogusow, Kolloid Z. u. Z. Polymere **250**, 945 (1972)

[9] Gurov, A.N., E.S. Vainerman and W.B. Tolstogusow, Stärke **26**, 172 (1974)

[10] Tolstogusow, W.B. and E.S. Vainerman, Nahrung **19**, 45 (1975)

[11] Thompson, L.U., P. Allum-Poon and C. Procope, Can. Inst. Food Sci. Technol. J. **9**, 15 (1976)

[12] Schwenke, K.D., D. Augustat and W. Wagenknecht, Nahrung **32**, 393 (1988)

[13] Schwenke, K.D., D. Augustat and W. Bock, Sci. Aliments **8**, 97 (1988)

[14] Schwenke, K.D., K. Elkowicz and H. Kozlowska, Nahrung **23**, 967 (1979)

[15] Schwenke, K.D., R. Mothes, K. Marzilger, J. Borowska and H. Kozlowska, Nahrung **31**, 1001 (1987)

[16] Evans, W.J., E.J. McCourtney and K.I. Shrager, J. Amer. Oil Chemist's Soc. **4**, 189 (1982)

# PROTEIN INTERACTIONS WITH PROCYANIDINS

Barry G. Swanson[1] and William E. Artz[2]

**Abstract**

Thermodynamic analysis of the temperature dependence of procyanidin binding to bovine serum albumin (BSA) and bean (*Phaseolus vulgaris*) glycoprotein G-1 suggested predominantly hydrophobic and hydrophilic binding, respectively. Protein-procyanidin binding was analyzed with tritiated procyanidin by ultrafiltration to separate free ligand and protein-bound ligand. Binding constants were determined from Scatchard plots. Van't Hoff plots indicated procyanidin binding to BSA was spontaneous and entropy driven. Evidence with cis-parinaric acid supported hydrophobic interaction of procyanidin and BSA. Van't Hoff plots indicated procyanidin binding to native bean globulin G-1 was also spontaneous but, in contrast to BSA, enthalpy driven. Analysis with cis-parinaric acid confirmed the hydrophilic character of procyanidin binding to G-1. Evaluation of procyanidin binding to heat denatured G-1 with cis-parinaric acid indicated hydrophobic interactions. Procyanidin ingestion may be detrimental to the digestibility of food proteins, the activity of digestive enzymes, active transport of glucose, sodium and amino acid across the intestinal epithelium, and the absorptive capability of the intestinal mucosa.

## Introduction

Procyanidins, condensed tannins, are polymeric plant phenolics that reduce protein availability by interacting with protein (Feeny, 1969 and Aw and Swanson, 1985). The mechanism of procyanidin- protein interaction has received substantial research attention. Gustavson (1956), Loomis and Battaile (1966), Loomis (1974) and van Sumere et al. (1975) proposed procyanidin-protein interaction resulting from hydrogen bonding. Loomis and Battaile (1966) observed the interaction of condensed tannin with polymers like polyvinylpyrrolidone (PVP), gelatin, collagen and nylon and concluded hydrogen bonding was the probable mechanism. Haslam (1974) evaluated the association of proanthocyanidin dimer and trimer with glucosidase and concluded that hydrogen bonding occurred between phenolic hydroxyl groups and peptide bond carbonyl groups. Hagerman and Butler (1981) enhanced hydrogen bondig of condensed tannin to formamide by alkyl substitution on the amide N adjacent to the carbonyl Formamide has less affinity for condensed tannin than the substituted derivatives N-methyl formamide

[1]Food Science and Human Nutrition, Washington State University, Pullmann, Washington 99164-6330, USA
[2]Food Science, University of Illinois, Urbana, Illinois 61801, USA

or N,N-dimethyl formamide. Electron donating methyl groups on the N adjacent to the carbonyl increases the electronegativity of the oxygen on the carbonyl group and increases the strenght of the hydrogen bonds between the carbonyl and the procyanidin hydroxyl groups.

There is also evidence of hydrophobic interaction between procyanidin and protein. Detergents (Goldstein and Swain, 1965) as well as organic solvents (Loomis, 1969) can dissociate tannin from protein. Calderon et al. (1968) reported that ethanol decreased the affinity of tannin for protein, while NaCl increased the affinity of tannin for protein. Oh et al. (1980) indicated that interaction of procyanidin and protein was hydrophobic based on several observations: 1) protein was eluted with detergent solutions from a column of immobilized tannin, 2) interaction between tannin and protein was enhanced with increase ionic strength and temperature and 3) tannins were absorbed readily onto uncharged polystysrene columns. Butler et al. (1984) concluded that tannin bound to protein as a result of both hydrogen bonding and hydrophobic bonding.

To resolve the type of interaction(s) involved, thermodynamic analysis of the binding of protein to procyanidin was undertaken to determine the extent of hydrophobic and/or hydrophilic interaction.

Hydrophobic interactions are also called entropy-driven interactions because they are characterized by a positive change in entropy and enthalpy. On the other hand, hydrophilic interactions are characterized by a decrease in enthalpy. To obtain estimates for the entrophy and enthalpy changes upon binding, Van't Hoff plots can be used (Tinoco et al., 1978). The slope of the plot provides the enthalpic contribution while the intercept gives the entropic contribution (Lauffer, (1975).

**Materials and Methods**

Chemicals used were reagent grade unless otherwise specified. Dimeric and trimeric procyanidin were prepared by the reduction of dihyroquercetin with sodium borohydride in the presence of recrysstallized catechin (3x) under an atmoshere of nitrogen (Eastmond, 1974). The polymerization of dihydroquercetin and catechin was followed with silica gel TLC using an acetone:toluene:formic acid (60:30:10) solvent (Lea, 1978). Tritium labeled catechin dimer and trimer were prepared with tritiated sodium borohydride. Procyanidin dimer and trimer were separated on a column of Sephadex LH-20 with an ethanol:water (45:55) solvent. The eluent was monitored continuously at 280 nm with a Model SC-15 ISCO UV monitor (Lincoln, NE). The radioactivity of each labeled fraction was determined with a scintillation counter (Packard Model TR1-CARB 460 DC, Downers Grove, IL). Fractions eluted containing monomer, dimer or trimer were collected, the ethanol removed by roto-evaporation and the procyanidin fractions freez-dried. Purity of greater than 97 % for both the dimer and trimer was observed with silica gel TLC (Lea, 1978) and confirmed with HPLC (UV detector, 279 nm) using a reverse phase column (Microsorb, 3 m, E. Merck & Co.) isocratically with 4 % acetic acid in water.

Eastmond (1974) identified dimeric and trimeric catechin reaction products following reduction of dihydroquercetin with sodium borohydride in the presence of catechin, with paper chromatography, UV spectroscopy, gas liquid chromatography and mass spectroscopy. According to Eastmond (1974) only dimeric and trimeric oligomers containing C4-C8 carbon bonds were produced during the synthesis. Gradient elution with acetic acid and water according to the method of Jerumanis (1985) indicated only one major peak with both the dimer and trimer fractions.

## Protein Purification and Preparation

BSA was selected for the thermodynamic analysis since it is capable of hydrophobic binding, its primary function being lipid transport in the blood. Purified defatted BSA was purchased from Sigma Chemical Corp. (St. Louis, MO). The bean (*Phaseolus vulgaris L.*) glycoprotein G-1, the major storage protein in beans, (Romero and Ryan, 1978) was selected since it exists naturally in legumes with proanthocyanidin in colored legume seeds. G-1 was purified according to the method of Stockman et al. (1976), based on the reversible pH-dependent polymerization of G-1, with slight modifications. XAD-1 and PVP (3.5 g each) were added to 7 g of dehulled bean flour to bind free phenolic compounds. To extract the phenolics, the bean flour plus XAD-1 and PVP, was washed at 21°C for 5 min. with 150 ml of acetone water (80:20, v/v) containing 0.1 % (w/v) ascorbic acid in a 400 ml beaker with continuous stirring. The flour was washed for 5 min. in a Buchner funnel with a second aliquot (350 ml) of the same acetone water solvent. Next, G-1 was extracted at 21°C for 30 min. with 100 ml of 0.5 M NaCl, pH 8.5, 0.1 M bicarbonate buffer in a 400 ml beaker with continuous stirring. The G-1 was purified by affinity chromatography (Stockman et al., 1976). Discontinuous SDS slab gel electrophoresis [Laemmli as modified by Stockman et al. (1976)] indicated only three distinct bands corresponding to the three subunits of G-1 (Stockman et al., 1976). The G-1 isolate showed no trace bands of either the other major globulin or other impurities. After purification, G-1 was desalted and concentrated on an Amicon pressure filtration system with an Amicon PM-30 filter at 2°C. After desalting, the G-1 was freeze-dried and stored at 20°C.

## Binding Analysis

Binding constants of ligand (procyanidin dimer and trimer) to BSA and G-1 were determined by the method of Sophianopoulos et al. (1978) with an Amicon Micropartition System MPS-1. Binding was determerminded at pH

7.0 to maintain G-1 solubility, to keep G-1 in a monomeric form (G-1 polymerizes below pH 6.5) and to evaluate the interaction near the physiological pH of beans. Separation of the free ligand from the bound ligand was accomplished by convective filtration of free ligand through an anisotropic, hydrophilic YMT ultrafiltration membrane (Amioon Crop., Danvers, MA). Protein and protein-bound ligand were quantitively retained above the membrane while the low molecular weight ligand filtered through.

Procyanidin dimer concentrations were 23.89-1531.0 µg/ml in distilled water, while trimer concentrations were 9.3-111.6 µg/ml in distilled water for the BSA-binding study. The BSA concentration was 7 mg/ml in the dimer/ligand experiment and 1 mg/ml in the trimer/ligand experiment. For the G-1 and trimer experiment, the G-1 concentration was 1 mg/ml and trimer concentrations were 9.3-111.6 µg/ml in distilled water. BSA and G-1 were prepared in 0.2 M NaCl, pH 7.0, 0.01 M phosphate buffer.

Each MPS-1 system and membrane was pretreated with the addition of ligand at the same concentration, specific activity and temperature as for the respective binding analysis. To determine the efficacy of the pretreatment several aliquots of labeled procyanidin oligomer were added in sequence to the MPS-apparatus. The MPS-1 system was centrifuged after the addition of each aliquot. A slight reduction in the procyanidin oligomer concentration occurred in the first aliquot added to the MPS-1 containing the membrane. The addition of three more aliquots in sequence showed no increase in radioactivity indicating neither additional binding nor release of ligand. The pretreatment procedure for both the highest and lowest concentrations used in the binding analysis was evaluated.

Ligand solution (0.6 ml) was added to the protein solution (1.6 ml), mixed and allowed to equilibrate for 10 min. Temperatures of 19, 29 and 39°C were selected for the experiment. After equilibration, 0.6 ml of the protein-ligand mixture was added to each MPS-1 and centrifuged (2000 g for 8, 7 and 6 min. respectively, at 19, 29 and 39°C). Two replicates (100 µl) from each MPS-1 system were analyzed. The scintillation fluid used was Scinti Verse II (SO-X-12, Fisher Scientific Co.). All ligand concentrations were determined with a scintillation counter (Packard Model TRI-CARB 460CD, Downers Grove, IL). Free ligand concentration was determined from a standard curve.

Binding constants of BSA and procyanidin dimer and trimer were determined from Scatchard plot analysis for the three different temperatures 19°C (Figure 1), 29°C and 39°C (Weiland et al., 1979). The free ligand concentration is [L], while v is the moles of ligand bound/mole of protein. The equilibrium binding constant was equal to the negative slope of the corrected Scatachard plot curve.

Linear regression was used to determine the high-affinity binding. The nonspecific binding of the dual-component system was determined and corrected for by the method of Chamness and McGuire (1975) for a two-component system, where one component has a much lower affinity than the other. Nonspecific binding was determined as the y-axis intercept of the lower affinit binding line. Chamness and McGuire (1975) state that the ratio of bound ligand to free ligand will reach a limiting value after saturation of the high-affinity sites. The slope of the line corresponding to the limiting value for nonspecific binding is zero (Chamness and McGuire, 1975). To correct for the nonspecific binding, according to the method of Chamness and McGuire (1975), the limiting ratio of $\underline{v}/[L]$ is determined and then multiplied by the free-ligand concentration, [L], for each $\underline{v}$ to determine nonspecific binding at that point. Nonspecific binding is subtracted from the total binding, $\underline{v}_{total}$, to determine the specific or high-affinity binding $\underline{v}_{sp}$.

$$\underline{v}_{sp} = \underline{v}_{total} - [L] \lim_{v \to \infty} (\underline{v}/[L])$$

The $\underline{v}_{sp}$ is plotted against $\underline{v}_{sp/[L]}$ to produce the corrected binding line or corrected Scatchard plot curve.

## Fluorescence Analysis

The surface hydrophobicity of a protein can be evaluated with the fluorescent surface probe, cis-parinaric acid (Nakai et al., 1980, Kato and Nakai, 1980). A large increase in the fluorescence quantum yield of cis-parinaric acid occurs when cis-parinaric acid partitions from a polar environment into a nonpolar environment, e.g. from an aqueous solvent to the lipid binding domain of BSA (Sklar et al., 1977). The method of Kato and Nakai (1980) for determining protein surface hydrophobicity was adapted for evaluating procyanidin dimer binding to BSA and G-1. BSA and G-1 were prepared in buffer (0.2 M NaCl, pH 7.0, 0.01 M phosphate) at four concentrations (0.005 %, 0.01 %, 0.02 % and 0.04 % (w/v). Procyanidin dimer was prepared in water (25 mg/ml). Aliquots (0.5 ml) of procyanidin were added to two of the four test tubes containing 2 ml of protein solution and allowed to
equilibrate for 10 min. Cis-parinaric acid (10 µl, $3.6 \cdot 10^{-3}$ M in absolute ethanol) was added to all four test tubes. The fluorescence was determined in an Aminco-Bowman spectrophotofluorometer (Silver Spring, MD) at an excitation wavelength of 325 nm and an emission wasvelength of 420 nm. The fluorescence of each individual component was subtracted from the fluorescence of the mixture of protein, procyanidin and cis-parinaric acid at each concentration of added procyanidin. The difference in fluorescence indicated the effect of procyanidin on the binding of cis-parinaric acid to BSA and G-1. The equation used to correct for the fluorescence due to each component was:

$$F_{corrected} = F_{cp,p,o} - F_{p,o} - (F_{cp,o} - F_o)$$

where $F_{cp,p,o}$ = the fluorescence of the combination of protein, cis-parinaric acid and procyanidin oligomer; $F_{p,o}$ = the fluorescence of protein and procyanidin oligomer; $F_{cp,o}$ = the fluorescence of cis-parinaric acid and procyanidin oligomer; and $F_o$ = the fluorescence of procyanidin oligomer.

## Results and Discussion

### Procyanidin Binding to BSA

Binding constants of BSA and procyanidin dimer and trimer were determined from Scatchard plot analysis for three different temperatures (19, 29 and 39°C) and are presentesd in Table 1. Figure 1 is the Scatchard plot for BSA proxyanidin dimer at 19°C. Thermodynamic analysis of the binding constants of BSA and procyanidin dimer indicated a temperature dependence (Figure 2); i.e., the binding constants increased with increased temperature. The binding constants at 19, 29 and 39°C are, respectively, 2400, 3100 and 4100 $m^{-1}$.

Table 1. Equilibrium Association Constants for Protein and Procyanin Oligomers

| | 19°C | 29°C | 39°C |
|---|---|---|---|
| BSA x dimer | 2,400[a] ± 440[b] | 3,100 ± 430 | 4,100 ± 920 |
| BSA x trimer | 48,000 ± 4,000 | 66,000 ± 4,000 | 83,000 ± 3,000 |
| G-1 x trimer | 68,000 ± 5,000 | 48,000 ± 4,000 | 17,000 ± 3,000 |

[a]Units $M^{-1}$
[b]Standard deviation of regression

The integrated Van't Hoff equation (Weiland et al., 1979) is

$$\ln K = \Delta H/RT + \Delta S/R.$$

The equilibrium binding constant is <u>K</u>, the change in enthalpy is $\Delta H$, the change in entropy is $\Delta S$. <u>R</u> is the gas constant and <u>T</u> is the absolute temperature. The slope of a plot of 1/<u>T</u> vs ln <u>K</u> is $-\Delta H/R$. The enthalpy change of the binding of procyanidin dimer to BSA was equal to 4.9 kcal/mol. From the Van't Hoff equation, the entropy change was 32.1 eu. The change in free energy ($\Delta G$) can be determined from:

$$\Delta G = -RT/\ln K$$

and was equal to -4.5 kcal/mol. The Van't Hoff plot indicates, therefore, a reaction with a positive entropy change, a positive enthalpy change and a negative free energy change i.e. a spontaneous reaction that is totally entropy driven. This indicates the binding of BSA to procyanidin dimer is hydrophobic in nature (Weiland et al., 1979).

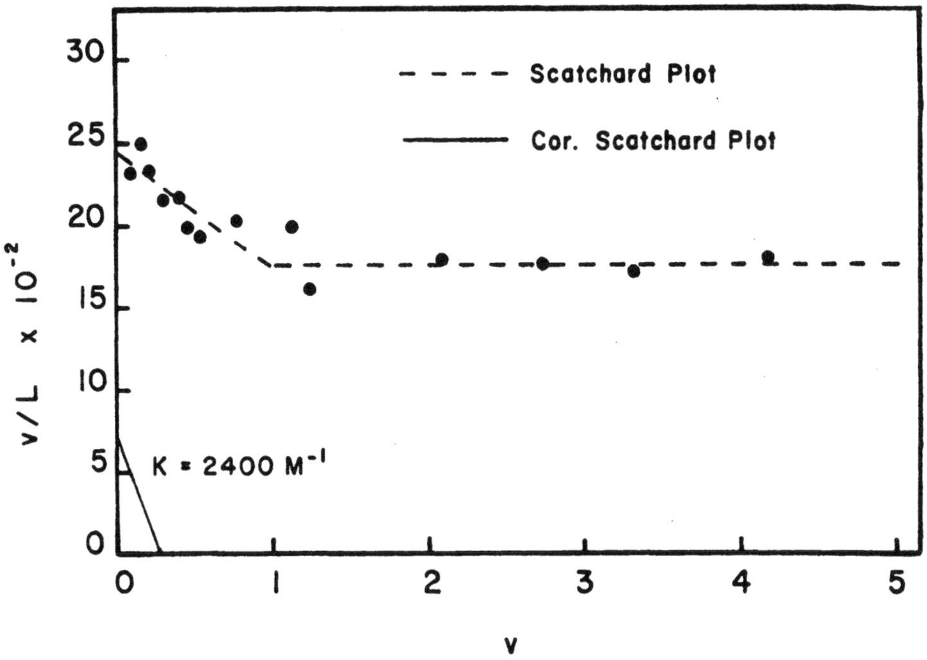


Figure 1 Scatchard plot of BSA and proanthocyanidin at 19°C

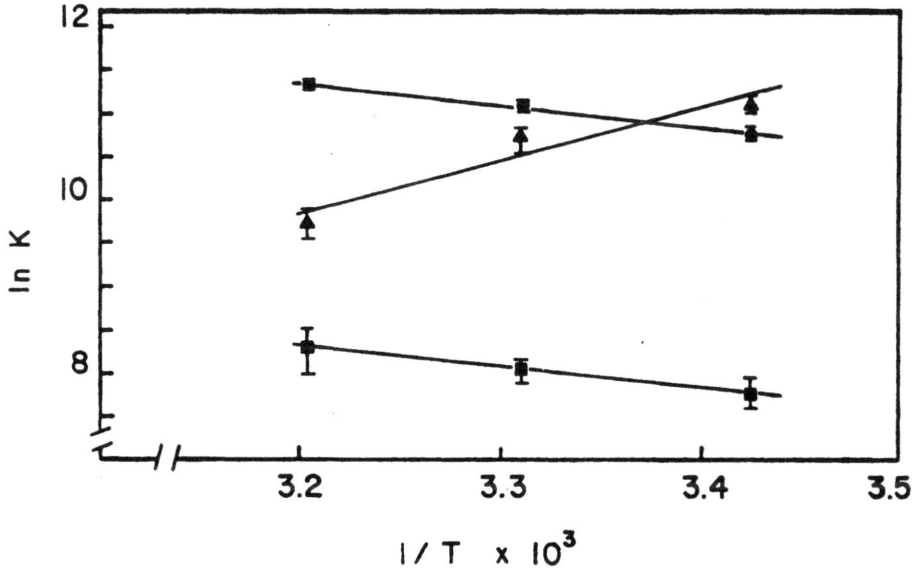


Figure 2 Van't Hoff plots of the dependence of K on temperature. Circles indicate BSA and proanthocyanidin trimer and triangles indicate G-1 and trimer, while squares indicated BSA and dimer. The slope of the line is equal to $-\Delta H/R$. The error bars indicate the standard deviation of regression as determined from the statistical analysis of the slope of the Scatchard plots.

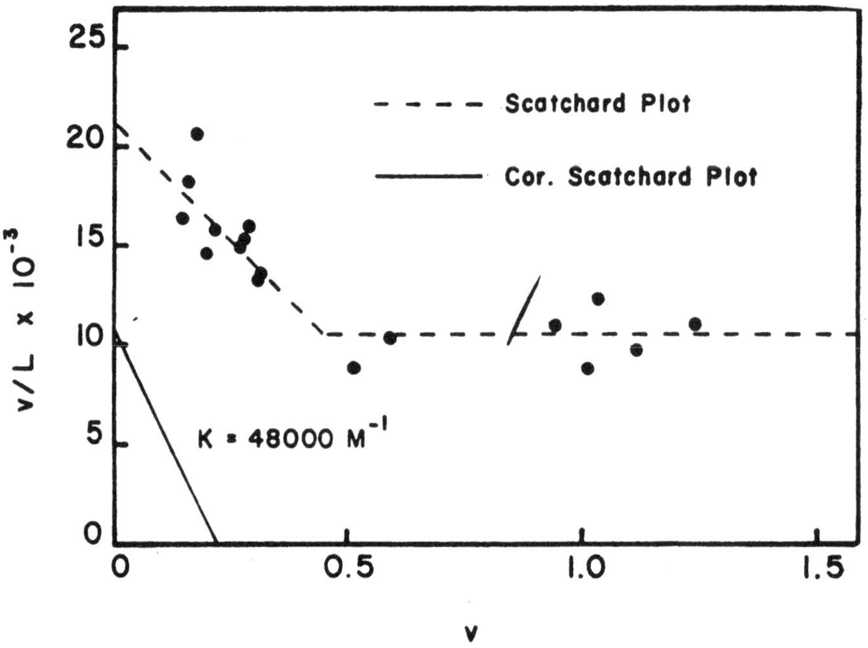


Figure 3 Scatchard plot of BSA and proanthocyanidin trimer at 19°C

Scatchard plots of the binding of procyanidin trimer to BSA were plotted at temperatures of 19 (Figure 3), 29 and 39°C. The equilibrium binding constants were 48,000, 66,000 and 83,000 $M^{-1}$, respectively. As with the dimer, thermodynamic analysis indicated binding of procyanidin trimer to BSA was temperature dependent (Figure 2). Increased reaction temperature resulted in an increased binding constant. The enthalpy change was equal to 5.0 kcal/mol, S was equal to 38.4 eu and G was equal to 6.3 kcal/mol. The negative free energy change and positive change in both entropy and enthalpy indicated the binding of procyanidin trimer to BSA was spontaneous and hydrophobic in nature.

The binding of procyanidin dimer and trimer to BSA was driven by the increase in entropy that resulted when water molecules, ordered around the nonpolar ligand binding site on BSA, were displaced (Weiland et al., 1979). Therefore, the driving force for the hydrophobic interaction was the increase in entropy when the ordered water was released to the bulk water. The term entropic union may be more appropriate for the procyanidin-protein situation than hydrophobic bond (Lauffer, 1975).

A stronger bond exists between procyanidin trimer and BSA than between procyanidin dimer and BSA. Previous research by Haslam (1974) indicated less proanthocyanidin trimer than dimer was needed to precipitate and inactivate amylase, implying stronger binding of the trimer.

Previous investigators have observed that cis-parinaric acid, an 18-carbon polyunsaturated fatty acid, binds to serum albumin similar to other 18-carbon fatty acids with respect to mole ratio, binding strength and specificity (Sklar et al., 1977; Berde et al., 1979; Hsia and Kwan, 1981). The binding has also been characterized as a hydrophobic association with entropy as the major driving force (Berde et al., 1979).

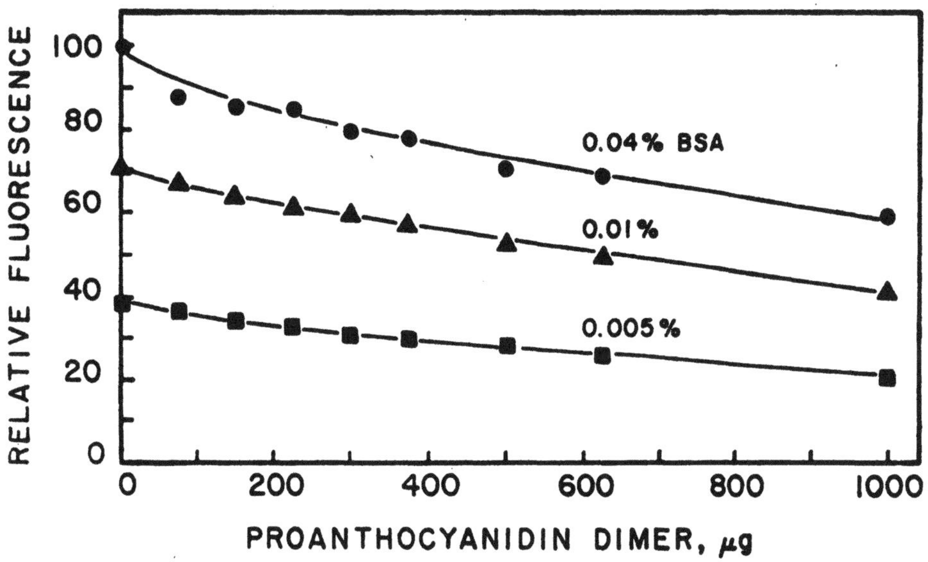


Figure 4 Fluorescence of BSA, proanthoxyanidin dimer and cis-parinaric acid.

The fluorescence of cis-parinaric acid was reduced as more procyanidin dimer (Figure 4) or trimer was added to BSA prior to the addition of cis-parinaric acid suggesting that procyanidin competes with hydrophobic compound, cis-parinaric acid, for the binding site on BSA, a competition that suggests that interaction is hydrophobic. Although procyanidin may be hydrogen bonding to the protein and sterically hindering the cis-parinaric acid from reaching the site, thermodynamic analysis indicates that procyanidin was bound to the hydrophobic domain of BSA. The results of the fluorescent analysis support the thermodynamic analysis that indicates the binding of procyanidin dimer and trimer to BSA is hydrophobic, rather than hydrophilic, in character.

Procyanidin Binding to G-1

Scatchard plots (Figure 5) were used to determine the binding constants of the procyanidin trimer to G-1. The binding constants were 68,000, 48,000 and 17,000 $M^{-1}$, respectively, at 19, 29 and 39°C.

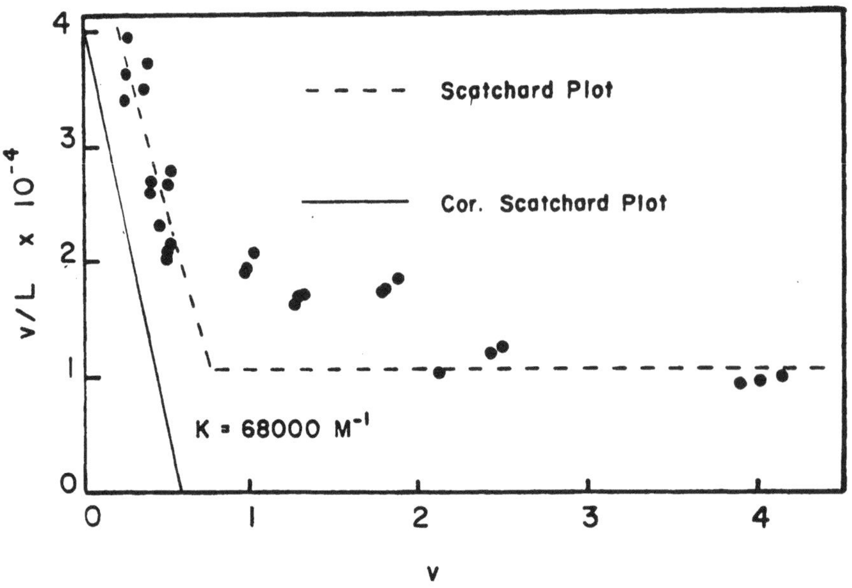


Figure 5 Scatchard plot of G-1 and proanthocyanidin trimer at 19°C

The binding constant of procyanidin trimer binding to G-1 decreases with an increase in temperature. The enthalpy change was -12.5 kcal/mol and the entropy change was -20.8 eu, while the free energy change was -6.5 kcal/mol, based on the Van't Hoff plot. Procyanidin trimer binding to G-1 is spontaneous and hydrophilic. The binding is driven by the negative enthalpy, which, along with the negative entropy, indicates hydrophilic interactions, van der Waal's interactions and/or a hydrogen bonding (Ross and Subramanian, 1981).

Heat-denatured G-1 had a surface hydrophobicity grater than that of native G-1. The increase was not unexpected since hydrophobic groups are usually oriented toward the center of the protein in aqueous solvents. Heat denaturation reorients hydrophobic groups. Fluorescence of **cis**-parinaric acid bound to heat-denatured G-1 decreased considerably with prior addition of procyanidin dimer (Figure 6). The fluorescence data suggested that the binding of procyanidin to native G-1 is different from procyanidin binding to denatured G-1. The effect of procyanidin addition on denatured G-1 and **cis**-parinaric acid fluorescence was similar to that of BSA and **cis**-parinaric acis. Binding of procyanidin dimer to denatured G-1 appears to be hdrophobic in character, while the interaction of procyanidin and native G-1 appears to be polar or hydrophilic in nature.

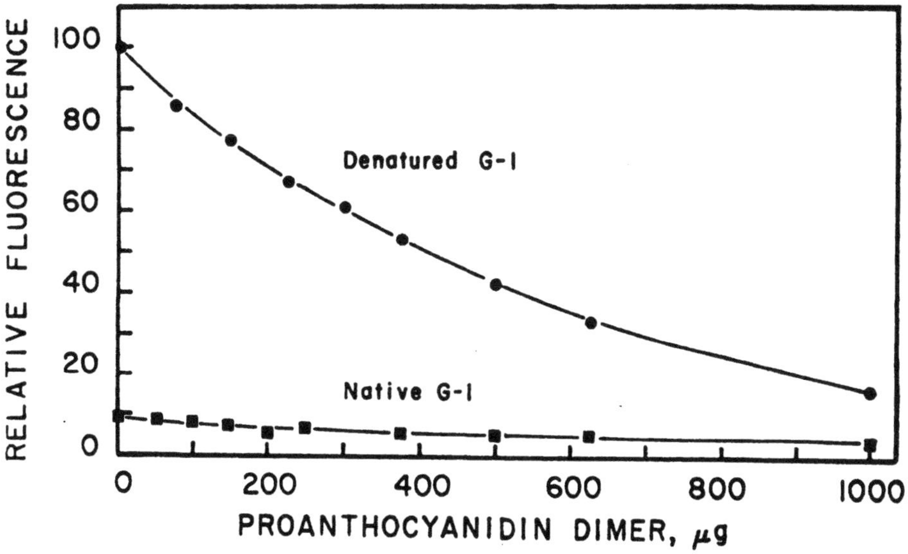


Figure 6 Fluorescence of G-1 (0.04 %), proanthocyanidin dimer and cis-parinaric acid.

Apparently, procanidin oligomers are capable of both hydrophobic and hdrophilic interactions with protein as suggested previously by other researchers. Hagerman (1980) observed tannin-protein complexes stabilized by both hydrogen byonds and hydrophobic forces.

**Conclusions**

Analysis of the equilibrium binding constants of procyanidin oligomer to BSA with respect to temperature indicates the major driving force for the association is positive entropy. Fuorescent analysis of the interaction indicates that the procyanidin oligomer competes with the cis-parinaric acid for the hydrophobic domain on BSA, and supports the thermodynamic analysis.

The binding of native G-1 and the procyanidin trimer is an enthalpy-driven reaction. The results of thermodynamic and fluorescent analysis indicate hydrophilic interactions are favored for binding of native G-1 and procyanidin dimer. However, fluorescent analysis suggests that hydrophobic interactions are favored for binding of denatured G-1 and the procyanidin dimer. With denatured G-1, nonpolar amino acids normally oriented internally to the protein, were aparently exposed. Therefore, the procyanidin-protein interaction is dependent on the types of protein sites available, which may be altered during denaturation of the protein.

**Acknowledgement**

Partial financial support for this research was provided by USAID Title XII Bean/Cowpea CRSP. Project No. 0560, Agricultural Research Center, College of Agriculture and Home Economics, Washington State University, Pullman, Washington 99164-6330.

**Literature**

[1] Aw, T.L. and B.G. Swanson: J. Food Sci. **50** (1985) 67-71.
[2] Berde, C.R., BS. Hudson, R.D. Simoni and L.A. Sklar. J. Biol. Chem. **254** (1979) 391.
[3] Butler, L.G. Riedl, D.G. Lebrysk and H.J. Blytt. J. Am. Oil Chem Soc. **61** (1984) 916-920.
[4] Calderon, P., J. Van Buren and w.B. Robison. J. Agric. Food Chem. **16** (1968) 479-482.
[5] Chamness, G.C. and W.L. McGuire. Steroids **26** (1975) 538-542.
[6] Eastmond, R. J. Inst. Brewing **80** (1974) 192-200.
[7] Feeny, P.P. Phytochem. **8** (1969) 2119-2126.
[8] Goldstein, J. and T. Swain. Phytochem **4** (1965) 184-192.
[9] Gustavson, K.H. in "The Chemistry of Tanning Prooess" Academic Press, NY. (1956) 156.
[10] Hagerman, A.E. Diss. Abstr. Int. **42** (1980) 180-181.
[11] Hagerman, A.E. and L.G. Butler. J. Biol. Chem. **256** (1981) 4494-4497.
[12] Haslam, E. Biochem. J. **139** (1974) 285-288.
[13] Hsia, J.C. and N.H. Kwan. J. Biol. Chem. **256** (1981) 2241.
[14] Jerumanis, J. J. Inst. Brewing **91** (1985) 250-252.
[15] Kato, A and S. Nakai. Biochem. Biophys. Acta **624** (1980) 13-20.
[16] Lauffer, M.A. In "Entropy Driven Processes in Biology". Springer-Verlag, NY (1975).
[17] Lea, A.G.H. J. Sci. Food Agric. **29** (1978) 471-477.
[18] Loomis, W.D. Methods Enzymol. **13** (1969) 555-563.
[19] Loomis, W.D. Methods Enzymol. **31** (1974) 528-544.
[20] Loomis, W.D. and J. Battaile. Phytochem. **5** (1966) 423-428.
[21] Nakai, S., L. Ho, H. Helbig, A. Kato and M.A. Tung. Can. Inst. Food Sci. Technol. J. **13** (1980) 23-27.
[22] Oh, H.I., J.E. Hoff, G.S. Armstrong and L.A. Hoff. J. Agric. Food Chem. **28** (1980) 394-398.
[23] Romero, J. and D.S. Rysn. J. Agric. Food Chem. **26** (1978) 784-788.
[24] Ross, P.D. and S. Subramanian. Biochem. **20** (1981) 3096-3102.
[25] Sklar, L.A., B.S. Hudson and R.D. Simoni. Biochem. **16** (1977) 1500.

[26] Sophianopoulos, J.A., A.J. Durham A.J. Sophianopoulos, H.L. Ragsdale and W.PJ. Cropper. Arch. Biochem. Biophys. 187 (1978) 132-137.

[27] Stockman, D.R., T.C. Hall and D.S. Ryan. Plant Physiol. 58 (1976) 272-275.

[28] Van Sumere, C.V., J. Albrecht, A. Dedoner, H. DePooter and I. Pe. In "The Chemistry and Biochemistry of Plant Proteins". J. B. Harbourne and C.F. Van Sumere, Eds. Academic Press, NY. (1975).

[29] Weiland, G.A., K.P. Minneman and P.B. Molinoff. Nature (London) 281 (1979)

Figures Reprinted from:

Artz, W.E., P.D. Bishop, A.K. Dunker, E.G. Schanus and B.G. Swanson. J. Agrc. Chem. 35 (1987) 417-421.

## INTERACTIONS BETWEEN N-COMPONENTS AND CARBOHYDRATES

Günter Westphal und Lothar Kroh[1]

In line with the general topic of this symposium we should like to mean by nitrogen or N-components generally derivatives of ammonia and, in a more specific sense, amino acids, peptides and proteins - while, with regard to carbohydrates we will especially deal with their reduction representatives, mainly with aldohexoses and derivatives derived from them.

| carbohydrates | amino acids |
|---|---|
| ß-D-Glc(p)NAc | $NH_2$-amido in Asn |
| ß-D-Gal(p)NAc | HO in Ser/Thr |
| ß-D-Xyl(p) | HO in Ser |
| ß-D-Gal(p) | HO in 5-HO-Lys |
| ß-L-Ara(f) | HO in Hypro |

(nach H. Kristen, Ch. Vogel, Mitt.CG 34 (1987) 266)

Fig. 1: Frequent carbohydrate components and bonding amino acids in glycoproteins [4]

In the bonding between carbohydrates and N-components the first provide, at least primarily, the glycolic OH group, while the latter provide alcoholic or amino groups, respectively. We know that the kind of components involved as well as the stata of bonding between them, i.e. essentially the kind and the sequence of the bonds and their spatial arrangement, frequently affect decisively the biological activities under certain reaction conditions, and this is true to speak of nitrogen-carbohydrate compounds as well. According to VOGEL and VOGEL [4] in glycoproteins the sugar components generally are considered to be responsible for the respective conformative arrangement and physicochemical properties, this regards especially also their hydrophilic and hydrophobic properties.

It has been especially SCHWENKE who in his works has pointed out the influence of carbohydrates, for instance, on the gelation properties of native or modified proteins. Yet, there has not been reached

[1] Humboldt-Universität zu Berlin, Sektion Nahrungsgüterwirtschaft/ Lebensmitteltechnologie, Invalidenstr. 42, Berlin 1040

absolute clarity so far about the significance of carbohydrates for the reception, storage and transmission of information in natural symplexes.

CERAMI et al. [2] proved experimentally a year ago tha reactions between sugars and amino acids within a human organism in general lead to their netting and, specifically, to the ageing of that organism.

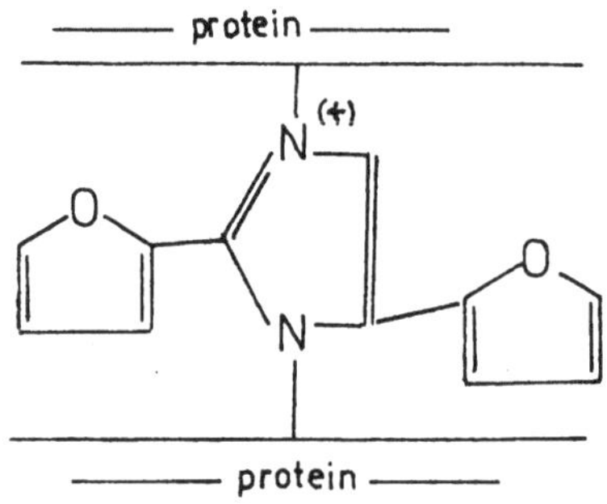


**(nach A. Cerami, H. Vlassara, M. Brownlee)**

Fig. 2: Crosslinking of body proteins by glucose, or glucosylamino acids or proteins, respectively [2]

Figure 2 shows the hitherto existing concept of the formation of noxious high-molecular compounds. These findings of CERAMI et al. served as a further motivation for our own experimental work on non-enzymatic browning reactions, especially for our work on the MAILLARD reactions, which have been known for more than 75 years and have been researched into again and again - in the following I should like to concentrate on this topic.

The significance of the above-mentioned reactions for the storage, preservation, processing and treatment of agricultural raw materials and foodstuffs since long has been known, and still today new findings are made in this field. Besides the multifarious aromatic substances and melanoidines, which are products of one or more reaction mechanism, more and more intermediate compounds get known, which may be used for the assessment of an immediate state of natural or processed raw materials.

Non-enzymatic browning reactions have proceeded since nitrogen and carbohydrat components came into existence; the respective kind, intensity and speed of such reactions depend on the structure of reactants involved and on the environmental conditions.

Browning reactions based on amines, amino acids, peptides and proteins, respectively, and reducing sugars were discovered by MAILLARD in 1912 [5].

MAILLARD's observations at a glucose/glycine system in boiling water have been confirmed several times subsequently - in general the frequently requested aromatic and dye substances are generated within a finite period of time. The structure and properties of these final

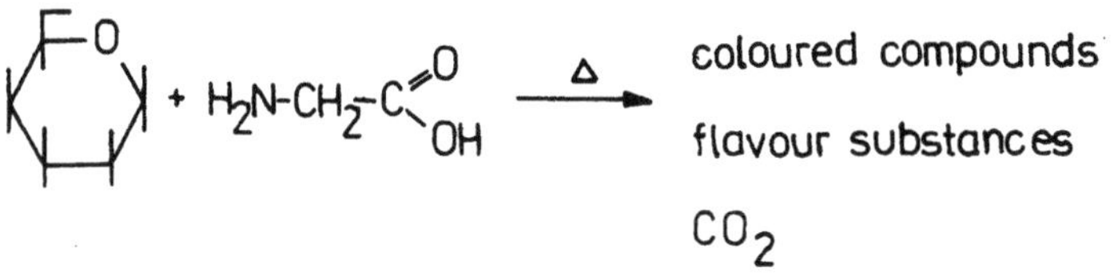


Fig. 3: MAILLARD reaction (1912)

products depend on internal and external parameters of such reactions. The internal factors comprise the constitution and spatial arrangement as well as the concentration of the respective reactants, on which comparably little has been reported yet. Whereas quite a number of findings are available on the influence of external factors on the MAILLARD reactions, i.e. on the time-depending impact of e.g. temperature, pH-value, solvents or combinations of these.

The increasing knowledge of the relationship between cause and effect has improved opportunities to empirically promote and, which is more difficult, to inhibit MAILLARD reactions.

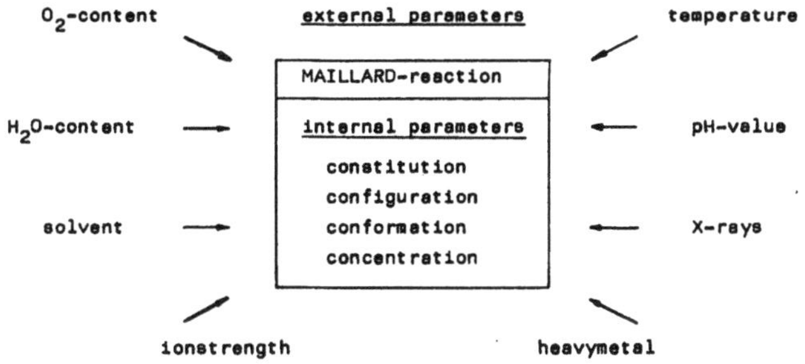


Fig. 4: Internal and external paraeters influencing the MAILLARD-reactions

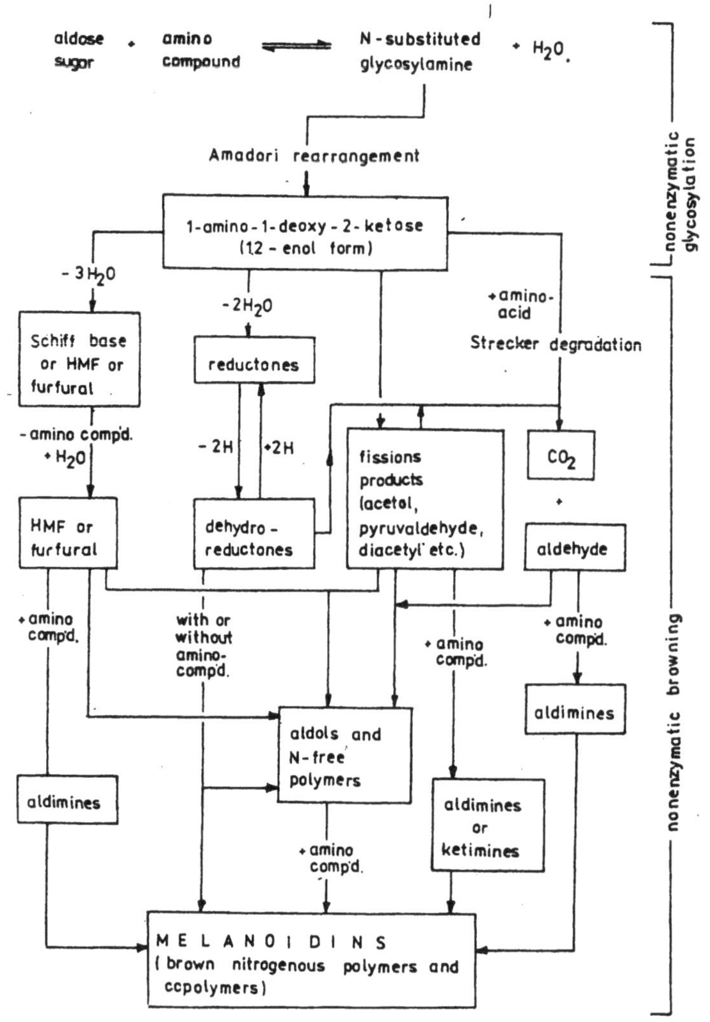


Fig. 5: Mechanism of MAILLARD reaction, according to HODGE

To do this more carefully directed means to research into the complex reaction mechanisms, i.e. to clarify the kind and series of the individual reactions phases, linked with the detection and, if possible, the isolation of idividual intermediate compounds.
The mechanism of the MAILLARD reaction as formulated by HODGE [3] 25 years ago has proven until today a workable interpretation for many findings and experiences from laboratories, factories and kitchens. According to the so-called HODGE pattern rearranged carbonyl compounds are formed in the first phase, i.e. the non-enzymatic glycosidation, via glycorylamino acid. The AMADORI-compounds [1] lead to the second phase of the MAILLARD reaction, the non-enzymatic browning reaction. The latter will be introduced by the formation of at least be-functional carbonyl compounds from which finally with or without the presence of amino acids polymeric melanoidines are formed.

Nearly ten years ago further systematic researach into individual phases of the MAILLARD reaction has led to the formulation of a three-phase mechanism by MAURON [6]. According to him desoxy-carbonyl compounds which keep the carbon structure of a saccharide, are formed in the introducing or early phase from nitrogen compounds and reducing carbohydrates via N-substituted amino sugars. At the saccaride there are with or without the insertion of N-components highly volatile aromatic substances formed and, in polar solvents, soluble reactive synthesis components, from which in the final phase the melanoidines which solve only hard in water.
Which recent findings on the process of the MAILLARD reaction have been made over the past ten years?
In answering this question I should like to concentrate especially on the introductory steps of the MAILLARD reaction and their being influenced by internal parameters. During our researach work we often employed glucose and phenylalanine as reactants.

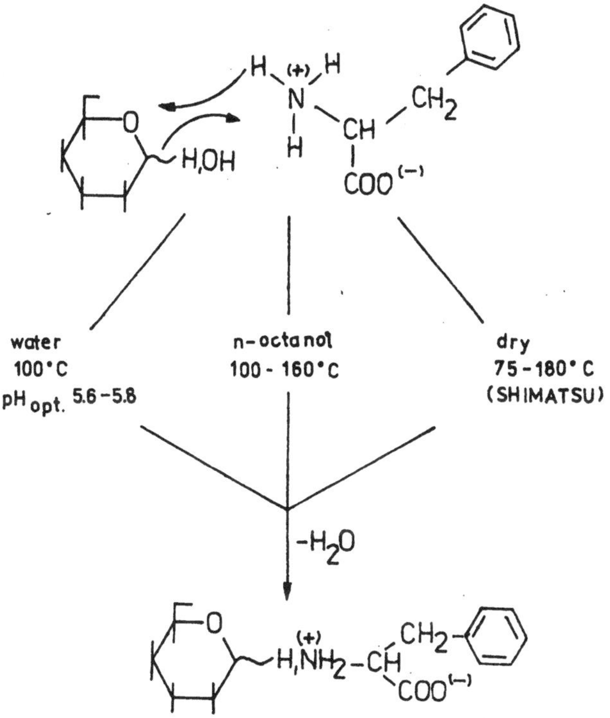


Fig. 6: Reactions between D-glucose and DL-phenylalanine in water, n-Octanol and without solvent

The hitherto unisolable is formed at both components in water, n-octanol or without a solvent in a reversible nucleopilic' reaction, generally acid-catalyzed, i.e. under an ionic mechanism. In accordance with Fig. 6 ß-D-glucose reacts stereoselectively, possibly even stereospecifically - and this statement may also be applied to other saccharides of the D-series - with the amino components under a detectable elimination of one mole water. The isolable N-glycosides of aromatic amines or amino acids often occur in ß-anomeric forms.

In the subsequent reaction step the aldosyl amino acids underly valency isomerizations, again generally acid-catalized. On the way towards metastable ketosyl amino acids, the AMADORI compounds, I formulate, in accordance with OBRETENOV, the doubtlessly very reactive enaminols [7], which may not only be regarded as control agents in the MAILLARD mechanism but also as points of intersection with other types of nonenzymatic browning reactions.

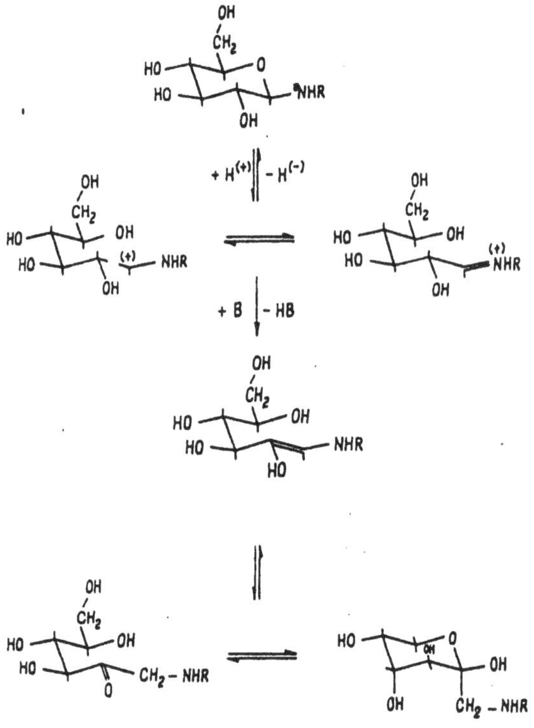


Fig. 7: AMADORI rearrangement of N-glucosides [1]

The AMADORI compounds are accessible at their nitrogen atom for further electrophilic and their glycosidic C-atom for further nucleophilic reactions; then diketosylamino or diaminoketosyl, respectively, are formed. 1-, 3- or 4-desoxyoson is formed from the N-carbohydrate molecules of ratios 2:1, 1:1 and 1:2. The very reactive 1-desoxyoson of the reduction type is only accessible via non-enzymatic browning reactions of the MAILLARD reaction type. The elimination of the nitrogen compound means in effect that its catalyzing function in the rearranging and isomerization reactions of the carbohydrate components has ceased. On the one hand the above-mentioned dicarbonylic compounds may generate STRECKER aldehydes and carbon dioxide as well as heterocyclic compounds, on the other hand the 1.2- 1.3-dicarbonyl compounds supply the known 1C-, 2C- and 3C-decomposition pieces, and as well dicarbonyl compounds. The carbonyl compounds that have been formed in

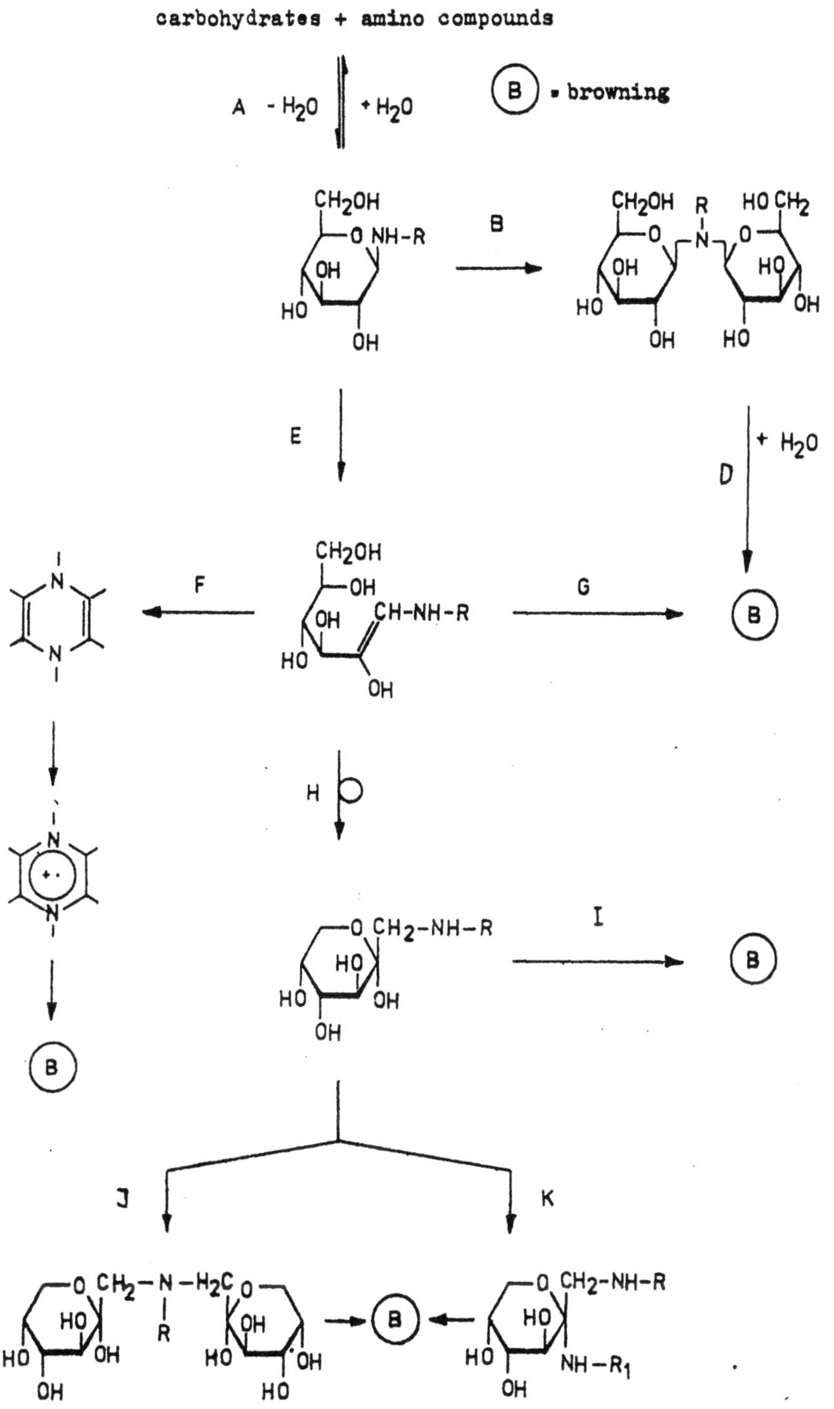


Fig. 8: Subsequent reactions of AMADORI compounds

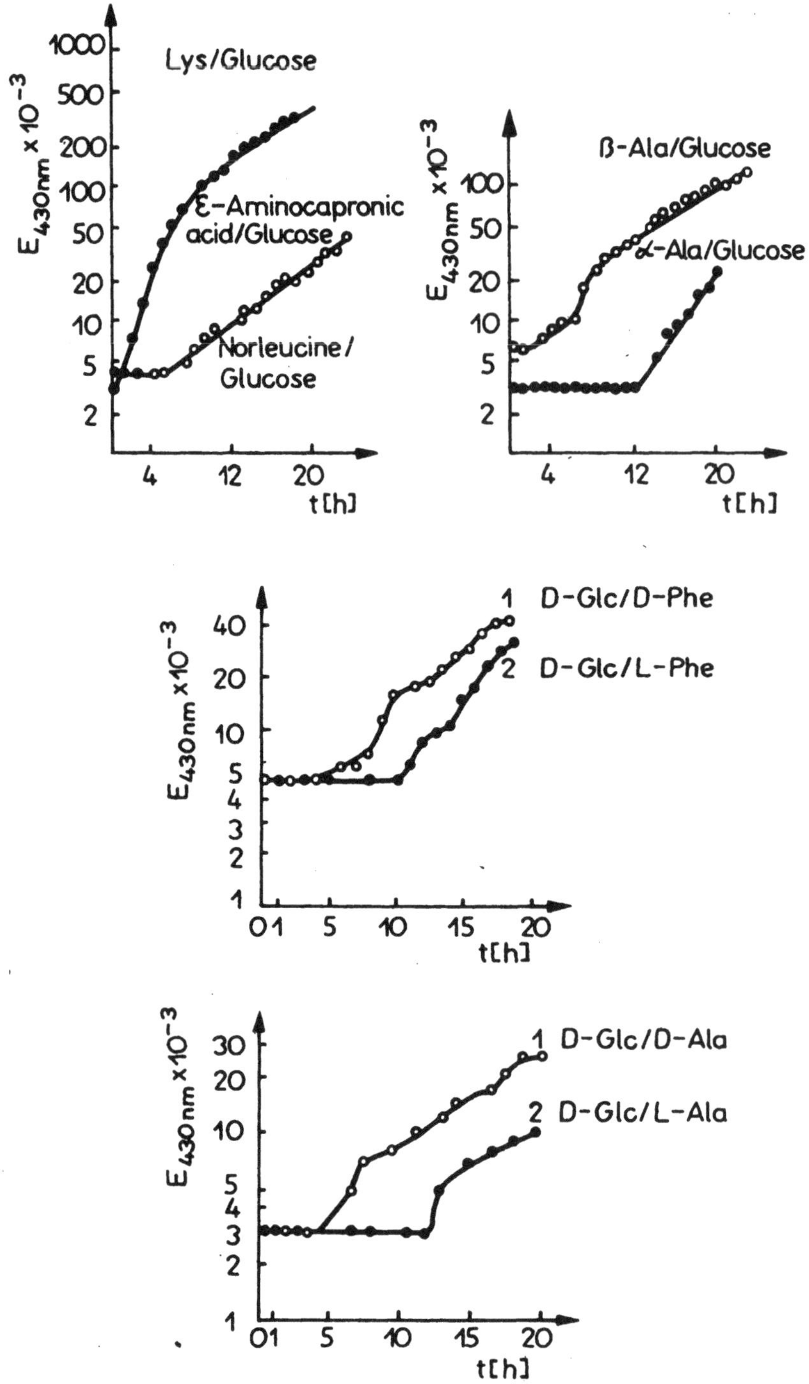


Fig. 9: Influence of the constitution and configuration of amino acids on browning in the presence of glucose in water

several different ways are mostly aromatic, likewise the heterocyclic components derived from them.

The numerous monomeric and oligomeric, mostly low-molecular compounds, polymerize or polycondense, respectively, into melanoidines of different molecule sizes and structures. In case one wants to generate purposefully melanoidines, e.g. beacause of their often detected antioxidative effect, one should employ for the generation of model melanoidines D-amino acids and amino acids with final-positioned amino groups or one extracts them from baked, roasted or grilled foodstuffs. The browning curves in Fig. 9 will speak for themselves.

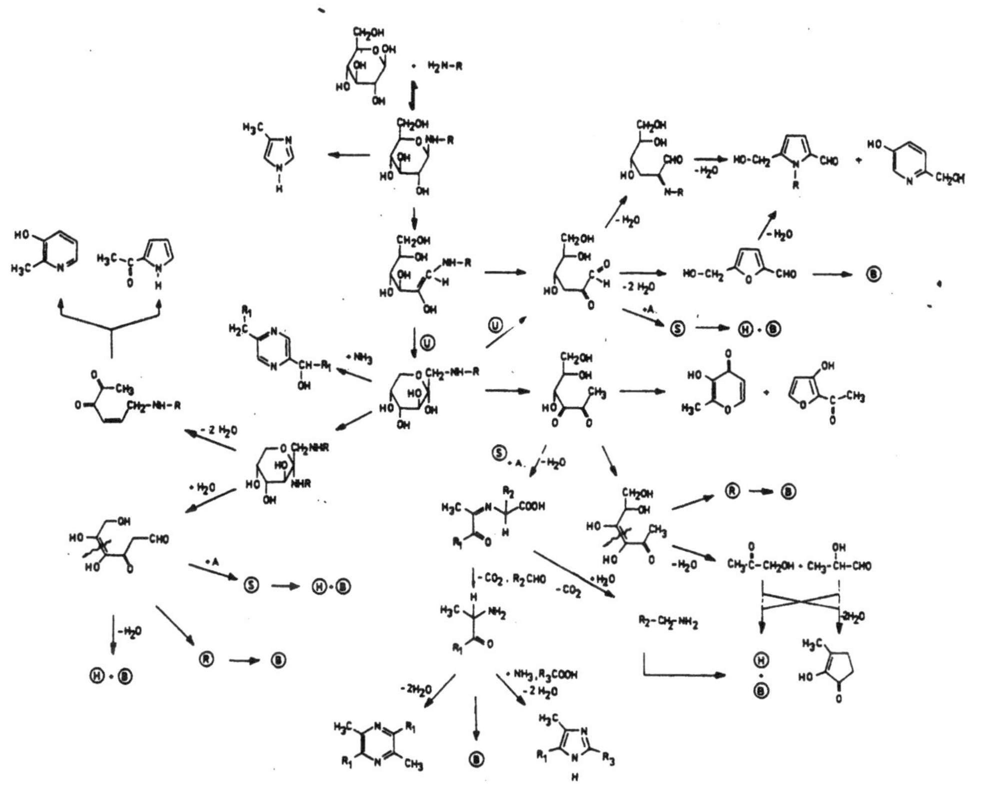

Fig. 10: Mechanism of the MAILLARD reaction, according to MAURON and PAULSEN [6]

$R_2$ - side chain A
$R_3$ - aliphatic residue
A - amino acid

U - rearrangement
S - STRECKER degradation
R - reductones
H - heterocycles
B - browning

After going into some details we should like to deal, in conclusion, again with some recent findings on the mechanism of the MAILLARD reaction (Fig. 10). In the early phase of the complex reaction there is at first the glycosidation of nitrogen components, subsequently the glycosides lay into the AMADORI compounds, in accordance with the LOBRY-DE-BRYN-VAN-ECKENSTEIN rearrangement, during these reaction steps as well as during the following elimination of amino compounds from the amino-carbonyl compounds the sequence of the C-atoms in the carbohydrate will be maintained. Their rearrangement as well as the splitting of the C-chain will be carried out in the advanced phase of the MAILLARD reaction, then volatile carbonyl compounds and nitrogen and sulphur compounds derived from them will be generated; the latter as well as the low-molecular soluble compounds polymerize or polycondense into melanoidines of different molecular weights and different properties. Apart from this series of reactions which preferably proceeds in an ionic manner, according to the most recent findings by NAMIKI, also reactions of short might happen. Here these free radicals appear at a very early stage, i.e. even prior to the AMADORI rearrangement, and lead to the detected formation of di-alkylpyrosines which, on their part, take part in the above-mentioned formation of melanoidines.
If the mechanism of the non-enzymatic browning of the MAILLARD reaction type and the fact that its typical products are also generated under physiological conditions are considered then analogies might be drawn with enzymatic metabolism of carbohydrates, as for instance during glycolysis, because also this case is an example of a primary interaction between the substratum glucose and the enzymatic protein, followed by the valency isomerization of aldose into ketose, than in general 3-carbon-carbonyl compounds are generated via a number of intermediate stages etc. It goes without saying that the differences between comparable enzymatic and non-enzymatic reaction are maintained, with regard to their selectivity and specialness, respectively. It remains to further findings on the individual elementary reactions of the very complex mechanisms to show analogies between these types of reaction - this is not only interesting in theoretical terms but should also be of very high practical significance.

**Literatur**


[1] Amadori, M., Atti R. Accad. Naz. Lincei; Mem. Cl. Sci. Fis. Nat. **13** (1931) 6, 72

[2] Cerami, A., H. Vlassara and M. Brownlee, Spectr. Wiss. **7** (1987) 44

[3] Hodge, J.E. and C.E. Rist, J. Am. Chem. Soc. **74** (1952) 1494

[4] Kristen, H. and Ch. Vogel, Mitt. Chem. Ges. **34** (1987) 12, 266

[5] Maillard, L.C., C. R. hebd. Seances Acad. Sci. **154** (1912) 66

[6] Mauron, J., Prog. Food Nutr. Sci. **5** (1981) 5

[7] Obretenov, T., Dokt.-Diss., Plovdiv 1987, 137

**SOME CHANGES IN THE HYDROPHOBIC INTERACTIONS OF WHEAT PROTEINS DURING GRAIN MATURATION**

J. Kaczkowski, S. Kos and H. Piór[1]

## Introduction

Since several years we are carrying out investigations on the changes of some properties of storage proteins during wheat grain development. One of those properties being of high interest because of its practical, as well as theoretical importance is the protein hydrophobicity, as it is suggested to be one of features affecting flour baking quality. Therefore many analytical methods for indirect determination of flour protein hydrophobic intractions were developed, such as hydrophobic interaction chromatography [4, 5, 7], protein aggregation under the influence of sodium salts of lyotropic series [13, 19, 20], as well as the protein solubility in long chain fatty acid sodium salts (soaps) of various concentrations [10, 11, 12]. However most promising and direct hydrophobicity evaluation, simultanous to protein precise separation was found to be the reversed-phase high-performance liquid chromatography (RP/HPLC), which was introduced to cereal protein analysis some years ago by Bieth and his group [1, 7, 8] and developed by some other authors [16].

Using wheat grains of two varieties: Cheyenne and Zeta of various maturity, we wanted to demonstrate in this paper the changes in protein properties bound with their hydrophobicity, occuring during grain development. We used one indirect method based on protein solubility in soap and the direct one - RP-HPLC separation.

## Material and methods

### Material

Two winter wheat varieties Cheyenne and Zeta were used as the experimental material. They were grown in the 1985/86 season in the Institute fields on the gray-brown podsolic soil formed on glacial drift. Plants were harvested six times during grain maturation, starting 10 - 12 days after anthesis, when the grain dry matter reached approximately 27 %. Next harvests were performed each 7 - 10 days (depending on wheater conditions), the last one being at full grain maturity. Grain dry matter of the successive harvests [1 to 6] amounted approximately 28, 35, 48, 57, 75 and 80 % respectively. Cheyenne variety was found in technolocial analysis to be of high quality, but Zeta one - of medium quality.

[1]The University of Agriculture, Dept. of Biochemistry,
02 528 Warsaw, Rakowiecka 26/30, Poland

## Methods

The kernels were threshed out of spikes by hand immediately after the harvest, weighed and stored at -18°C till further analysis. Dry matter and 1000 kernel weight were determined according to the Polish Standard [17] and total nitrogen estimated automatically in Kjell-Foss equipment (Foss-Electric, Kopenhagen). The reversed-phase high-performance liquid chromatography (RP-HPLC) separation of gliadins and glutenin subunits were carried out according basically to the procedure of Huebner and Bietz [8] and in their Laboratory at Peoria, IL. The procedure was as follows. Gliadins were extracted from flour samples (50 mg) in 10 ml capped polypropylene tubes for 60 min in 70 % ethanol (2 ml) with continuous agitation on a Vortex at room temp. After extraction samples were centrifuged for 15 min at 30 000 g in a Beckman L8-70M centrifuge. Glutenin was prepared by sequentially extracting albumins, globulins and gliadins first with 0.4 M NaCl and then with 70 % ethanol. The residue was suspended in 70 % ethanol containing 0.1 M acetic acid for 30 min and agitated. The suspension was then adjusted to pH 6.5 to precipitate glutenin and remove non-glutenin proteins. Remaining glutenin was reduced with 0.1 % (w/v) dithiothreitol for 1.5 hr in 4 M urea and 0.05 M phosphate buffer pH 7.6, but not alkylated.

RP-HPLC was performed using the equipment described by Huebner and Bietz [8] with the Vydac column 4.1 x 250 mm. Column temp. was kept constant at 60°C. Eluted components were detected at 210 nm at 0.1 absorbance units full scale (AUFS)/10 mV. Gradients were generated from solvents A (water containing 0.06 % trifluoracetic acid - TFA) and B (acetonitrile-ACN, containing 0.04 % TFA). Before use solvents were filtered through a 0.45 μm (HVLP) Millipore filter, deaerated under vacuum and sparged with a rapid flow of helium for 10 - 15 min. During use the slow sparging with helium was continued to provide slight back presure in solvents. Samples of 15 - 35 μl were analysed at 1 ml/min and 60°C with linear gradient in the limits 28 - 57 % ACN during 55 or 65 min for glutenin and gliadin, respectively.

Experiments on sodium laurate extraction were carried out using the method described earlier [15]. The solubilisation potentiality of wheat proteins in sodium laurate of various soap concentrations (5, 10, 20 and 40 mg per 1 g meal dry matter and 10 ml water) was investigated. In other experiments the fractional composition of proteins solubilised successively in NaCl. Na laurate (of concentrations mentioned), in 1 % SDS and insoluble residue, was analysed.

## Results and discussion

The RP-HPLC separations of gliadins and glutenin subunits of 6 maturation stages were carried out using the corresponding extracts of Cheyenne and Zeta varieties. As the examples of separations the patterns of gliadins and glutenin subunits of Cheyenne are presented in figure 1 and 2.

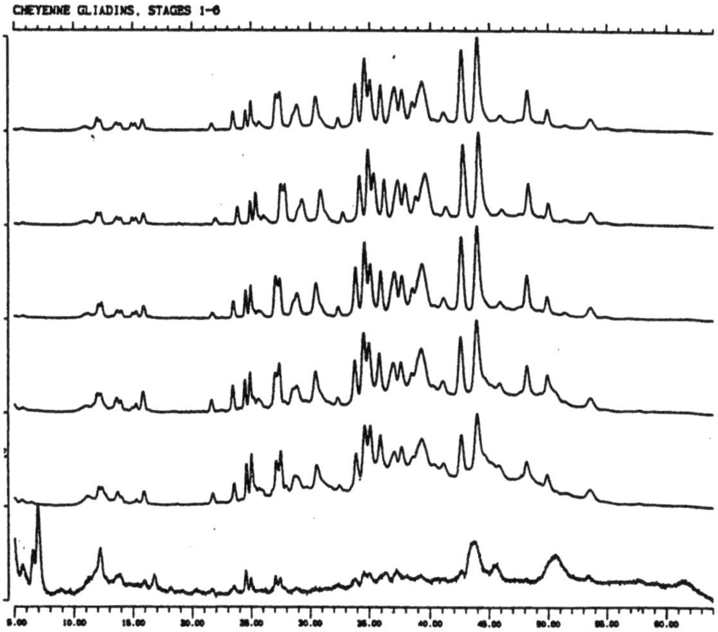


Figure 1: Comparison of RP-HPLC patterns of gliadin proteins extracted from the meal of wheat variety Cheyenne of successive maturation stages 1 to 6 counting from the bottom upwards;
figures at the bottom - retention times in minutes
separation conditions - see methods

It can be seen from both figures, that already about 12 days after anthesis the synthesis of at least some fractions of gliadins, as well as glutenin subunits is advanced. In case of gliadin fractions of the retention times (RT) 15, 25 - 28 and 44 - 45 min are very well visible in the extract of the 1-st stage; those fractions are developing further on during maturation. In this stage also other fractions are visible, which next are disappearing; those are of RT 5 - 8, 12 and 51 min. As was announced by Burnouf and Bietz [2], the most important fractions, whibh can be bound with quality, are those of RT 43 - 45 min, having the positive influence, as well as those of RT 50 - 55 min of negative one. The comparison of gliadin patterns presented for Cheyenne with that of Zeta variety, of much lower baking quality (not presented here) show the presence of high peaks at RT 54 min in the latter case, as well as the lack of those at RT 6 - 7 min. As those two varieties are differentiated in quality, there could be assumed, that some peaks mentioned should correspond to components responsible for high or low bread-making potentiality. Therefore the gliadin patterns of particular varieties can demonstrate their industrial value. On the other hand the comparison of gliadin patterns, extracted from the successive maturation stages can demonstrate the synthesis sequence of selected protein fractions. The case demonstrated in fig. 1 shows, that most changes upon gliadin composition occur between the 1-st and 4-th maturation stages and later on they are very small only, if any. Therefore it could be assumed also, that since that time, i.e. when grain dry matter amounts to 62 %, the maximum baking quality could be observed. This is similar to the old observation of Finney [6].

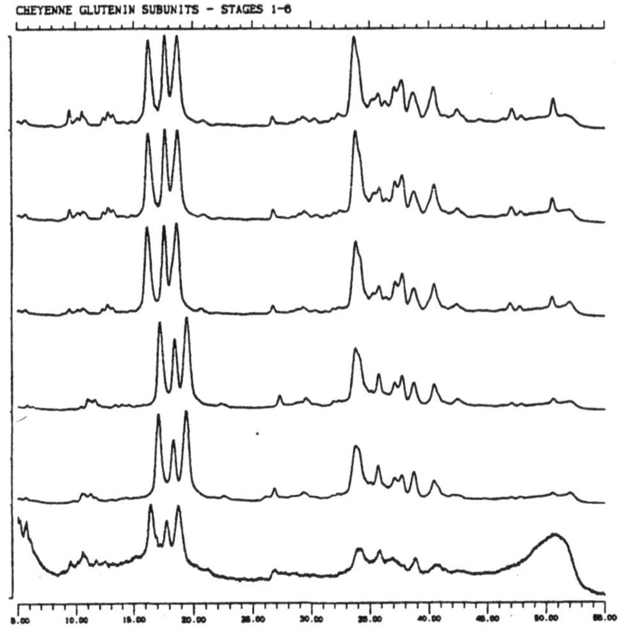


Figure 2: Comparison of RP-HPLC patterns of glutenin subunits extracted from the meal of wheat variety Cheyenne of successive maturation stages 1 to 6 counting from the bottom upwards;
figures at the bottom - retention times in minutes
separation conditions - see methods

Fig. 2 presents the glutenin subunit RP-HPLC patterns of Cheyenne veriety of six maturation stages. When those patterns are compared to those of Zeta (not presented here), only few differences can be observed. They concern only the peak group of RT 16 - 20 min and those of 36 - 38 min. The former ones correspond to the high molecular weight subunits [3] and the latter ones were found to be those of low molecular weight. Of high interest seems to be the peak group of RT 16 - 20 min composed of three separate, well destinguished peaks, which are synthesized earlier in case of Cheyenne, than in that of Zeta variety, having in that of former one the higher relative area. Contrary to the gliadin patterns, those of glutenin subunits demonstrate some changes also in the later maturation stages, not only in case of peaks mentioned, but also in that of group of RT 10 - 12 min, were some protein groups were synthesized between 4-th and 6-th maturation stages, particularly at Cheyenne variety. This last group could also be of significance in the complexing of gluten particles, as those proteins seem to be of high molecular weight, although of low hydrophobicity (eluted at 25 % ACN).

There were also calculated the per cent contributions of relative areas of some selected protein fractions, as compared to the total areas in case of all maturation stages and two varieties investigated. In the following tables 1 and 2, the results concerning gliadin and glutenin fractions, respectively, for Cheyenne variety, are demonstrated.

Table 1: Relative areas (in per cents of total area) of selected gliadin peaks extracted from meal of Cheyenne variety of successive maturation stages

| Stage | Retention times of separate protein peaks | | | | | | | | | | Total |
|---|---|---|---|---|---|---|---|---|---|---|---|
| | 12.0 | 27.1 | 28.9 | 30.5 | 33.8 | 34.6 | 37.1 | 39.3 | 42.6 | 44.3 | area |
| 1 | 7.5 | 3.8 | - | - | 3.5 | - | 2.3 | 2.1 | 1.4 | 18.3 | 0.51 |
| 2 | 1.6 | 2.5 | 2.8 | 4.0 | 3.1 | 3.6 | 3.9 | 7.7 | 4.9 | 8.3 | 15.56 |
| 3 | 2.2 | 2.6 | 3.1 | 4.2 | 3.3 | 4.5 | 4.5 | 8.1 | 8.9 | 8.7 | 15.43 |
| 4 | 1.6 | 4.9 | 3.4 | 4.3 | 3.9 | 5.3 | 5.2 | 10.0 | 7.8 | 11.5 | 18.77 |
| 5 | 1.3 | 5.2 | 3.5 | 4.7 | 3.9 | 5.5 | 5.2 | 9.5 | 7.9 | 11.3 | 15.16 |
| 6 | 1.4 | 5.2 | 3.8 | 4.7 | 4.0 | 5.8 | 5.4 | 8.9 | 8.4 | 12.0 | 12.92 |

In case of gliadins (table 1) the increase of total area of all peaks seems to be finished very early during maturation (at 2-nd stage). But in this case the increase of some fraction contribution takes place almost till the end of the process; this concerns fractions of RT 28.9, 34.6 or 42.6 min. But in general fractions of lower RT are revealed by Marchylo [14] be ω-gliadins; they seem to be synthesized rather early and parallelly to total protein increase.

Table 2: Relative areas (in per cents of total ones) of selected glutenin subunit peaks extracted from meal of Cheyenne variety of successive maturation stages

| Stage | Retention times of separate protein peaks | | | | | | | | | | Total |
|---|---|---|---|---|---|---|---|---|---|---|---|
| | 10.6 | 16.3 | 17.7 | 18.7 | 32.4 | 33.7 | 34.1 | 37.7 | 40.4 | 50.6 | area |
| 1 | 4.0 | 12.6 | 6.6 | 12.2 | - | 4.0 | 1.3 | 1.3 | - | 38.0 | 0.82 |
| 2 | 1.2 | 12.6 | 7.5 | 15.1 | 0.9 | 15.5 | 6.1 | 3.2 | 3.4 | 1.9 | 7.14 |
| 3 | 1.1 | 12.2 | 8.5 | 15.1 | 0.8 | 16.7 | 6.1 | 4.0 | 5.4 | 2.0 | 10.87 |
| 4 | 1.1 | 13.5 | 10.5 | 16.0 | 0.8 | 9.9 | 5.7 | 4.7 | 4.7 | 3.0 | 9.98 |
| 5 | 1.2 | 10.5 | 8.6 | 12.5 | 1.0 | 9.8 | 5.0 | 4.6 | 4.7 | 2.8 | 11.51 |
| 6 | 1.0 | 10.9 | 9.1 | 13.2 | 1.5 | 11.1 | 5.4 | 5.0 | 5.3 | 3.1 | 10.04 |

As can be seen from table 2, the total area of all glutenin protein peaks increases during maturation till the 3-rd stage, i. e. when the grain dry matter reaches 50 %. Similar behaviour of most fractions selected can be also observed, although some exceptions occur, particularly in case of the very interesting group of peaks of RT 16.3, 17.7 and 18.7 min, the contribution of which does not change since the start of experiment. Fractions mentioned are the highmolecular weight subunits [3, 9], which could be of importance in the formation of gluten complex.

Summarising this part of experiment we would like to mention, that RP-HPLC method of protein characterisation is very useful in many directions of their investigations, for example in ours, as it makes possible to detect changes in their relationships during maturation, as well as to present the behaviour of most important ones for quality formation during this process.

The other approach to the hydrophobocity characteristics of gluten proteins is their solubility in sodium salts of long chain fatty acids, e. g. laurate. We are presenting here the results of experiments, in which proteins were extracted using Na laurate of various concentrations, from meals, following the NaCl extraction, when the material of different maturation stages, was used; they are presented in table 3.

Table 3: Gluten protein contents in mg per 1 g meal dry matter in Na laurate extracts of various concentrations

| Stage | Zeta | | | | Cheyenne | | | |
|---|---|---|---|---|---|---|---|---|
| | Na laurate concentrations | | | | | | | |
| | 5 mg | 10 mg | 20 mg | 40 mg | 5 mg | 10 mg | 20 mg | 40 mg |
| 1 | 2.08 | 2.80 | 9.47 | 16.69 | 1.71 | 3.04 | 10.83 | 20.52 |
| 2 | 2.37 | 3.63 | 8.72 | 24.05 | 2.02 | 4.56 | 11.02 | 44.58 |
| 3 | 2.84 | 4.55 | 14.08 | 40.49 | 0.95 | 3.42 | 12.03 | 37.52 |
| 4 | 1.71 | 4.17 | 13.38 | 33.62 | 3.04 | 3.04 | 23.00 | 42.00 |
| 5 | 3.02 | 2.84 | 11.20 | 32.30 | 1.14 | 3.80 | 22.04 | 44.08 |
| 6 | 2.26 | 5.12 | 19.57 | 36.12 | 2.85 | 5.32 | 32.11 | 44.65 |

The data constitute mean values of three replications

The results of table 3 demonstrate the different action mechanisms of wheat protein solubilisation in case of low (5 and 10 mg) and high (20 and 40 mg) laurate concentrations. The former caused rather limited and nonspecific protein solubilisation, as the amounts extracted were only slightly differing between the successive stages and varieties investigated. On the other hand, the latter soap concentrations (20 and 40 mg) caused much higher and specific protein solubilisation and the amounts extracted are differing in case of maturation stages and varieties. We concluded, that the solvents of low soap concentrations are acting on proteins by means of their carboxyl groups of hydrophylic character, but those of high soap concentrations are acting hydrophobically - by means of their alyphatic chains [12]. The results presented here indicate, that during grain maturation the hydrophobicity of storage proteins inceases, which can make possible the complexing of their subunits to form the high molecular weight gluten components. Of both varieties investigated, that of higher baking quality - Cheyenne - seems to expose more hydrophobicity. The increase of protein hydrophobicity is taking place on the highest rate during grain maturation of both varieties investigated until the 3-rd or 4-th stage, but also in the end of maturation it is proceeding to some extent. This indicates, that also in the last period of grain development the gluten complexing processes are possible.

**Acknowledgements:**

The authors are indebted to thank to Drs J. A. Bietz and F. R. Huebner from the NRRC ARS Peoria IL for their very kind cooperation in analysing the samples in RP-HPLC.

This work was carried out under the partial financial support of the US Dept. of Agriculture: Grant No J-MOA/USDA-17.

**Literature**

[1] Bietz, J.A.; Separation of cereal proteins by Reversed-phase High-performance liquid chromatography. J. Chromatography **255** (1983) 219

[2] Burnouf, T., J.A. Bietz; Reversed-phase high-performance liquid chromatography of durum wheat gliadin: relationships to durum wheat quality. J. Cereal Sci. **2** (1984) 3

[3] Burnouf, T., J.A. Bietz; Chromosomal control of glutenin subunits in aneuploid lines of wheat analysis by reversed-phase high-performance liquid chromatography. Theor. Appl. Genetics **70** (1985) 610

[4] Charbonnier, L., Th. Terre-Laforgue, J. Mosse; Some physicochemical properties of Triticum vulgare ß-, γ- and ω-gliadins. Ann. Technol. agric. **29** (1980) 175

[5] Chung K.H., Y. Pomeranz; Acid-soluble proteins of wheat flour. II Binding to hydrophobic gels. Cereal Chem. **56** (1979) 196

[6] Finney, K.F.; Contributions of the hard winter wheat quality laboratory to wheat quality research. Trans. Amer. Cereal Chem. **12** (1954) 127

[7] Huebner, F.R., J.A. Bietz; Detection of quality differences among wheats by high-performance liquid chromatography. J. Chromatography **327** (1985) 333

[8] Huebner, F.R., J.A. Bietz; Improvments in wheat protein analysis and quality prediction by Reversed-phase high-performance liquid chromatography. Cereal Chem. **64** (1987) 15

[9] Huebner, F.R., J.A. Bietz, J. Kaczkowski; Quantitative protein variation of wheat kernels during development and among locations on the spike. Abstr. presented at the 73 Annual Meeting of AACC, San Diego, CA Oct. 9 - 13 (1988)

[10] Kaczkowski, J., D. Dojczew, J. Gruszczynski; Rapid evaluation of technological properties of wheat flour based on the protein extractability in sodium laurate. Abstr. of 7-th Congress: Cereal 82, Prague, No 326

[11] Kobrehel K.; Extraction of wheat proteins with salts of fatty acids and their electrophoretic characterisation. Ann. Technol. agric. **29** (1980) 125

[12] Kobrehel, K.; Sequential solubilisation of wheat proteins with soaps; protein-protein and protein-lipid interactions. 2-nd Workshop on Gluten Proteins, Wageningen 1984, Eds: A. Graveland and J.H.E. Moonen.

[13] Kos, S., J. Kaczkowski, H. Piór;
Turbidity test using sodium salts of lyotropic series for measurement of gluten protein hydrophobicity.
Die Nahrung **32** (1988) 275

[14] Kruger, J.E., B.A. Marchylo;
Selection of column and operating conditions for reversed-phase high-performance liquid chromatography of proteins in canadian wheats. Can. J. Plant Sci. **65** (1985) 285

[15] Kurowska, E., J. Kaczkowski;
the short-term extraction of flour gluten proteins using the solvents acting on hydrophylic bonds as the method of studying their properties. Bull. Polish Acad. Sci. **31** (1983) 1

[16] Lookhart, G.L., L.D. Albers, J.A. Bietz;
Comparison of polyacrylamide gel electrophoresis and high-performance liquid chromatography analyses of gliadin polymorphism in the wheat cultivar Newton.
Cereal Chem. **63** (1986) 497

[17] Polish Standard PN-86, A-74011 (1986)

[18] Popineau, Y., B. Godon;
Application de la chromatographie hydrophobe au fractionement des prolamines du blé tendre.
C.R. Hebd. Sceances Acad. Sci. ser. C **283** (1976) 1051

[19] Preston, K.B.;
Effects of neutral salts upon wheat gluten proteins.
I Relationship between the hydrophobic properties of gluten proteins and their extractability and turbidity in neutral salts. Cereal Chem. **58** (1981) 317

[20] Preston, K.R.;
Gel filtration and characterisation of neutral salt extracted wheat gluten proteins varying in hydrophobic properties.
Cereal Chem. **61** (1984) 76

# LIPID-PROTEIN INTERACTIONS IN WHEAT GLUTEN: A RENEWAL

D.Marion (1), C.Le Roux (2), C.Tellier (3), S.Akoka (3), D.Gallant (1) J.Gueguen (1), Y.Popineau (1), and J.P.Compoint (1).
(1) Centre de Recherches Agro-Alimentaires Institut National de la Recherche Agronomique 44072 Nantes cedex, (2) Générale Biscuits 91207 Athis-Mons cedex, (3) Laboratoire de Résonance Magnétique Nucléaire et de Réactivité Chimique UA CNRS 472 Université de Nantes 44072 Nantes cedex.

Decrease in the extractibility of lipids by apolar solvents on wheat flour hydration is a well known phenomenon which is currently attributed to the binding of lipids to the gluten proteins (1). The so-called "bound lipids" are essential to the expression of the physical properties of gluten and baked products . To explain their role most of the investigations were carried out on lipid-protein interactions and have been devoted essentially to the search for lipoprotein complexes formed between lipids and either storage proteins (2-4) or specific lipid binding proteins (5,6).

However, these studies were generally conducted with a methodology implying multistep extraction of lipid and protein fractions by various solvents followed by a chemical characterization of the extracts. From a molecular point of view, the results of these experiments are difficult to interpret in terms of specific lipid-protein interactions, as these fractiomations are quite denaturing for lipoproteins and have been performed on freeze-dried gluten or doughs whilst it is well known that lipid-protein interactions are water dependent (7).

Furthermore it is important to note that lipids, especially polar lipids, are not discrete molecules but forms liquid-crystalline aggregates structure of which is influenced by hydration and other physico-chemical parameters (temperature, ionic strenght...) as it was shown for wheat lipids (8,9). Therefore, gluten appears to be a polyphasic system, in which three dependent types of interaction occur : protein-protein, lipid-lipid and lipid-protein. The studies of lipid-protein interactions must inevitably take into account the situation in the whole hydrated gluten and can only be appoached by means of physical techniques and mild biochemical methods allowing preservation of native lipid structures.

Owing to the use of such techniques especially as freeze-fracture electron microscopy and phosphorus NMR we have got in the last two years (10-14) some new information on lipid-protein and lipid-lipid interactions in wheat flour, dough and gluten.

**Polymorphic behavior of lipid from wheat flour to dough and gluten: water dependent lipid-lipid interactions in wheat flour.**

Freeze-fracture electron microscopy is one of the most suitable techniques to observe native lipid liquid-crystalline phases (15) and we have used it to observe the organisation of lipids in wheat endosperm, flour, doughs and gluten. For low hydrated samples such as endosperm and flour pure glycerol has to be added not to avoid damages during freezing but as an embedding medium to ensure good fracture of these solid samples. In highly hydrated gluten and doughs, glycerol was necessary to avoid freeze damage due to ice crystal growth and was added to give a final concentration of 30%. However, wheat samples were incubated in glycerol just before freezing in an ice-liquid nitrogen slush in order to minimize the effects on lipid structures. It is effectively well established that polyols prevent formation of hexagonal phases and other non-bilayer phases during dehydration of biomembranes (16, 17).

In these experimental conditions large isolated polymorphic aggregates are observed in flour (figure 1b-d), exhibiting packing tubes and granular aggregates surrounded by vesicules which are the well known patterns of the polar lipid in hexagonal, cubic and lamellar liquid-crystalline phases (10, 15). Such aggregates were also observed near starch granules in wheat endosperm (figure 2). In wheat flour as in endosperm numerous vesicles were present in the areas where glycerol has diffused (figure 1a and 2a).

Hydration of wheat flour and resting during 15 min. imply the appearance of numerous vesicles and large granular structures surrounded by vesicles. The latter are more abundant when the amount of water added is only 30% (figure 3a and 3b) and rare when it is of 60% (figure 3c and 3d). Some of the formed vesicles fusioned with oil droplets (figure 3d) and are inserted in the gluten network (figure 3c). Whatever the water content only vesicles were observed when doughs were rested for 2 hours (figure 3e). In gluten only vesicles are observed (figure 3f).

The granular structures supposed to be lipid cubic liquid-crystalline phases are considered as an intermediate step in the bilayer to hexagonal phase transition of polar lipids (18, 19). This seems to be the case for wheat lipids since these structures appears mainly on hydration near starch granules where hexagonal phases are observed in endosperm and they disappear during a long resting time of doughs. This is also consistent with the fact that vesicles are the unique lipid structure observed in dough and gluten. This hexagonal to lamellar phase transition is induced by hydration and also by glycerol as evidenced by freeze-fracture micrographs of flour and endosperm. Thus, it is difficult to know the real proportion of polar lipids organized in non bilayer phase in wheat flour and endosperm. From the aqueous phase diagram of extracted wheat lipids obtained by Carlson and coworkers (8,9) it might be assumed that all polar lipids are in hexagonal phases at the water content of wheat flour and endosperm.

On a physiological point of view these results suggest that dehydration of wheat grain during maturation induces a transition of lamellar biomembranes to an hexagonal structure as it was suggested for other seeds (18).

**Wheat lipid vesicles are lipoprotein structures.**

In any way these results show that a large part of lipid vesicles stems from membranes remnants. Therefore it was expected these vesicles contain proteins, i.e; membrane proteins. To characterize them we have developed a method allowing isolation of lipid vesicles from wheat flour by sequential sucrose density flotation ultracentrifugation. The vesicles isolated by this method exhibit freeze-fracture pattern similar to this embedded in gluten except some more evident details on vesicle surface (figure 4). Especially small particles (0.5 to 0.8 nm) are visible on the external part as well as on the internal part of the vesicles. These intramembrane particles might be membrane proteins according to work on biomembranes (21,22).SDS-PAGE under reducing conditions (figure 5) show a pattern quite different from the main wheat gluten proteins. These proteins are rich in low molecular weight proteins and their amino acid composition (table 1) is quite different from prolamins in regard to the low level of Glx and Pro residues and high amount of basic amino acids. It is noteworthy that these characteristics are similar to these of proteins of the spherosome layer of the maize scutella agreeing with the membrane nature of the proteins present in wheat lipid vesicles (23).

SDS-PAGE under reducing conditions (figure 5) show a pattern quite different from the main wheat gluten proteins. These proteins are rich in low molecular weight proteins and their amino acid composition (table 1) is quite different from prolamins in regard to the low level of Glx and Pro residues and high amount of basic amino acids. It is noteworthy that these characteristics are similar to these of proteins of the spherosome layer of the maize scutella agreeing with the membrane nature of the proteins present in wheat lipid vesicles (23).

Table 1 - Amino acid composition of membrane fractions FI and FII, and of purified 16500 Molecular Weight membrane protein (in mole per cent of total amino acids)

(a) : aspartic + asparagin, (b) : glutamic + glutamin ; tryptophan was not determined; N.D.: not determined.

| | FI | FII | LMW |
|---|---|---|---|
| ASX[a] | 6.0 | 8.3 | 10;0 |
| THR | 4.7 | 3.7 | 3.7 |
| SER | 8.2 | 5.0 | 10.0 |
| GLX[b] | 10.0 | 20.6 | 13.6 |
| PRO | 6.5 | 7.5 | 5.2 |
| GLY | 10.3 | 5.0 | 10.4 |
| ALA | 6.6 | 5.2 | 6.7 |
| VAL | 5.6 | 6.8 | 6.4 |
| MET | 3.7 | 1.0 | N.D. |
| ILE | 4.7 | 4.2 | 3.8 |
| LEU | 9.2 | 8.7 | 5.9 |
| TYR | 2.2 | 1.9 | 1.0 |
| PHE | 3.9 | 4.4 | 3.3 |
| LYS | 6.6 | 6.1 | 9.2 |
| HIS | 1.4 | 2.7 | 2.2 |
| ARG | 5.7 | 6.4 | 8.8 |
| CYS | 4.7 | 2.4 | N.D. |

On account of the rearrangements affecting wheat biomembranes during maturation it may be asked if all membrane proteins are associated with gluten lipid vesicles. It has been effectively shown that during the lamellar to hexagonal phase transition of biomembranes during dehydration, lateral segregation of lipids and some proteins occurs (24). This phenomenon might lead to the expulsion of protein from membranes into the protein matrix formed by wheat storage protein. Works are in progress in our group to elucidate the mechanisms of membrane dehydration.

**Dynamic of lipoprotein vesicles in wheat gluten.**

Interaction of the lipoprotein vesicles with the protein gluten network were followed by phosphorus NMR. The phospholipid present on the vesicle gives rise to a symmetric peak width of which was modified during an heating-cooling cycle (figure 6a and 6b). The symmetric shape of the signal is the resultant of the small size of lipid vesicles and of the low residual chemical shift anisotropy of the main specific wheat phospholipids, the N-acylphosphatidylethanolamines (13).

During heating up to 50°C the NMR peak becomes broader. This was a surprising result since the mobility of the phosphate head group and the tumbling rate of the vesicles will increase at higher temperatures as reported for membranes. This phenomenon may be explained by a proton-phosphorus dipolar broadening due to an increase in motional correlation time on account of the adoption by phospholipids of the motional characteristics of the larger proteins or by an increase in the residual chemical shift anisotropy if less freedom of motion is available when protein is interacting with the phospholipids. Whatever the cause of resonance broadening, it probably arises as a consequence of the interactions between proteins and phospholipids. However, the line width of the signal decreased from 50 to 70°C and during cooling from 70 to 25°C. This decrease by heating above 50°C is supressed by a reducing agent (figure 6b), dithiothreitol which allow line width increase up to 70°C. This decrease in line width is related to the expulsion of lipoprotein vesicles in the aggregated protein network into large aqueous pockets. These aqueous zones are not present in reduced gluten (figure 7). It has been shown that sulphydryl-disulphide interchange reactions begin after 50°C and that up to 75°C glutenins are the most affected proteins (25). These rearrangements leading to the formation of large disulphide-linked protein aggregates, are not reversed on cooling and might be responsible for the lipid vesicles expulsion from the protein network and decrease in NMR line width.

**Conclusion**

The results obtained show that wheat lipids are organized in lipoprotein vesicles mobility of which is influenced by interactions between wheat prolamins. Such an organization and a dynamic of wheat lipids is quite different from the previously proposed models of protein-lipid interaction in dough and gluten (2-4).

It is noteworthy that the organisation of lipids in vesicles favours their dispersion in dough and the high surface area so produced may allow an optimization of the stabilisation of air/water or oil/water interfaces during baking process. It is also important to note that membrane proteins are enzymes, activity of which may be important for the structure and aggregation of prolamins (especially the oxydo-reductase activities).

Finally it may be noted that the water dependent lipid phase transitions occuring in wheat grain and technological products are probably not limited to wheat. Such events might occur in other dried plant material and might account for the modification of the foaming and emulsifying properties of some plant protein isolates.

**References**

1- Chiu C.M., Pomeranz Y. J.Food Sci. 31 (1966) 753-758.
2- Hoseney R.C., Finney K.F., Pomeranz Y. Cereal Chem. 47 (1970) 135-140.
3- Wehrli M.P., Pomeranz Y. Cereal Chem. 47 (1970) 135-140.
4- Chung O.K., Pomeranz Y. Baker's Dig. 5 (1977) 32-45
5- Frazier P.J., Daniels N.W., Russel-Eggirr P.W. J.Sci.Food Agric. 32 (1981) 877-891.

6- Zawistowska U., Bekes F., Bushuk W. Cereal Chem. 62 (1985) 284-289.
7- Edelhoch H. Horizons Biochem.Biophys. 5 (1978) 241-280.
8- Carlson T.L-G, Larsson K., Miezis Y. Cereal Chem. 55 (1978) 168-179.
9- Carlson T.L-G., Larsson K., Miezis Y., Podvarodom S. Cereal Chem. 56 (1979) 417-419
10- Al-Saleh A., Marion D., Gallant D. Food Microstruct. 5 (1986) 131-140.
11- Marion D., Le Roux C., Akoka S., Tellier C., Gallant D. J.Cereal Sci. 5 (1987) 101-115
12- Akoka S., Tellier C., Le Roux C., Marion D. Chem. Phys. Lipids 46 (1988) 43-50
13- Le Roux C, Marion D., Gallant D. Lebensm. -Wiss. Technol. (in press)
14- Le Roux C., Marion D., Gallant D., Compoint J.P. J.Sci. Food Agric. (in press).
15- Verkleij A.J. Biochim.Biophys.Acta 779 (1984) 43-63.
16- Crowe L.M., Crowe J.H. Arch.Biochem.Biophys. 217 (1982) 582-587
17- Crowe L.M., Mouradian R., Crowe J.H., Jackson S.A., Womersley C. Biochim.Biophys.Acta 769 (1984) 141-150.
18- Vail W.I., Stollery J.G. 551 (1979) 74-84.
19- Verkleij A.J., Van Echteld C.J.A., Gerritsen W.J., Cullis P.R., De Kruijff B. Biochim.Biophys.Acta 600 (1980) 620-624
20- Toivio-Kinnucan M.A., Stushnoff C. Cryobiology 18 (1981) 72-78
21- Deguchi N., Jorgensen P.L., Maunsbach A.B., J.Cell Biol. 75 (1977) 619-634
22- Gulik-Krzywicki T. in " Physical methods on Biological Membranes NATO ASI Series, Plenum Press 1985.
23- Qu R., Wang S.M., Lin Y-H., Vance V.B., Huang A.H.C. Biochem. J. 235 (1986) 57-65.
24- Gordon-Kamm W.J., Steponkus P.L. Proc. Natl.Acad. Sci.USA 81 (1984) 6373-6377.
25- Schofield J.D., Bottomley R.C., Timms M.F., Booth M.R. J.Cereal Sci. 1 (1983) 241-253.

## MYOSIN - PLANT PROTEIN INTERACTIONS

Lásztity, R.[1], A. Salgó[1], M. Ember-Kárpáti[1] and E. Ungár[1]

### Abstract

Different plant protein preparations are widely used in food industry mainly in production of meat products. The great variety of protein preparations and the properties they posses necessitate to determine precise technological procedures which are to be applied in the particulare products in order to utilize their potential functionality. This is an indispensable condition for obtaining the final products with appropiate desirable properties to be accepted by consumers. The realization of purposes mentioned above needs a deeper knowledge of the protein - protein interactions at a molecular level.

Experiments were made with different model systems containing myosin, actomyosin and plant protein preparations (soy glycinin, sunflower seed globulin, gliadin and glutenin). Textural properties of heat treated samples were determined using INSTRON Typ 1140 apparatus. Surface hydrophobicity and sulfhydryl group content of proteins was also measured. Sausages were also prepared using as extenders soy isolate, vital gluten and sunflower seed isolate.

Generally it can be stated that the strength and character of interactions are slightly different of that in meat protein systems causing lower cohesivity and consistency in comparison with pure meat protein systems. The role of disulfide bonds and hydrogen bonds is limited in the interactions, and a significant role of hydrophobic interactions is suggested.

### Introduction

Non-meat proteins derived from a variety of plant sources are used extensively as fillers, binders, and extenders in meat systems. A lot of specific sausages or similar products is produced using non-meat proteins as additives.

It is typical for such type of products that they have a considerable amount of fat, which must be uniformly distributed in the mass of the product. Concerning the texture generally the desire is to have a product which would most likely cut with a knife. The concept of restructuring meat and poultry products come into wide use in the past decade. Research and development work was conducted in many laboratories. The word restructuring as it is used with respect to red

[1]Department of Biochemistry and Food Technology Technical University, Budapest, H-1502 Pf. 91. Budapest, Hungary

meat and poultry meat refers to taking the raw material - the soft tissue, including lean, fat and connective tissue - and change the colloidal properties, the texture of the chopped components and their form.

This restructuring adds value and can upgrade raw materials which would not normally be a part of steak-like product. Typically these raw materials are used for ground meat systems.

In last period also in Hungary considerable interest has developed in restructuring poultry products because the processor can increase the value of specific primal cuts, utilize lean timmings and produce specific new products. The processor can also tailor the composition of products to consumer specific needs. From this point of view the composition of raw materials is the most important. The most problematic is the fat content. From one side fat is a major contributor to juiciness and flavor of finished meat product. Complaints about dry and tasteless products can often be corrected with closer attention to fat content. There is also the economic implication of formulating to higher fat contents. From other side there is a pressure to reduce the fat content. Nevertheless it is true that through formulation, consistent fat content, and thus consistent texture are more obtainable in restructured products than in the intact muscle products with lowered fat levels.

The properties of ground meat systems containing considerable amount of fats are generally discussed based on the meat emulsion phenomenon. It is suggested that the finely comminuted meat systems are emulsions where in continuous hydrophilic phase (solution of proteins, mineral components and some water soluble minor components) fat globules are dispersed coated with a protein layer. Among the factors influencing the stability of such colloidal system the properties and mechanical strength of the protein layer at the surface of the fat globules and the viscosity of the continuous phase are the most important. The highest stability may be achieved if the continuous phase is gelified. In relation to the textural properties of the system the interaction of the proteins during heat treatment is the most important.

Myofibrillar proteins play a major functional role in production of processed meats and myosin is generally considered as the most effective protein. Binding junctions that would develop between meat pieces in sectioned and formed products were shown to be strongest when formed with myosin. It is understandable that addition of non-meat plant proteins would change the conditions due to the new protein-protein interactions between myofibrillar meat proteins and plant proteins. There is a need from side of technologists to predict the functionality of these non meat proteins in meat systems. Although determination of such functional properties as water binding capacity, emulsifying capacity, gelling ability etc. give valuable information for the producer, quantitative estimates of the performance of non-meat proteins in meat emulsions have not been developed.

The prerequisit of a better prediction is a deeper knowledge of the protein-protein interactions. Theoretically, among formation of new disulfide bonds, three main forms of interactions are possible: forming of new hydrogen bonds, ionic binding and hydrophobic interactions. Studying the muscle-protein structure - functionality relationships Li Chan et al. [1] have found that generally samples with superior thermally induced functionality possessed higher protein content, lower fat and pH in mince, higher solubility and sulfhydryl group content and lower hydrophobicity in unheated salt - extractable proteins and finally greater decrease in solubility and increase in hydrophobicity after heating. These observation suggest that the process of heat denaturation combined with structural changes of protein molecules play also significant role in the interactions.

In the framework of the investigations in our laboratory protein model systems and sausages (frankfurter type) prepared with different plant protein addition were investigated.

## Materials and methods

Soy glycinin, wheat gliadin and glutenin, sunflower globulin, actomyosin and myosin were used in model experiments. For the preparation of sausages beef meat, fat non meat proteins such as soy isolate, sunflower seed isolate and vital gluten were used.

In model experiments a suspension containing 2.2 g myosine or actomyosine, 0.5 g sodium chloride, 0.05 g $Na_4P_2O_7$ and 7.25 g water was prepared and filled in test tubes (26 mm Ø, 12 mm height). To study the effect of plant protein preparations in the suspension mentioned above 0.2 g, 0.4 g and 0.6 g of myosin resp. actomyosin were substituted by glycinin, gliadin, glutenin and sunflower seed globulin.

The suspensions were heated at 80°C for 40 minutes. Sausages were prepared according following recipe:

Beef meat 95.8 g, fat 40.0 g, NaCl 3.8 g, nitrite 0.2 g,
$Na_4P_2O_7$ 0.6 g, water 59.6 g.

To study the effect of plant protein preparations 2.0 g of the meat protein were substituted with soy isolate, sunflower seed isolate and vital gluten, resp.

For the characterization of textural properties of model systems the test pieces (26 mm Ø, 12 mm height) were tested in an Instron Type 1140 apparatus using double-compression test with constant rate (25 %) of deformation. Three replications were made and the texture profile curves were evaluated. The surface hydrophobicity of meat protein preparations was determined using 1-anilinonaphtalen-8-sulfonic acid according to Li Chan et al. [2] and hydrophobicity of gluten proteins and sunflower seed globulin using alfa-p-toluidinyl-naphtalene-6-sulphonate according to Greene and Kasarda [3]. Sulfhydryl content of protein preparations was determined amperometrically.

Table 1: Textural properties of the model systems

| Sample | Myosin | Acto-myosin | Myosin-gliadin | Myosin-glutenin | Myosin-glycinin | Myosine-sunflower seed globulin |
|---|---|---|---|---|---|---|
| Work of 1-st compression $A_1/mm^2$ | 1350 | 1180 | 1220[1]<br>1170[2]<br>1040[3] | 1310[1]<br>1290[2]<br>1270[3] | 1210[1]<br>1150[2]<br>1030[3] | 1150[1]<br>1030[2]<br>970[3] |
| Work of 2-nd compression $A_2/mm^2$ | 240 | 210 | 205[1]<br>195[2]<br>190[3] | 190[1]<br>185[2]<br>176[3] | 187[1]<br>179[2]<br>1172[3] | 185[1]<br>175[2]<br>169[3] |
| Hardness (H) | 73.4 | 73.3 | 60[1]<br>58[2]<br>55[3] | 72.5[1]<br>71.5[2]<br>70.2[3] | 69.5[1]<br>68.2[2]<br>67.9[3] | 64.2[1]<br>63.8[2]<br>61.9[3] |
| Elastsicity (E) | 22.0 | 16.0 | 18.0[1]<br>16.0[2]<br>13.0[3] | 20.2[1]<br>19.3[2]<br>18.8[3] | 17.9[1]<br>17.5[2]<br>16.8[3] | 17.6[1]<br>17.3[2]<br>16.5[3] |
| Cohesivity (C) $[A_2/A_1]$ | 0.180 | 0.178 | 0.1682[1]<br>0.166[2]<br>0.182[3] | 0.145[1]<br>0.143[2]<br>0.137[3] | 0.154[1]<br>0.155[2]<br>0.166[3] | 0.160[1]<br>0.169[2]<br>0.17[3] |
| Gumminess (G) [CxH] | 13.2 | 13.0 | 10.08[1]<br>9.628[2]<br>10.01[3] | 10.51[1]<br>10.25[2]<br>19.61[3] | 10.703[1]<br>10.571[2]<br>11.27[3] | 10.272[1]<br>10.78[2]<br>10.77[3] |
| Chewiness (Ch) [GxE] | 190.6 | 208.7 | 181.44[1]<br>154.048<br>130.13[3] | 212.302[1]<br>197.825[2]<br>180.668[3] | 191.58[1]<br>184.99<br>189.336[3] | 180.78[1]<br>186.494[2]<br>177.705[3] |

[1] - 2.0 g myosin + 0.2 g added protein
[2] - 1.8 g myosin + 0.4 g added protein
[3] - 1.6 g myosin + 0.6 g added protein

Table 2: Textural properties of sausages propared with addition of different protein preparations

| Sample | Control | Control + soy isolate | Control + sunflower seed isolate | Control + vital gluten | Control + myosin |
|---|---|---|---|---|---|
| Work of 1-st compression $[A_1]$ | 1192 | 1135 | 970 | 950 | 1220 |
| Work of second compression $[A_2]$ | 202 | 170 | 160 | 150 | 205 |
| Hardness [H] | 73.3 | 68.6 | 70.0 | 60.0 | 70.0 |
| Elasticity [E] | 15.0 | 15.0 | 13.5 | 15.0 | 18.0 |
| Cohesivity [C] $[A_2/A_1]$ | 0.178 | 0.164 | 0.165 | 0.157 | 0.168 |
| Gumminess [G] [CxH] | 13.04 | 11.27 | 11.55 | 9.47 | 11.76 |
| Chewiness [Ch] [GxE] | 195.6 | 169.0 | 155.9 | 142.1 | 211.68 |

## Results and discussion

The results of the measurement of textural properties of model systems are summarized in the Table 1. On the basis of the data included in the table it could be stated that the samples containing only myosin as protein component possess the best textural properties. Substitution of myosin with other proteins results always to a smaller or greater extent in a decrease especially in hardness and elasticity but changes in cohestivity are small. Glutenin results in a practically unchanged hardness and elasticity. The substitution of a part of myosin with soy glycinin and sunflower seed globulin results in a slight decrease in textural parameters. The trend of changes is very similar and slight advantage of glycinin may be observed in comparison with globulin of sunflower seed.

No significant effect of quantity of sulfhydryl groups on the textural properties was observed. Desamidation of gliadin caused only slight decrease in cohesivity and hardness of samples. The results suggest the conclusion that the role of disulfide and hydrogen bonds is limited in the formation of gel during heat treatment. Although the differences in hydrophobicity are not to big between different protein preparations, neverheless the role of hydrophobic interactions might be the most important. The denaturation of the proteins and structural changes probably increase the number of apolar groups being able to interact. Such views were expressed also by Foeding et al. [4].

In the Table 2. textural parameters of sausages prepared with addition of different protein preparations are shown. Myosin addition resulted in slight improvement of the textural properties as seen from the data included in the table. A decrease of textural quality of product was observed in the case of other protein preparations. Soy isolate was relatively the best extender.

## Literature


[1] Li Chan, E., S. Nakai and D.F. Wood;
J. of Food Sci. **52** (1987) 1, 31 - 41

[2] Li Chan, E., S. Nakai and D.F. Wood;
J. of Food Sci. **49** (1984), 2, 345 - 349

[3] Greene, F.C. and D.D. Kasarda;
Cereal Chem. **48** (1971), 5, 601 - 608

[4] Foeding, E.A., W.R. Dayton and C.E. Allen;
J. Food Sci. **51** (1986), 1, 104 - 108

# PROTEIN-DYE INTERACTION: A POWERFUL PRINCIPLE FOR PURIFICATION OF PROTEINS

Gerhard Kopperschläger[1], Gerd Birkenmeier and Jürgen Kirchberger

The development of group specific affinity adsorbents in which the immobilized ligand interacts specifically and reversibly with many complementary proteins has proved to be a valuable addition to the methods available for protein purification. In recent years some of the most widely used ligands for application in this type of affinity chromatography have been a variety of reactive textile dyes. Reactive dyes were introduced to the textile trade for the dyeing of the cellulose fibres, cotton and viscose to enable dyeing of high fastness to washing. They achieve this effect by formation of covalent bond between the dye and the matrix.

Immobilized dyes also appear to be especially effective adsorbents for the purification of enzymes like oxidoreductases, phosphotransferases, ligases and other coenzyme-dependent enzymes, oligo- and polynucleotide-dependent enzymes, hydrolases, esterases and a host of blood proteins [1-4]. In addition, affinity chromatography and related techniques become significant because genetic engineering has provided a tool for the production of large quantities of diagnostic and therapeutic proteins.

The use of synthetic textile dyes as biomimetic media offers significant advantages over the more conventional immobilized biological ligands. For example, the protein binding capacity of immobilized dye adsorbents exceeds those of natural biological media by 10 to 100 fold and the low capital cost, the commercial availability and the ease of coupling to a variety of solid supports offer prospects for affinity chromatography in large scale. Furthermore, synthetic dyes are chemically and biologically stable and display a remarkably broad specificity of reversible interaction with proteins.

Most of the reactive dyes employed in protein purification are polysulphonated aromatic molecules. In Fig. 1 different basic structures of reactive dyes are displayed. The reacting group to a nucleophile is either the mono- or dichlorotriazinyl ring - this type of dyes are designated as triazine dyes - or the vinylsulphone group which is generated during the reaction from a sulphatoethylsulphonic precursor by elimination of sulphonic acid. The latter are trade named as Remazol dyes. It appears that the charged chromophores of these dyes mimic more

---

1) Karl-Marx-Universität Leipzig, Institut für Biochemie, Bereich Medizin, Liebigstrasse 16, 7010 Leipzig, GDR

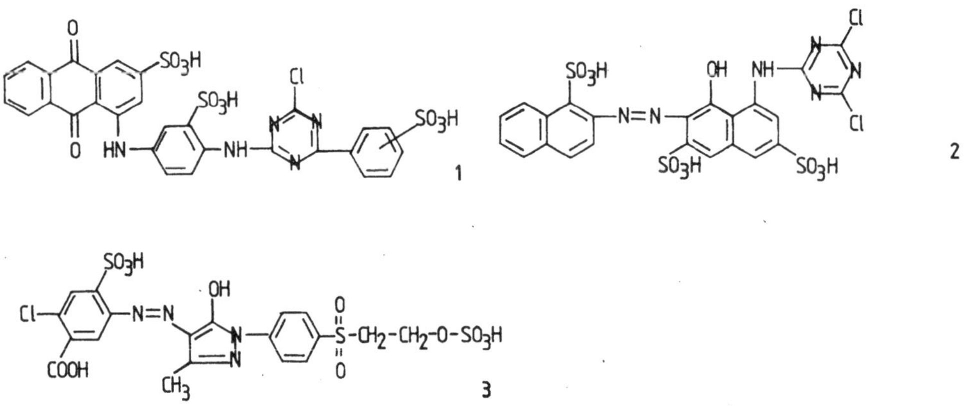

Fig. 1: Structure of reactive dyes
(1) Cibacron Blue F3G-A, (Reactive Blue 2; Anthraquinone-dye; Monochlorotriazine-dye)
(2) Procion Red MX-8B, (Reactive Red 11; Azo-dye; Dichlorotriazine-dye)
(3) Remazol Yellow GGL, (Reactive Yellow 13; Azo-dye; Vinylsulphone generating dye)

or less the binding to complementary structures of proteins of the natural occurring anionic heterocycles such of the coenzyme $NAD^+$, $NADP^+$, ATP, coenzyme A and other nucleotides and polynucleotides.
Recently also cationic dyes have been found to interact specifically to a number of proteases like trypsin, thrombin and carboxypeptidase B [5]. Some work has been done to understand the chemical basis and the conformational requirements of the protein-dye interaction but the existing results are not consistent enougn to generalize a theoretical concept [2].
Various methods have been elaborated for studying protein-dye interaction. Difference spectral titration provides evidence for both hydrophobic and ionic contributions to dye-protein binding in many cases [6]. However, to interprete spectral changes in the dye in association with different polar and apolar binding sites the spectral characteristics of the respective dyes with the organic solvent, salt etc. and the model protein have to be examined. One example is given in Fig. 2 in which the difference spectra of Procion Red HE-3B in the presence of sodium chloride, ethylene glycol, L-arginine and the enzyme alkaline phosphatase are drawn [7]. The similarities of the shape of the spectra in the

presence of salt and arginine respectively to the spectrum in the presence of alkaline phosphatase indicate that electrostatic interactions between the enzyme and the dye seems to be dominant.
In addition, great caution should be exercised in interpretation spectral titrations to get quantitative data because some dyes are able to form stacked states at greater concentrations.

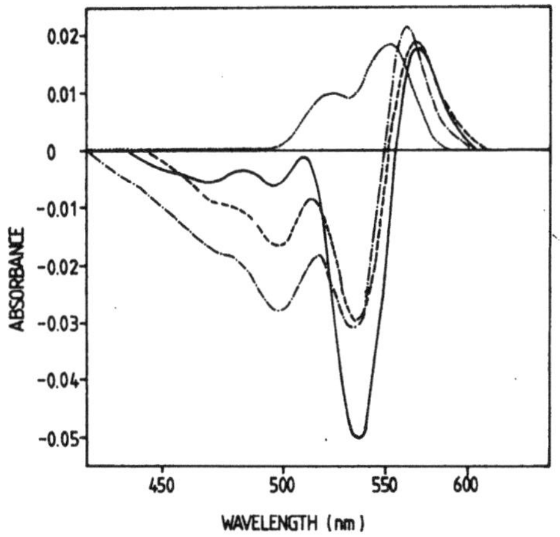


Fig. 2: Difference spectra of Procion Red HE-3B in the presence of NaCl (———), L-arginine (—•—), ethylene glycol (········) and alkaline phosphatase (– – –).

Kinetic analyses by following the inhibitory action of the dyes to a certain enzyme and the studies of reversibility of inhibition after addition of natural ligands are frequently performed to give compelling evidences for the presence and nature of dye binding site of enzymes. For example, the comparison of the inhibition constants of dyes with different structures allows to evaluate the significance of the charged groups and of their spatial arrangement within the chromophore for the binding to the protein. The results of this study can be confirmed by affinity chromatographic techniques providing improvements of the application in preparative scale.
Affinity labelling with reactive dyes has yielded more definite information on the protein-dye interaction. By using this technique the dye is covalently bound to the protein and behaves as irreversible active site-directed affinity label. For this investigation the more reactive dichlorotriazine dyes have to be selected. Studies with horse liver alcohol dehydrogenase [8] and carboxypeptidase G-2 [9] have been published. The exact number of dye molecules bound per mole of subunit and the amino acid residue within a peptide sequence to which the dye has been covalently attached are obtained. Thus, structural features of

the protein-dye interaction are deducible particularly, if the spatial structure of the protein is known.

In the case of horse liver alcohol dehydrogenase the binding of Cibacron Blue F3G-A to orthorhombic crystals of the enzyme has been examined by X-ray diffraction analysis [10]. This study has defined the binding characteristics for the different rings of the dye but not the precise orientation nor conformational details of the rings were resolved especially of the terminal ring D of the dye. Therefore, modification of the terminal ring of Cibacron Blue F3G-A were considered the most likely to produce significant variations in binding affinity to the enzyme [11]. In Fig. 3 the apparent $K_d$-values in dependence on the substituent in the terminal ring are presented. The data demonstrate that small substituents bind more tightly than more bulky species and especially so if substituted in the o- or m-position on the terminal ring. From this study improvements of protein binding to the ligand for application in chromatographic techniques can be deduced.

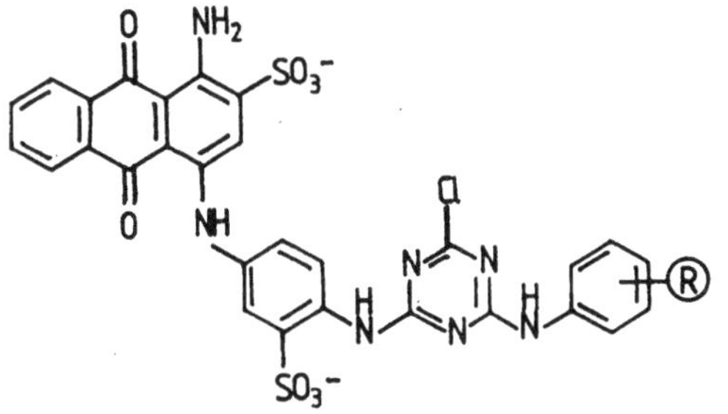


| R | APPARENT $K_d$ (/uM) |
|---|---|
| m-COOH | 0.06 |
| H | 0.2 |
| o-COOH | 0.2 |
| o-$SO_3H$ | 0.4 |
| m-$SO_3H$ | 1.6 |
| m-$CH_2OH$ | 4.5 |
| m-$CONH_2$ | 5.7 |
| p-COOH | 5.9 |
| p-$SO_3H$ | 9.3 |
| p-$PO_3H_2$ | 10.5 |
| p-$N^+(CH_3)_3$ | 172 |

Fig. 3: Apparent affinities of terminal ring analoques of Cibacron Blue F3G-A for horse liver alcohol dehydrogenase

In the last decade the technique of affinity partitioning becomes attractive for studying protein-dye interaction. The principle of this method is drawn in Fig. 4. Generally, proteins are partitioned in two aqueous phases of a system composed for instance, of the polymers dextran and poly(ethylene glycol) (PEG) and water. The properties of liquid/liquid-phase systems and the widespread application for the separation of biological macromolecules has been described by Albertsson and coworkers [12 ]. The partition of a protein between the PEG-rich upper phase and the dextran-rich lower phase is expressed by the partition coefficient, K, defined as the ratio of the protein concentration in the upper and in the lower phase.

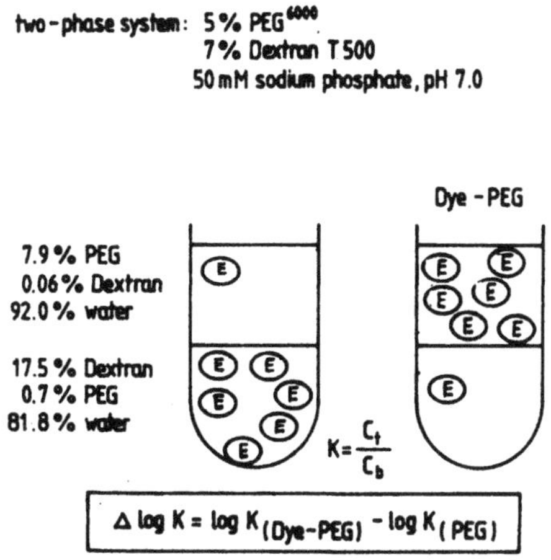


Fig. 4: Principle of affinity partitioning

The partition of proteins depends on a large number of external factors and shows great individual response to these parameters. Of particular interest is the change of the partition of proteins if one of the phase-forming polymers is substituted with a biospecific ligand, e.g. with a reactive dye. In affinity partitioning the protein of interest with affinity for a certain dye can be extracted into the ligand-containing phase leaving the other proteins in the opposite phase. The effectiveness of extraction is usually expressed as $\Delta \log K$, i.e. the difference in the logarithm of the partition coefficients in systems with and without the ligand.

The dependence of the affinity partitioning effect on the concentration of the polymer-bound ligand give rise to a saturation curve in many cases from which the maximum of extraction ($\Delta \log K_{max}$) and the half saturation point at $0.5 \times \Delta \log K_{max}$ are obtained (Fig. 5).

The $\Delta \log K_{max}$ is assumed to be related to the number of binding sites of the ligand of the protein and can be regarded as a measure of the strength of extraction power whereas the affinity of the ligand to the protein correlates with the value of $0.5 \times \Delta \log K_{max}$.

Both parameters are of interest for employment extractive procedures of liquid/liquid phases for the purification of proteins. For instance, if the affinity partition effect $\Delta \log K_{max}$ is about two and the volumes of both phases are approximately equal the conditions for extractive procedures can be adjusted that around 90 % of the target protein which binds to the ligand are transferred into those phase where the ligand is present, whereas other proteins without affinity to the ligand are not affected. Some practical applications are summarized in the last section of this paper.

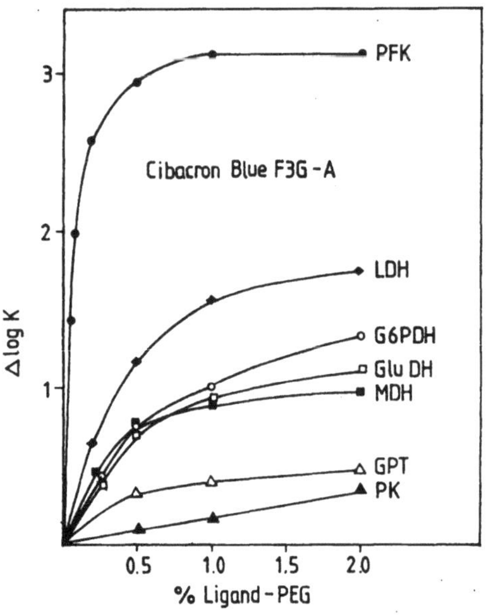


Fig. 5: Dependence of the affinity partitioning effect (Δ log K) on the concentration of dye-ligand PEG for different enzymes

Affinity partitioning is also excellently suited for recognizing small differences in the strength of protein-dye interaction. Thus, the method gives rise to screen protein-ligand interaction in a simple manner by varying a number of parameters like the chemical structure of the dye-ligand, the buffer composition, the pH-value, the temperature, competing effectors etc. to obtain the following data:

1. Selection of an optimum dye ligand for a certain protein
2. Selection of optimum conditions for association/dissociation of the protein-dye complex (i.e. metal-ion promoted protein-dye interaction)
3. Selection of corresponding effectors to compete with protein-dye interaction
4. Elucidation of the chemical basis of protein-dye interaction

As a rule, data obtained by this technique are valid also for other affinity-ligand techniques like affinity chromatography and affinity electrophoresis.

In Fig. 6 the influence of competing effectors at constant concentration of the dye-polymer ligand on the effect of affinity partitioning of lactate dehydrogenase (LDH) and pyruvate kinase (PK) is demonstrated. For instance, the binding of LDH to Cibacron Blue F3G-A is diminished by increasing amounts of $NAD^+$ but seems to be not completely abolished at 2 mM of the effector. However, addition of sodium sulphite reduces the affinity partition effect completely at rather low concentration of $NAD^+$. This component is known to form a ternary enzyme/$NAD^+$/sulphite complex exhibiting an extremely low dissociation constant. In the case of PK the affinity partitioning effect was diminished partially by ATP. If $Mg^{++}$-ions are supplemented which are known to form a stable MgATP complex being the actual substrate of the enzyme, the competitive action did not increase. In contrast, the $Mg^{++}$-ions seem to promote the protein-dye interaction as indicated by the curve of the Fig. 6.

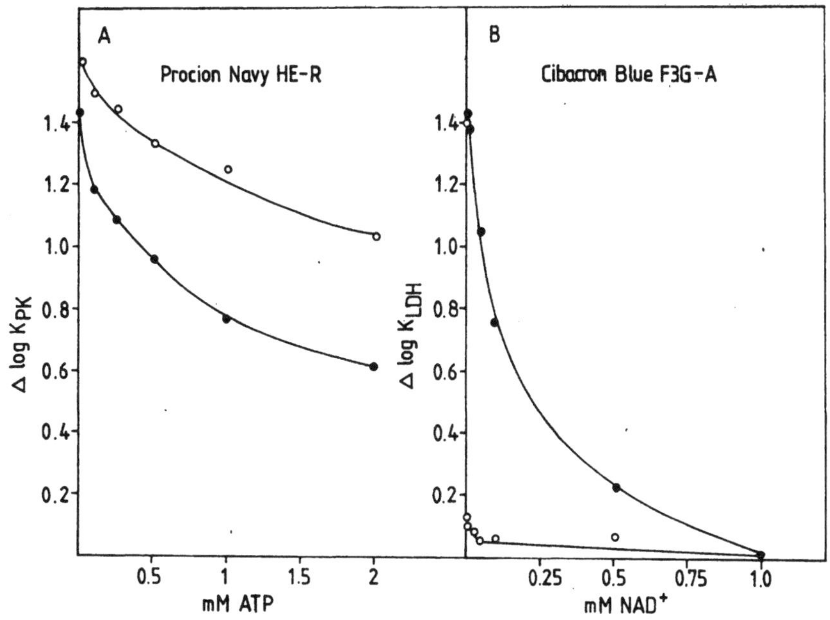


Fig. 6: Dependence of the affinity partitioning effect of pyruvate kinase and lactate dehydrogenase on the concentration of competing effectors
A) ATP (●—●), MgATP (○—○)
B) $NAD^+$ (●—●), $NAD^+$/Sulphite (○—○)

Fig. 7 shows that NADPH competes differently with the dyes Procion Green H-4G, Procion Yellow HE-3G and Procion Blue MX-G for the binding sites of glucose 6-phosphate dehydrogenase (G6PDH) although the extent of the affinity partitioning effect by using these three dyes are similar.
A sreening of ten PEG-bound dyes for the interaction with pre-albumin and albumin is demonstrated in Fig. 8. Albumin shows strong affinity for Cibacron Blue F3G-A as well as for several other dyes. Pre-albumin, in contrast, displays binding predominantly to Remazol Yellow GGL but not to the other dyes indicating a high selectivity in dye-protein interaction. This behaviour in binding has been exploited for the purification of pre-albumin from human serum by application dye-ligand affinity chromatography as summarized in Table 1 [13].

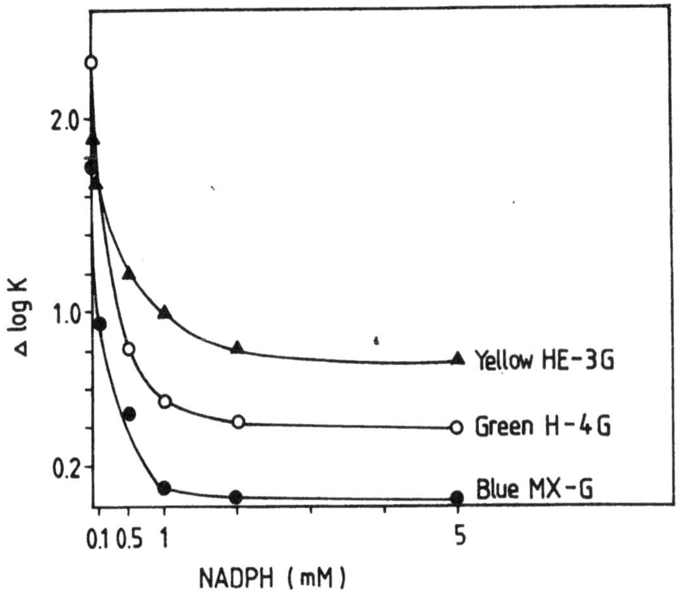


Fig. 7: Dependence of the affinity partitioning effect of glucose 6-phosphate dehydrogenase on increasing amounts of NADPH

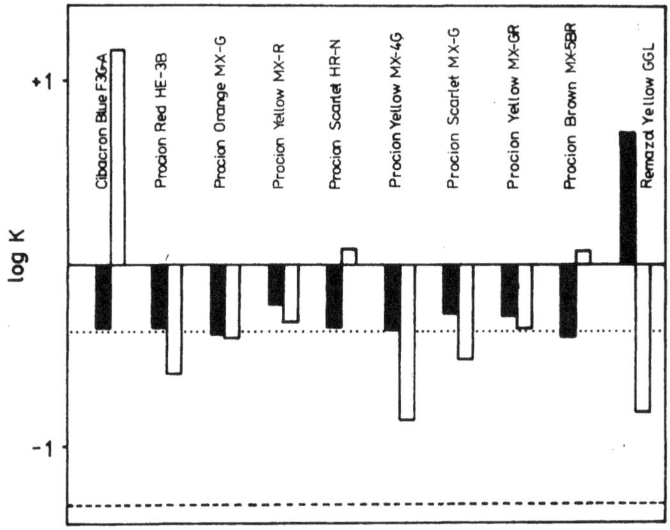


Fig. 8: Effect of different dye-PEG derivatives on the partitioning of pre-albumin (black bars) and albumin (white bars), 1) Cibacron Blue F3G-A, 2) Procion Red H-3B, 3) Procion Orange MX-G, 4) Procion Yellow MX-R, 5) Procion Scarlet HR-N, 6) Procion Yellow MX-4G, 7) Procion Scarlet MX-G, 8) Procion Yellow MX-GR, 9) Procion Brown MX-5BR, 10) Remazol Yellow GGL Partitioning of pre-albumin (— — —) and albumin (·······) in absence of dye-PEG

TABLE 1: PURIFICATION OF PRE-ALBUMIN

| Fraction | Total protein[a] (mg) | Pre-albumin[b] (mg) | Yield (%) |
|---|---|---|---|
| Serum[c] | 33 750 | 105 | 100 |
| Ammonium sulphate fraction | 17 550 | 52 | 49 |
| Remazol Yellow GGL chromatography | 76 | 41 | 39 |
| Cibacron Blue F3G-A chromatography | 34 | 36 | 34 |

a) Measured according to LOWRY

b) Measured by rocket electroimmunodiffusion

c) When plasma was used similar results were obtained

Affinity partition is also suited to analyze the dependence of the flexibility of the structure of a dye-ligand on the strength of binding. This has been exemplarily demonstrated with alkaline phosphatase from calf intestine and several Procion dyes (Fig. 9) [14].

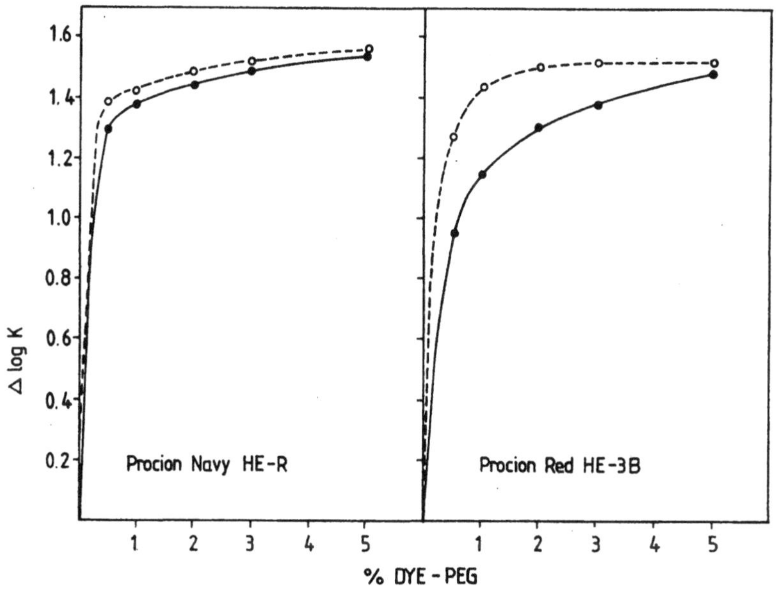


Fig. 9: Affinity partitioning of alkaline phosphatase by using chemically modified dye-PEG derivatives
The percentages of dye-PEG refer to the total amount of PEG, unmodified dye-PEG (●—●), the dye-ligand was modified by reduction of the azo-linkages with sodium borohydride (○—○).

To increase the flexibility azo-linkages of certain dyes were reduced to form hydrazino-bridges. The hydrogenation of those dyes exhibiting high affinity and a great $\Delta$ log $K_{max}$ like Procion Navy H-ER had no influence on the partition effect. In the case of Procion Red HE-3B, however, the affinity markedly increased without change in the $\Delta$ log $K_{max}$.

Affinity chromatography and affinity partitioning using dye-ligands have been extensively developed over the last decade in response to greater demands placed on protein purification technology. The number of papers published has been increased rapidly and at present time more than 100 proteins have been purified employing this principle of biorecognition. Many chromatographic procedures have been elaborated by coupling the dye covalently to supports such as agarose, cellulose, cross-linked dextran, silica and organic polymers yielding water insoluble affinity adsorbents.

Recently, the technique of affinity partitioning becomes more attractive for preparative purposes because of the simple technical manipulation to extract proteins in large scale. In Table 2 some enzymes purified by using this technique are listed.

TABLE 2: PURIFICATION OF ENZYMES BY MEANS OF AFFINITY PARTITIONING

| Protein | Dye-ligand | Purification-factor (n-fold) | Reference |
|---|---|---|---|
| Phosphofructokinase (yeast) | Cibacron Blue F3G-A | 10 | 14 |
| Glucose 6-phosphate dehydrogenase (yeast) | Procion Yellow HE-3G<br>Procion Olive MX-3G | 25<br>40 | 15<br>15 |
| Lactate dehydrogenase (muscle) | Procion Yellow HE-3G<br>Cibacron Blue F3G-A | 30<br>25 | 16<br>16 |
| Formate dehydrogenase (candida boidinii) | Procion Red HE-3B | 6 | 17 |
| Alkaline phosphatase (calf intestine) | Procion Red HE-3B | 13 | 18 |

The improvement of the binding properties of dyes to act as highly specific biomimetic ligands, particularly by employing the potential of computer-aided ligand design will increase the significance of affinity-ligand separation techniques for downstream processing in biotechnology.

References


[1] Dean, P.D.G. and Watson, D.H., in: Affinity Chromatography, (Hofmann-Ostenhof, O. et al., Eds.), 25 (1978) 25-46.

[2] Kopperschläger, G., Böhme, H.-J. and Hofmann E., in: Advances in Biochemical Engineering ( Fiechter, A., Ed.), 25 (1982) 101-138, Springer Verlag, Berlin, Heidelberg, New York.

[3] Lowe, C.R., in: An Introduction to Affinity Chromatography; Laboratory Techniques in Biochemistry and Molecular Biology, (Work, T.S., Work, E., Eds.), North-Holland, Amsterdam 1979.

[4] Subramanian, S.: Critical Rev. Biochem. 16 (1984), 169-205.

[5] Clonis, Y.D., Stead, C.V. and Lowe, C.R.: Biotechnol. Bioeng. 30 (1987), 621-627.

[6] Subramanian, S.: Arch. Biochem. Biophys. 216 (1982), 116-123.

[7] Kirchberger, J., Seidel, H. and Kopperschläger, G.: Biomed. Biochim. Acta 46 (1987), 653-663.

[8] Small, D.A.P., Lowe, C.R., Atkinson, T. and Bruton, C.J.: Eur. J. Biochem. 128 (1982), 119-123.

[9] Hughes, P., Sherwood, R.F. and Lowe, C.R.: Eur. J. Biochem. 144 (1984), 135-142.

[10] Biellmann, J.-F, Samama, J.-P., Bränden, C. and Eklund, H.: Eur. J. Biochem. 102 (1979), 107-110.

[11] Lowe, C.R., Burton, S.J., Pearson, J.C. and Clonis, Y.D.: J.Chromatogr. 376 (1986), 121-130.

[12] Albertsson, P.-A.: Partition of Cell Particles and Macromolecules, 2nd Ed. Almqvist & Wiksell, Stockholm 1971.

[13] Birkenmeier, G.,Tschechonin, B. and Kopperschläger, G.: FEBS-Lett. 174 (1984), 162-166.

[14] Kopperschläger, G., Kirchberger, J. and Kriegel, T., in: Die Makromolekulare Chemie (Höcker, H., Ed.), Hüthig & Wepf-Verlag, Basel, Heidelberg, New York 1988, in press.

[15] Kopperschläger, G. and Johansson, G.: Anal. Biochem. 124 (1982), 117-124.

[16] Johansson, G. and Joelsson, M.: Enzyme Microbiol. Technol.7 (1985), 629-634.

[17] Johansson, G. and Joelsson, M.: Appl. Biochem. Biotechnol.: 13 (1986), 15-27.

[18] Cordes, A. and Kula, M.-R.: J. Chromatogr. 376 (1986), 375-384.

[19] Kirchberger, J. unpublished result.

STUDY OF THE ACTIVE SITE OF PROTEASES BY MEANS OF SPIN-LABELED INHIBITORS

W. Damerau[1)], N. Genov[2)] and S. Fittkau[3)]

## Introduction

Proteases are nowadays used in a large scale in food processing e.g. for meat tenderization, soya sauce fermentation and protein degradation in general (1). A great part of protease production is applied as additives for detergents. With the increasing interest in proteases an interest has been grown in inhibitors of these enzymes. One very practical aspect is the use of inhibitors for the control of proteolytic action. Another point of view is the investigation of the active site of proteases in order to get a deeper insight in the mechanism of enzymatic action. The improved knowledge of the structure and function of active sites in proteases may be helpful for the design of enzyme derivatives with optimized properties.

For the study of the active site of proteases oligopeptide derivatives as substrate analogous inhibitors have been designed and synthesized. Thus, for thermitase, oligopeptide methylketones X - $Ala_nPheCH_3$ (with X = carbobenzoxy or other groups) have been described (2) which allow to derive information about the sterical and electronical requirements of the active site when the determined $K_i$ values are taken in account. Information about the active site can be extended when the potential inhibitor is additionally equipped with a reporter group able to inform about dynamical processes in or near the active site. Reporter groups may be fluorescence labels (3,4) or spin labels (5) in position X of the inhibitor mentioned above.

Spin-labeling of biomacromolecules means the introduction of a stable free nitroxide radical as a paramagnetic reporter group (spin label, SL) and the exploitation of advantages of the electron spin resonance (ESR) method:

1) Academy of Sciences of GDR, Central Institute of Molecular Biology, DDR-1115 Berlin-Buch, GDR

2) Bulgarian Academy of Sciences, Institute of Organic Chemistry, Sofia, Bulgaria

3) Martin Luther University, Institute of Biochemistry, Halle, GDR

- only the spin label is measured whereas the diamagnetic components of the system studied are ESR-silent
- high sensitivity (under favourable conditions even $10^{-8}$M SL are measurable)
- optical transparency is not required
- from the ESR spectra the motion of the SL group can be measured quantitatively and information about the influence of the surrounding protein on the mobility of the label is derived, thus giving information about dynamic processes occuring in the protein region where the SL group is located (6).

Strategies for the spin-labeling of active sites are discussed in (7,8) and consist in

- selective covalent binding of the label to special amino acid residues (e.g. Ser, Cys) by functional groups of the spin label
- introduction of the label by SL-coenzymes (9)
- introduction of the spin label by substrate analogous inhibitors which may be attached to the enzyme A) covalently or B) nonconvalently.

Advantages and disadvantages of mode A) and B), respectively, are discussed in detail in (8). An advantage of A) may be the seperation of unreacted label. On the other hand, with B) equilibria between bound and unbound inhibitor are measured directly and $K_i$ as well as the number of binding sites can be determined without any assumptions.

## Active sites in leucine aminopeptidase

An example for the usefulness of spin labeling active sites in proteases is the investigation of active sites in leucine aminopeptidase (LAP) by oligopeptides of different chain length, spin labeled at the C-terminus (10). Using tert.-butyl-ThrPhe$_n$-SL (n = 0, 1, 2, 3) we were able to show that there exist 2 classes of binding sites: 1 binding site with $K_i$ = 2,6 x $10^{-5}$M and 12 binding sites with $K_i$ = 9 x $10^{-4}$M, 6 of them being catalytically active as elucidated from comparison with kinetic measurements. It seems very probable that the hexameric LAP is an allosteric enzyme, although kinetic measurements could not give any answer to this question due to the high excess of substrate necessary in these measurements. Thus, allosteric behaviour of LAP may be overlooked. On the other hand, in the ESR experiments even molar ratios for enzyme and inhibitor of 1 : 1 were measured and the two classes of binding sites are demonstrated by the different ESR spectra as well as independently by the Scatchard plot.From combined ESR and biochemical data the description of a model for the active site of LAP was possible: i) the substrate is fixed by 2 hydrophobic subsites in a spacious pocket, ii) the substrate is additionally fixed by a strongly polar subsite outside this pocket, iii) a 'bottle-neck'-like aperture of this pocket can be passed only by molecules with a diameter < 8 Å, iv) the 3 subsites and this aperture avoid nonproductive binding of other compounds.

## Study of thermitase by noncovalently binding SL-inhibitors

A similar approach was applied to thermitase. For this enzyme the following N-terminally spin-labeled inhibitors

SL - $Ala_nPheCh_3$ with n = 0, 1, 2, 3

and SL = 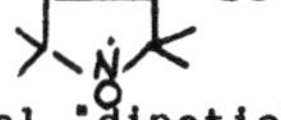

were synthesized (5) and used as a potential 'dipstick' for the active site of thermitase. Depending on the chain length, subsites S3, S4 or S5 can be 'explored' by the SL group once tetrahedral intermediate between the C-terminus and the Ser-225 inside the active site has been formed:

S5 ~ S4 ~ S3 ~ S2 ~ S1 ~ Ser-225

SL - Ala - Ala - Ala - $PheCh_3$

The derivatives with n = 2 and n = 3 exhibit high inhibition of the activity of thermitase as well as of subtilisin BPN' and their reversible binding to thermitase has been demonstrated by their ESR spectra (5). From the ESR spectra it is concluded that the access of the SL group to S3 is restricted as a consequence of its bulkyness, whereas S4 and S5 are located in a spacious part of the active site. An argument in favour of a narrow entrance, limiting access to S3 - S1 for molecules or residues with a diameter < 8 Å, is seen in the finding that SL - HgCl does not bind to the Cys-68 inside the active site pocket. Assuming formation of a half-ketal between Ser-225 and the methylketone group, a distance of 16 Å between the NO moiety of SL $Ala_2PheCH_3$ and $C_\beta$ of Ser - 225 has been evaluated (12). For SL - $Ala_3PheCH_3$ the corresponding value is 19.6 Å. Thus, a depth of about 20 Å for the active site of thermitase seems to be plausible (12). This value is near the value of 18 Å proposed for subtilisin BPN' by Morihara et al (13).

Study of serine proteases by covalently binding SL-inhibitors

Studies on thermitase were extended with irreversibly binding inhibitors SL - $Ala_nPheCh_2Cl$ (with n = 1, 2, 3) synthesized very recently (Fittkau et al.). ESR spectra reveal that the mobility of the SL moiety is diminuished with decreasing chain length. Decreasing mobility is expressed by the increasing splitting constant 2 $A'_{zz}$ which can be depicted from Fig. 1 for the 3 SL-inhibitors bound to thermitase.

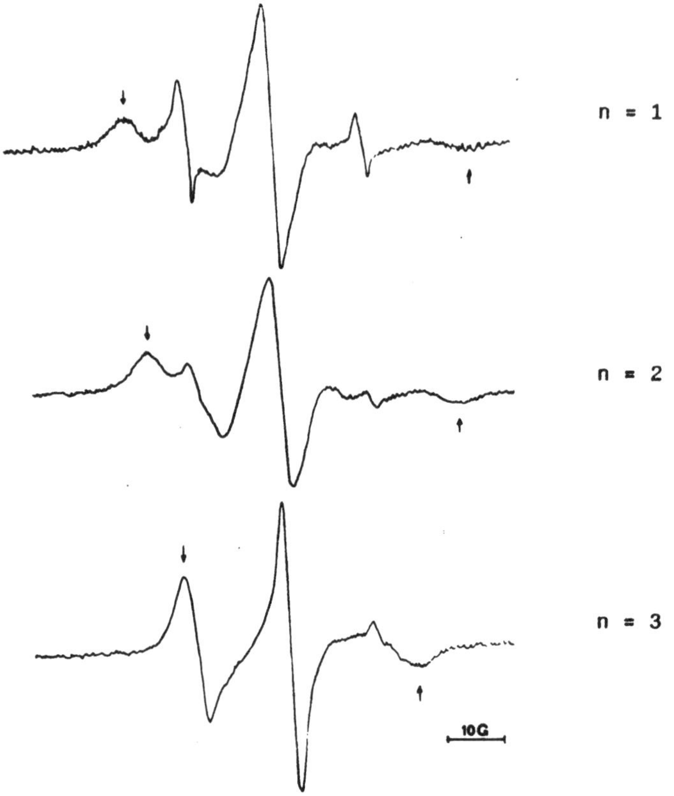


Fig. 1: ESR spectra for SL - $Ala_nPheCH_2Cl$ covalently bound to thermitase (modulation 2 G, power 20 mW, different gain)

From these values a rotational correlation time $\tau_c$ = 11,4 nsec has been estimated for the SL - $Ala_2PheCH_2Cl$/thermitase complex. This value is very near to the value evaluated for thermitase from quasielastic light scattering data (Zirwer and Gast, unpublished data) and means that the SL group is tightly bound to the enzyme molecule.

The SL-inhibitors mentioned before are bound irreversibly to serine proteases related to thermitase. The corresponding 2 $A'_{zz}$ values are compiled in table 1 and demonstrate differences in the structure of the active sites of these enzymes.

Table 1: 2 $A'_{zz}$ values for SL-$Ala_n PheCH_2Cl$ bound to proteases

| enzyme | n = 1 | n = 2 | n = 3 |
|---|---|---|---|
| proteinase K | 60.7 | 39.6 | 40.2 |
| thermitase | 61.2 | 53.8 | 42.5 |
| subtilisins BPN' | 58.5 | 59.0 | 41.1 |
| DY | 60.2 | 59.0 | 40.8 |
| Carlsberg | 59.0 | 59.0 | 39.9 |
| α-Chymotrypsin | 39.5 | 70.0 | 45.5 |

Remarkably is the very high value 2 $A'_{zz}$ for SL-$Ala_2PheCH_2Cl$/α-chymotrypsin which is assumed to be the consequence not only of tight binding but also by the accomodation of the SL group in a very strong polar region of the active site pocket of α-chymotrypsin. Similar, large splittings have been observed only in a few cases (11,14).

The mobility of the label is altered by addition of urea or guanidine-HCl giving information about changes in the conformation of subsites S3, S4 and S5, respectively, during denaturation. Preliminary ESR results suggest that the active site of thermitase is remarkably stable against 8M urea or 6M guanidine-HCl. High stability of the active site against 8M urea has been found also for subtilisin DY and points to the close structural relationship between thermitase and the subtilisins. On the other hand, the active site of α-chymotrypsin was found to be unfolded even with 4M urea within a time of shorter than 1 minute.

## Conclusions

Design and synthesis of substrate analogous SL-inhibitors and investigation by means of ESR may give information about

- number of binding sites
- dissociation constants
- mobility of the SL group inside the active site
- structural changes during denaturation
- polarity/hydrophobicity inside the active site

and may be helpful to characterize the active sites and subsites of enzymes. The approach to apply acceptable spin labeled ligands can be extended to complicated protein complexes and has been demonstrated even in the case of ribosome/mRNA complexes (15).

## References


1 Wisemann, A.: "Handbook of Enzyme Biotechnology", Ellis Horwood Ltd., Wiley and Sons, Chichester 1985, p. 355

2 Fittkau, S., K. Smalla and D. Pauli: Biomed. Biochim. Acta 43 (1984) 887-899

3 Peters, K., O. Bätz, W.E. Höhne and S. Fittkau: Biomed. Biochim. Acta 43 (1984) 909-918

4 Genov, N.Ch., and R.N. Boteva: Biochem. J. 238 (1986) 923-926

5 Fittkau, S., D. Pauli, Ph. Bouavarong and W. Damerau: Biomed. Biochim. Acta 45 (1986) 877-886

6 Berliner, L.J.: "Spin Labeling. Theory and Applications", Vol.1, Academic Press, New York 1976

7 Damerau, W.: "Characterization of Active Sites by Spin Labeling", Chapter 14, p. 137-146, in A. Schellenberger and R.L. Schowen: "Thiamine Pyrophosphate Biochemistry" Vol.II, CRC Press, Boca Raton 1988

8 Damerau, W., and S. Fittkau: Z. exper. Physik (in press)

9 Wenzel, H., and W. Trommer: FEBS Lett. 78 (1977) 184

10 Fittkau, S., and W. Damerau: J. prakt. Chem 322 (1980) 1032

11 Damerau, W., and S. Fittkau: studia biophys. 96 (1983) 177-186

12 Damerau, W., P. Herrmann, K. Peters and S. Fittkau: Proceedings of the 2nd Internat. Meeting "Molecular and Cellular Regulation of Enzyme Activity", Halle 1986 (in press)

13 Morihara, K., T. Oka and H. Tsuzuki: Biochem. Biophys. Res. Commun. 35 (1969) 210-214

14 Humphries, G.M.K., and H.M. Mc Connell: Biophys. J. 16 (1976) 275

15 Damerau, W., A.I. Petrov, J. Stahl, B.I. Sukhorukov and H. Bielka: Biomed. Biochim. Acta 45 (1986) 727-736

# INTERACTIONS OF LECTINS WITH MICROORGANISMS

Ch. Flemming [1)]

## Introduction

Lectins are proteins or glycoproteins of non-immune origin that agglutinate cells or precipitate soluble carbohydrates. They are characterized by their specific reactions with carbohydrates. The agglutination or precipitation activities are usually inhibited by mono- or oligosaccharides. Lectins do not posses enzymatic activities. They are isolated from a wide variety of natural sources, including seeds, plant roots and leaves, fungi, bacteria, body fluids of vertebrates and invertebrates and from mammalian cell membranes.

Due to their ability to recognize definite receptors on the cell surface lectins are an important tool in medicine, microbiology, pharmacology, and histology. The first results of therapeutic success in bone marrow transplantation using soybean lectin /1/ inaugurated a further area in which to use lectins. As far as we know lectins have more than one biological function.

Examples of application in medicine, microbiology, biochemistry, and histology:

- Precipitation of polysaccharides and glycoconjugates
- Agglutination of blood cells
- Agglutination of microorganisms
- Selective agglutination of tumor cells
- Visualization of glycoconjugates in the periphery of cells and organites
- Study of the structures of membranes and cell walls
- Determination of the number of receptor sites on the cell surface and the affinity of lectin binding
- Study of the dynamic of membranes
- Some lectins are very toxic (toxine), they inhibit the protein synthesis
- Blastic transformation of lymphocytes
- Mitosis induction
- Selective enzyme inhibition
- Serological grouping of bacteria
- Group specific agglutination of human erythrocytes.
- Specific fractionation and separation of cells
- Purification of glycoconjugates and polysaccharides by affinity chromatography

1) Institute of Biotechnology GDR-7050 Leipzig, Permoserstraße 15

- Crossed affino-electrophoresis

In this paper an easy to realize method is described which allows to quantify the interactions of lectins with microorganisms and the identification of microorganism strains.

## Results

### Determination of the agglutination rate

The velocity of cell agglutination is determined by measuring the optical density of a cell suspension with the aid of a continuously registrating photometer according to the method described by LINNEMANS et al. /2/ and completed by FLEMMING et al. /3/.
A lectin solution is added to the stirred cell suspension. The microorganism cells start to agglutinate immediately and the optical density of the stirred suspension decreases. The best results are obtained if the optical density on the starting point is E = 0.75 at 578 nm. 5 to 10 minutes are necessary for one agglutination reaction. The velocity of agglutination is expressed as change of optical density per time ($\Delta E/\Delta$ min) (by determining the slope of the tangent in the turning point).
The results are of good reproducibility and, therefore, the method is suitable to describe interactions between cellbound receptors and receptorspecific proteins in a qualitative and quantitative manner.

### Determination of lectin concentrations

As expected the velocity of cell agglutination depends on the concentrations of lectins. Small amounts of a lectin do not induce cell agglutination but at high lectin concentrations the agglutination rate reaches a constant value.
Measuring the velocity of cell agglutination it is possible to calculate unknown lectin concentrations. Using this method we can estimate both the association constants ($K_{ass}$) and the number of lectin molecules (n) bound to the cell surface. The first step is the incubation of the cells (e. g. blood cells) with the lectin and the separation of the lectin loaded cells. In the second step indicator cells (e. g. Saccharomyces cerevisiae cells) with known agglutination properties are added to the supernatant of the first incubation. Now, the amount of unbound lectin is determined from the velocity of the indicator cell agglutination. $K_{ass}$ and n were calculated according to the method of Scatchard or its modification to Steck and Wallach, respectively.
The advantage of this method: no labeling of the lectin is necessary.

Identification of microorganism strains by their agglutination velocity

Methods used in the taxonomy of microorganisms permit a determination of genus and species. But it is difficult to distinguish between different strains of one species. Production strains are characterized by their specific capabilities (for example the generation of products, growth rates). The determination of these properties needs time and it is not perfect.
Microbial strains of one species which can not (or only with difficulties) be distinguished by conventional methods may be differentiated by determining their specific agglutination kinetics. By working under standardized conditions each strain has a specific kinetic of cell agglutination. The method does not need a plenty of time and materials and can be used in routine examinations.
The strains to be tested are cultivated under standardized conditions, washed, and suspended in buffer. The microorganism cells are agglutinated by adding of lectin solution. The velocity of cell agglutination is determined by measuring the optical density as described above. The strains are identified or distinguished by their specific agglutination curves. The method can also be applied for the differentiation of mutants.

Literature

/1/ REISNER, Y. et al. Lancet, 327 (1981)

/2/ LINNEMANS, W. et al. Exp. Cell. Res., 101, 1084 a. 1091 (1976)

/3/ FLEMMING, Ch. et al. J. Basic Microbiol., 25, 493 (1985)

Review articles, Books

SHARON, N. and LIS, H., Science, 177, 949 (1972)

LIS, H. and SHARON, N., Ann. Rev. Biochem. 42, 541 (1973)

HART, D., Ann. J. Clin. Nutr. 33, 2416 (1980)

SHARON, N. "Advances in Immunology" F. DIXON and H. KUNKEL, eds., Academic Press, London and N. Y. p 213 (1983)

LIENER, I. et al., The Lectins, Academic Press, Orlando, Fl. 1986

# MECHANISM OF SEED PROTEINS PROTEOLYSIS; ITS IMPLICATION IN THE MODIFICATION OF THEIR FUNCTIONALITY

A.D. Shutov, J. Pineda, V.I. Senyuk, Do Ngok Lanh, and I.A. Vaintraub[1]

## Abstract

A "zipper" type proteolysis of 11S proteins brings about their consecutive changes: increase of negative charge, lowering of molecular mass, production of non-dissociated fragments of $\alpha$-chains, while the $\beta$-chains remain unaffected. This process is concluded by the formation of a relatively stable high-molecular mass product which is further hydrolyzed only by one-by-one mechanism. The analysis of the kinetic curves shows that the one-by-one hydrolysis proceeds from the beginning of proteolysis in parallel with the "zipper" process. The proteolysis of the 11S protein containing isolates appears to proceed in a way similar to that of the native proteins. A hypothetical scheme describing the formation of the fragments of two types of $\alpha$-chains and their localization in the initial chain is presented. Some conclusions pertinent to the proteolytic modification of the functionality of protein isolates are made. A method of superlimited proteolysis increasing the solubility of sunflower protein isolates is developed on their basis.

## Introduction

Limited proteolysis is one of the most promising methods of modifying the functional properties of protein isolates (5). Most of the investigations in this field, however, are empirical being confined to the study of the changes of the functional properties of isolates during proteolysis. This commmication is intended to provide an outline of the proteolysis mechanism of 11S proteins which are the main components of seed protein isolates. Some conclusions on the possibilities and limitations of the proteolytic modification of protein isolates are drawn thereof.

---

[1] Laboratory of Protein Chemistry, V.I.Lenin State University of Kishinev, Kishinev 277014, U.S.S.R.

General description of the proteolysis course of 11S proteins

Two consecutive stages are observed during the proteolysis of vetch and soybean 11S proteins. At the first stage which is relatively fast the following qualitative changes of the protein take place: increase in their negative charge, molecular mass reduction, formation of non-dissociating fragments of the $\alpha$-chains detected by SDS gel electrophoresis (10). During the second stage the hydrolysis rate is considerably lower and the qualitative composition and the ratio of polypeptides forming the molecule of partially hydrolyzed protein and its molecular mass remain unchanged. The changes of the 11S protein at the first stage are indicative of a "zipper" mechanism of hydrolysis (7). On the contrary, the decrease in the protein concentration without their qualitative changes gives evidence of the one-by-one process occuring during the second stage of hydrolysis.

The proteolysis regularities described are characteristic of seed 11S proteins of other dicotyledons and probably of 7S proteins, too (10). The overall electrophoretic pattern of the fragments formed during the "zipper" proteolysis of $\alpha$-chains being similar, different 11S proteins show some minor variations evidently due to differences in their structure. The proteinase specificity is displayed mainly in further cleavage by some proteinases of fragments being the end products of the "zipper" process when acted upon by some other proteinases. The proteinase specificity also affects the rate ratio of "zipper" and one-by-one processes (10). In all cases no qualitative changes of the basic $\beta$-chains of 11S proteins were detected during proteolysis.

The kinetics of vetch and soybean 11S proteins hydrolysis

The relationship $\ln P = f(t)$, where P denotes the mass concentration of the residual protein and t the proteolysis time, is linear at the second stage of vetch and soybean 11S proteins hydrolysis (Fig. 1). Thus, after the "zipper" process is completed the one-by-one degradation of the resulting modified 11S protein (m11S protein) may be regarded as a first-order reaction. This is consistent with the conception of one-by-one mechanism of proteolysis, which rate is limited by the cleavage of the first peptide bond in each protein molecule (7) and is, therefore, directly proportional to the concentration of the protein substrate if the latter is sufficiently low. The relationship $\ln P = f(t)$ is non-linear at the first stage of proteolysis since the "zipper" process is determined by a sequence of succesive reactions with rapidly decreasing rate constants (7).

The degradation of $\beta$-chains obeys the first-order kinetics during the whole course of proteolysis studied including the first stage (Fig. 1). Thus, the $\beta$-chains are hydrolyzed only by one-by-one mechanism. Evidently, the one-by-one breakdown of $\beta$-chains and consequently of the whole 11S protein proceeds from the very beginning of the proteolysis and the rate of this process is unaffected by the changes of the 11S protein conformation, which may be caused by the paralleling "zipper" proteolysis.

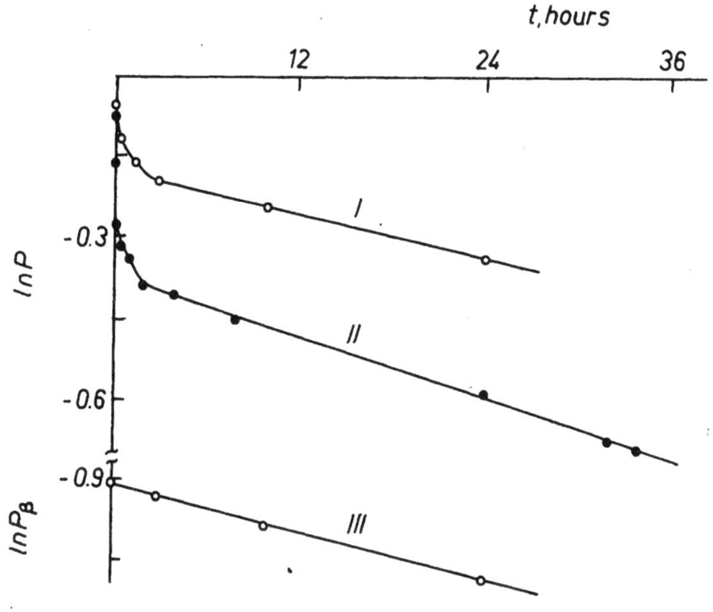


Fig. 1. The kinetics of 11S protein hydrolysis. I - pepsin hydrolysis of vetch 11S protein (1.5% suspension of protein in phosphate-citrate buffer pH 4.5 adjusted to the ionic strength 0.5 by adding NaCl, enzyme-substrate ratio 1:50, 30°). II - trypsin hydrolysis of soybean 11S protein (1% protein solution in tris-buffer pH 8.) adjusted to ionic strength 0.5 by adding NaCl, enzyme-substrate ratio 1:250, 30°). III - pepsin hydrolysis of $\beta$-chains. The same experiment as I; the $\beta$-chain mass concentration $P_\beta$ is calculated from the mass concentration of the residual protein and the relative content of $\beta$-chains determined by the densitomrtric evaluation of SDS-electrophoregrams. Only $P_\beta$ values at time zero and at the second stage of hydrolysis are given. At the first stage during the "zipper" process an intermediate $\alpha$-chain fragment having the electrophoretic mobility close to that of $\beta$-chains impairs the determination of $\beta$-chain concentration.

### The changes of the molecular mass of the vetch and soybean proteins

The molecular mass M(t) of vetch and soybean 11S proteins in the course of their proteolysis may be calculated from kinetical data (9). The relationship ln P = f(t) is expressed by the equation

$$\ln P(t) = \frac{P_o}{M_o} M(t) - kt,$$

where $M_o$ and $P_o$ denote the initial molecular mass and mass concentration of the protein, respectively, and k is the rate constant of the one-by-one hydrolysis. Hence

$$M(t) = \frac{P_o}{P(t)} M_o e^{kt} \qquad (1)$$

Another method of M(t) determination is based on the resistance of the $\beta$-chains of 11S proteins to the "zipper" proteolysis (11). Accordingly the molecular mass of the protein during hydrolysis is inversely proportional to the relative content of $\beta$-chains

$$M(t) = \frac{\beta_o}{\beta(t)} M_o \qquad (2)$$

In this equation $\beta_o$ and $\beta(t)$ denote the relative content of $\beta$-chains in the initial and partially hydrolyzed proteins determined by densitometric evaluation of SDS-electrophoregrams.

The value of M(t) calculated using the equation (1) during the first stage of pepsin hydrolysis of vetch 11S protein decreases from $M_o$ = 360 kD and reaches a constant value $M_m$ = 302 kD characteristic of the end product of "zipper" proteolysis (Fig. 2). The value $M_m$ = 305 kD obtained from the equation (2) is in good agreement with the former result. According to gel filtration on Sepharose CL-6B during the trypsin hydrolysis the molecular mass of vetch 11S protein also decreases to $M_m$ = 304 kD (4). A greater decrease of the molecular mass (from $M_o$ = 330 kD to $M_m$ = 227 kD) is observed during the trypsin hydrolysis of soybean 11S protein (Fig. 2).

### The scheme of the "zipper" type breakdown of vetch 11S protein

The course of the transformation of $\alpha$-chains was studied in detail in the case of pepsin hydrolysis of vetch 11S protein (9). The homology of seed 11S proteins (3) permits to compare these results with the structural data reported for other 11S proteins. According to the

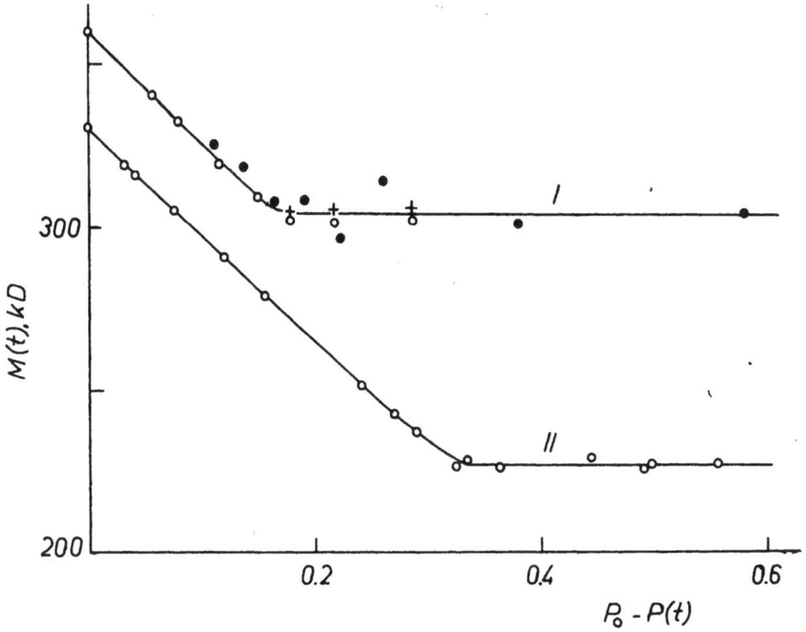


Fig. 2. The change of the molecular mass of 11S protein during proteolysis. The decrease of protein concentration is plotted on the abscissa. I - vetch 11S protein; o pepsin hydrolysis, M calculated by equation (1), + the same, M calculated by the equation (2), • trypsin hydrolysis, M evaluated by gel filtration on Sepharose CL-6B (4). II - soybean 11S protein; M calculated by the equation (1).

structural model of 11S proteins developed by Plietz et al. (6) the N-terminal regions of each pair of $\alpha$- and $\beta$-chains forms two domains linked by disulfide bridges which are radial-symmetrically arranged within the molecule. The strongly hydrophylic C-terminal $\alpha$-chain region is situated at the surface while the more hydrophobic $\beta$-chain C-terminal region is burried in the central part of the hexameric molecule.

It is quite possible that the $\beta$-chains are resistant to the "zipper" proteolysis because they are protected by the C-terminal region of $\alpha$-chains. The latter must evidently be attacked by proteinases in the first place.

As shown earlier (9) the increase in the negative charge of partially hydrolyzed vetch 11S protein at pH higher than their iso-electric point is due to the splitting-off of short terminal peptides with a high content of basic amino acids. The primary structure data (see (1) for references) show that such peptides may be split off only from the C-terminus of the $\alpha$-chain. The C-terminal region of $\alpha$-chains is highly variable (6). Nevertheless, in all dicots 11S proteins of a known primary structure the split-off of a limited number of peptides from the C-terminus of $\alpha$-chains will increase the negative charge of the protein. The fast raise of the negative charge at the very beginning of proteolysis (4,8) is a supporting evidence of the location of the C-terminal region at the surface of the 11S protein molecule.

It may be deduced from the results of quantitative analysis of the fragments formed during the "zipper" degradation (9) that the two types of $\alpha$-chains (methionine-rich type I or A and methionine-poor type II or B (3) are hydrolyzed in a different way (Fig.3). A longer sequence is split off from the C-terminus of type II $\alpha$-chain as short peptides. It includes not only the positive charged peptides, but also peptides from the adjacent region. The latter is characterized by a high content of acid amino acids so that as a whole the split-off sequence is acid or neutral. Thus, the increase in the 11S protein negative charge is probably due only to the splitting-off of C-terminal peptides from the type I $\alpha$-chains.

Further proteolysis brings about the cleavage of the type I $\alpha$-chain into two fragments (Fig. 3) which are retained within the molecule by non-covalent interactions and by a disulfide link (N-terminal fragment). The latter is an intermediate. By the hydrolysis of the C-terminal sequence it is transformed into the end product that probably corresponds to the $\alpha$-chain domain.

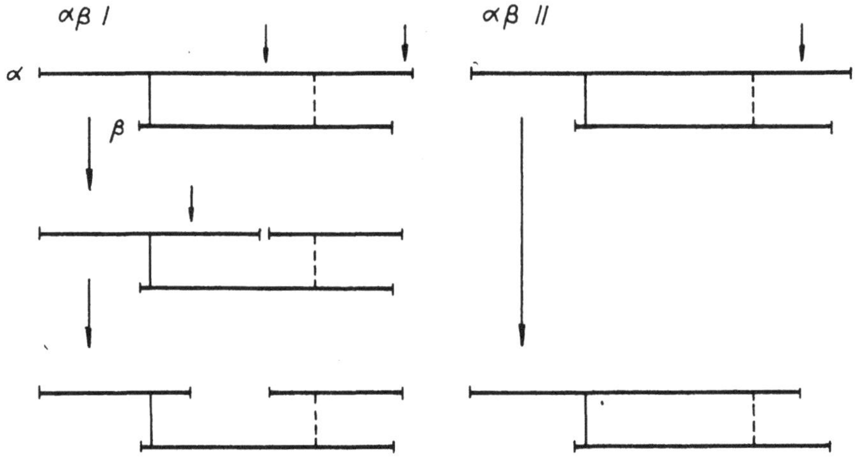


Fig. 3. Hypothetical scheme of transformations of $\alpha\beta$-subunits of vetch 11S protein during the "zipper" stage of pepsin hydrolysis. The continuous line - the disulfide bridge linking the $\alpha$- and $\beta$-chains, the dotted line - non-covalent linkages.

## Proteolysis of protein isolates

In protein isolates marked structural changes of proteins are expected, which may affect the course of their proteolysis. A preliminary study of the proteolysis course of sunflower isolates consisting almost entirely of 11S protein also shows the occurence of a mixed-type process. High-molecular intermediate fragments formed differ, however, from those formed during the proteolysis of native 11S protein. An increase in the negative charge of the protein was also observed at the beginning of the proteolysis. Thus, the proteolysis of isolates seems to proceed in a similar general way as that of the native protein.

## Conclusions pertinent to the proteolytic modification of protein functionality

The data stated above permit to draw the following conclusions concerning the possibilities and limitations of the proteolytic modification of the functionality of 11S protein containing isolates:

1. The changes of the functional properties of a protein may be reached only as a result of a "zipper"-type proteolysis. The one-by-one process brings about a complete degradation of protein molecules to peptides, i.e. to losses of protein. Thus, the proteolytical modification of functional properties is possible only for the proteins capable of "zipper"-type proteolysis.

2. The one-by-one mechanism is a widespread way of the proteolysis. Many proteins hydrolyzed by "zipper" process are likely to undergo a one-by-one degradation in parallel. This is true for 11S proteins.

3. The solubilization of 11S proteins is due in all probability to an increase in their negative charge. A sharp increase of the latter occurs at the very beginning of the 11S proteins proteolysis.

4. The course of the "zipper" proteolysis and the composition of the fragments formed is determined mainly by the structure of 11S proteins. The proteinase specificity may affect the ratio of "zipper" and one-by-one processes.

5. The general regularities of the proteolysis of native 11S proteins are retained by protein isolates consisting of 11S proteins.

6. To optimize the proteolytical modification of 11S protein such a level of hydrolysis must be found where the degree of the "zipper" process is sufficient for attaining the desired modification, while the protein losses brought about by the one-by-one proteolysis are minimum. The rate of the latter may be lowered by the selection of an appropriate enzyme.

Proteolytic modification of the functional properties of sunflower protein isolates

The use of the above-stated conclusions is illustrated by the study of the effect of the hydrolysis degree on the solubility and on the recovery of sunflower protein isolates (2). It was shown that a superlimited proteolysis (~0.1% splitting of peptide bonds) produces a 1.5-2-fold increase in the solubility, the losses of isoelectrically precipitable protein are unsignificant (2-5%). The enzyme treatment is of short-duration (15-30 minutes) and the enzyme-protein ratio is one order lower than that in the methods commonly used (5). Due to the solubility increase the modified isolates form thermotropic gels, while the unmodified ones are uncapable of gelation.

References


1. Borroto, K. and L. Dure III: The globulin storage proteins of flowering plants are derived from two ancestral genes. Plant Mol. Biol. 8 (1987) 2, 113-131.
2. Bulmaga, V.P., A.D. Shutov and I.A. Vaintraub: Modification of the functional properties of sunflower protein isolates by superlimited proteolysis. Nahrung 32 (1988) in press.
3. Casey, R., C. Domoney and N. Ellis: Legume storage proteins and their genes. Oxford Surveys Plant Mol. Cell Biol. 3 (1986) 1-95.
4. Do Ngok Lanh, A.D. Shutov and I.A. Vaintraub: The action of trypsin on vetch legumin: the changes of hydrolysis types. Biokhimiya 50 (1985) 4, 627-633.
5. Modification of proteins. Food, nutritional and pharmacological aspects: ACS Symp., Series No 198 (1982). R.E. Feeney, J.R. Whitaker (eds.).
6. Plietz, P., B. Drescher and G. Damaschun: Relationship between the amino acid sequence and the domain structure of the subunits of the 11S seed globulins. Int. J. Biol. Macromol. 9 (1987) 6, 161-165.
7. Rupley, J.A.: Susceptibility to attack by proteolytic enzymes. Methods in Enzymology 11 (1967) 905-917.
8. Shutov, A.D., V.P. Bulmaga, E.K. Boldt and I.A. Vaintraub: Study of modification of vetch seed reserve proteins during germination and limited proteolysis. Biokhimiya 46 (1981) 5, 841-850.
9. Shutov, A.D., J. Pineda, Le Tkhi Fu and Do Ngok Lanh: The action of pepsin on vetch legumin. The regularities of the proteolysis of 11S seed proteins related to their structure. Biokhimiya 54 (1989) in press.
10. Shutov, A.D. and I.A. Vaintraub: Degradation of storage proteins in germinating seeds. Phytochemistry 26 (1987) 6, 1557-1566.

# THE LEGUMIN-LIKE STORAGE PROTEIN SYSTEM IN LUPIN SEED AND ITS REGULATION BY PROTEOLYTIC ENZYMES

**Paolo Cerletti, Marcello Duranti, Daniela Giani, Nicoletta Guerrieri**

Department of Agrifood Molecular Sciences, University of Milan
via Celoria 2 - 20133 Milano, Italy

Legumins, the second largest storage protein of legume seeds, exist as oligomers of 15S, 12S, 7S while the subunits are 2S molecules. Little is known about the interrelations and possible interconversions between these molecules on a structural and physico-chemical basis, nor on their physiological significance and on the mechanisms that regulate their presence in seeds.

We studied the problem in Lupinus albus: here oligomers of 12S and 7S predominate and we found that they are in part interconvertible in an association-dissociation equilibrium displaced toward the 12S form by increasing ionic strength, but part of the 7S species does not associate (1). We shall indicate the interconvertible molecules as the 12 $\rightleftharpoons$ 7S component while molecules that do not associate are indicated as non associating or modified 7S component.

## Conformation, protomers and oligomeric transitions

Studies with circular dichroism (C.D.) and intrinsic fluorescence showed that transitions between oligomeric forms are related with changes in conformation. The native 12S $\rightleftharpoons$ 7S component has a lower alpha helix content than the non associating 7S oligomer. When titrated with urea its ellipticity increases. Also the intrinsic fluorescence of the 12S $\rightleftharpoons$ 7S component increase in 1 M urea, while modified 7S molecules are unaffected (FIG. 1). A significant decrease at 3-5 M urea is observed with both oligomers. Above 3 M urea also the wavelenght of tryptophan emission increases identically in both oligomers (FIG. 2). PAGE, C.D. and intrinsic fluorescence indicate that association to 12S molecules does not take place above 3M urea. At 6 M urea also 7S oligomers have disappeared (2).

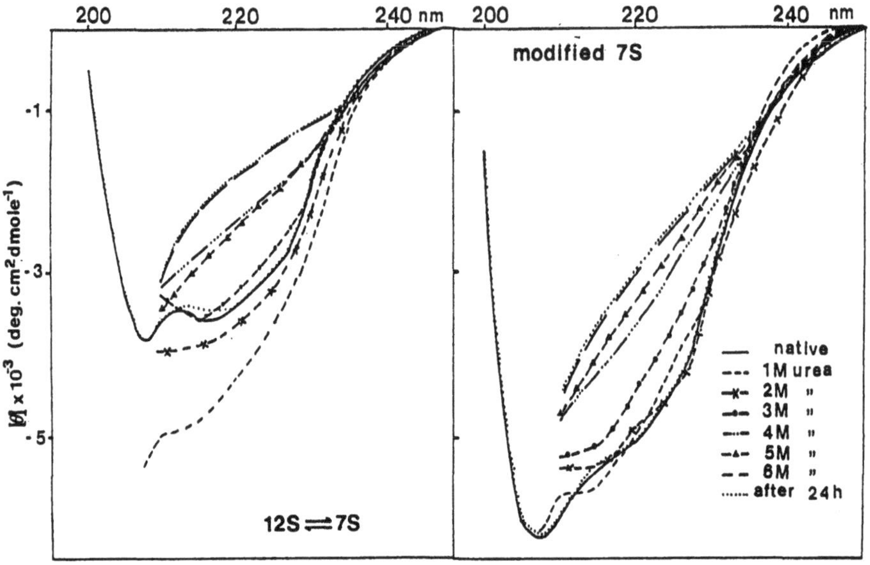


FIG. 1. C.D. **spectra** of the 12S⇌7S component and the modified 7S oligomer in 50 mM Pi, pH 7.5, 0.1 M NaCl and 1.3 mM EDTA. Protein 0.12 mg/ml. Spectra of the native and the 6 M urea treated proteins were measured also after 24 hours at 20°C (.....).

The stability and the modifications of the molecule in association processes were also studied by examining surface properties.

Presence of tryptophan and tyrosine residues on the surface of the molecule was detected by C.D. in the near ultraviolet, a situation similar to helianthinin, a legumin-like globulin of sunflower seeds (4).

Surface hydrophobicity of the oligomer, measured by titration with anilin naphtalene sulfonic acid (ANS), decreased on increasing the temperature (from 20 to 90°C) (5) or protein concentration, (from 0.8 to 3.4 mg $ml^{-1}$) while the affinity of the protein for the dye at first increased and then remained constant (2). This indicates that surface areas of moderate hydrophobicity are in regions of the protein that upon raising the temperature undergo conformational changes and that in associated molecules they belong to interacting domains: both these conditions make them unavailable to the dye in the course of the experiment. More hydrophobic areas are in more rigid regions that remain unmodified on heating and are not involved in the interactions occuring at association: structural adaptation is required in interacting domains, therefore rigid regions likely do not belong to them. Energetically association is driven also by removal of solvation water, which may be present in moderately hydrophobic regions but lacks in those of high hydrophobicity.

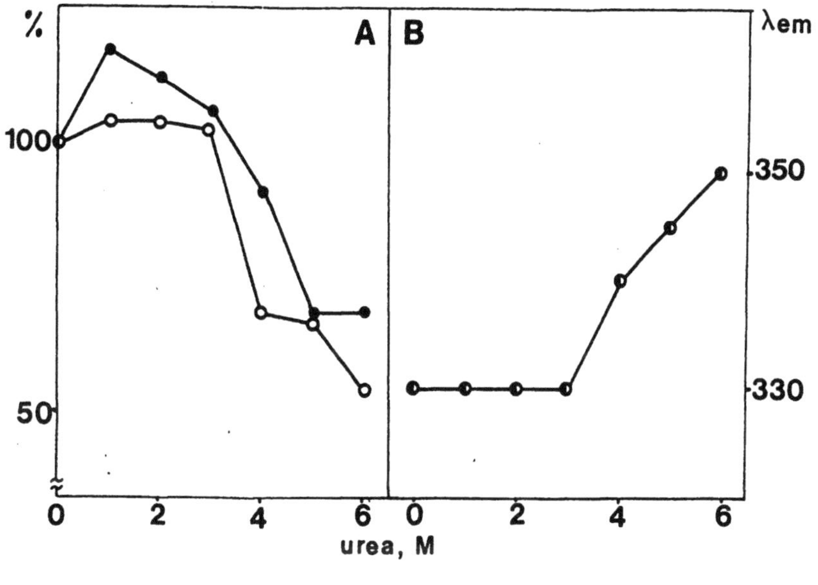


**FIG. 2.** A- **Intrinsic fluorescence** at increasing urea of the 12S⇌7S ( ● ), and the modified 7S ( O ) components in 50 mM Pi, pH 7.5, 0.1 M NaCl. Protein: 0.12 mg/ml. λex 290 nm, λem 330 nm. Slit: 5 nm. Results are given as % of intrinsic fluorescence of the native protein. **B-** Changes of the **emission wavelenght** upon increasing urea.

The non associating 7S oligomer lacks the protomers of 81-72 kD that are one major component of the 12S⇌7S species: this corresponds to absence of the acidic polypeptides of 52-50 kD and of 47 kD, the basic one being unchanged (2). A component at 63 kD (unreduced) or at

38 kD (reduced) becomes relevant. Size polymorphism of oligomers therefore relates also with the type of protomers, and not only to the environmental situation, e.g. ionic strenght. Likely assemblage of subunits in the oligomer is dictated by the distribution of polarity in the polypeptides and modification in the polypeptides as well as in the medium may act on conformation and/or association. Acidic chains have significantly lower average hydrophobicity, calculated according to Bigelow (6), than the basic chain (Table 1) and the covalently linked carbohydrate is bound to them (1): they are likely positioned to the exterior of the molecule, what makes them more susceptible to the action of proteinases.

**TABLE 1**

AMINOACID COMPOSITION AND AVERAGE HYDROPHOBICITY PER RESIDUE IN GLOBULIN 8 PROTOMERS

| | MOLES,% | | AVERAGE HYDROPHOBICITY,[+] (KCAL/RESIDUE) | |
|---|---|---|---|---|
| | Protomers | | | |
| | acidic | basic | | |
| ASX | 9.4 | 12.3 | globulin 8 | 0.95 (0.92)[*] |
| THR | 4.2 | 4.6 | acidic protomer | 0.87 |
| SER | 5.1 | 6.0 | basic protomer | 1.05 |
| GLX | 28.8 | 14.7 | | |
| PRO | 6.2 | 5.4 | | |
| GLY | 7.3 | 8.4 | glycinin | |
| ALA | 3.8 | 7.5 | (Glycine max) | 0.94 |
| VAL | 3.7 | 7.1 | legumin | |
| ILE | 4.6 | 5.2 | (Vicia faba) | 0.96 |
| LEU | 8.5 | 9.4 | legumin | |
| TYR | 3.7 | 4.4 | (Pisum sativum) | 0.93 |
| PHE | 2.6 | 4.5 | ribonuclease | 0.87 |
| HIS | 1.4 | 1.2 | catalase | 1.20 |
| LYS | 2.8 | 3.4 | | |
| ARG | 7.8 | 5.8 | | |

[+] calculated according to Bigelow (6)

[*] calculated from the separated contributions of the acidic and the basic polypeptide

Autolysis of legumin

Quite often in extensively purified preparations of globulin 8, that appear homogeneous on PAGE and SDS-PAGE, after a 36 hour or longer period at 37°C heavy protomers begin to slowly disappear: the one of 81 kDa is involved first and new ones of 63 and 50 kD are formed, the one of 75 kD being degraded later. The one of 69 kD at first increases and later disappears. The total area of stained protomers in a laser-scanned gel decreases in parallel with degradation; this indicates that small fragments not detected by SDS-PAGE are formed. The ratio of 12S⇌7S component to not associating 7S molecules changes in parallel with the mentioned modifications in protomeric pattern. Nonetheless in other preparations such self-degradation does not occur also upon prolonged incubation (90 hours) (7).

At least in early stages the time course of autolysis and the type of products speak for a stepwise endopeptidase cleavage of the acidic polypeptide while the basic one remains unmodified. This shows that protease(s) act preferentially on polar regions of the molecule.

De novo synthesis of proteinase e.g. during the initial incubation period is not in question. The proteolysis is likely due to proteases tightly associated with the protein that are not removed during purification of the legumin.

The 12S⇌7S component is less susceptible than the modified 7S oligomer to self degradation and, as will be described later, to proteolysis by added endopeptidases. One possible cause is that the 7S oligomer is a more relaxed and possibly more solvated molecule than the 12S form. Assembly of subunits into large oligomers and tight folding limit the sites available to the enzyme: dissociation and (local) changes in conformation allow a better access to proteases.

Because of its compactness and resistance to proteolysis the 12S oligomer appears the form of choice for deposition and storage under the conditions of water deficiency that exist in protein bodies of the resting seed; this view receives support by the equilibrium shift toward formation of 12S molecules at high ionic strenght (1). Water is by far too scarce in protein bodies (7-9%) to provide adequate solvation to proteins: direct interactions with other molecules become predominant and conformation as well as other properties of the protein may differ from those existing in a water rich medium.

Water acts seemingly as a mediator between the physiology of the seed and the molecular changes under discussion: indeed protein deposition terminates with seed dehydration while imbibition, that starts embryogenesis, makes the conversion of the 12S oligomer to a more relaxed molecule easier: this change becomes irreversible after limited proteolysis. In particular this prepares the protein to the action of proteolytic enzymes appearing at germination. Also activation of proteases is possibly related to changes in water content (see later).

<u>The agents of proteolysis</u>

In an attempt to identify the agents of the proteolysis, we have isolated from the albumin fraction of mature lupin seed two different endopeptidases which hydrolyze the acidic polypeptides of legumin and have no effect on the basic one. They are proteinase **1**, a cysteine-proteinase formed by a single polypeptide of $M_r$ 70,000 and proteinase **2**, a metalloendopeptidase formed by a polypeptide of 14-15 kD (7).

The two proteases share some of their properties. Several aspects of their behaviour are in common with autolysis of globulin 8 but this does not necessarily involve both enzymes. We shall consider each property in the various systems so as to allow an easier comparison.

**Substrate specificity**

Proteinase **1** acts on the synthetic substrate BAPA (benzoyl-D,L-arginine-p-nitroanilide) with an optimum at pH=8.0, and on lupin legumin with optimum at pH=7.4: here it splits preferentially the 81 kD protomer and the resulting protein has a protomer pattern similar to the modified 7S oligomer (FIG. 3) (8). Proteinase **1** also acts on jack bean vicilin and on the mature legumin and the 50,000 $M_r$ vicilin precursor of pea; partial aminoacid sequencing of fragments produced from the precursor indicated that cleavage occurs in a highly hydrophylic domain of the molecule in proximity of paired arginine residues (9): this is in agreement with inhibition by salmin, a protein that contains more than 70% arginine residues.

Proteinase **2** does not act on BAPA nor on globulin 4, a vicilin like protein of the lupin seed. Cleavage of globulin 8 is more extensive than by proteinase **1** (FIG. 3): all major polypeptides of the native protein disappear beginning with those of 81 and 75 kD. The major product is of 52 kD but polypeptides of 45 and 37 kD are also formed. They all contain the basic chain unmodified. A transient species of 12 kD, and at long incubations one of 9 kD appear that lack the basic chain: they are likely fragments of acidic polypeptides (7).

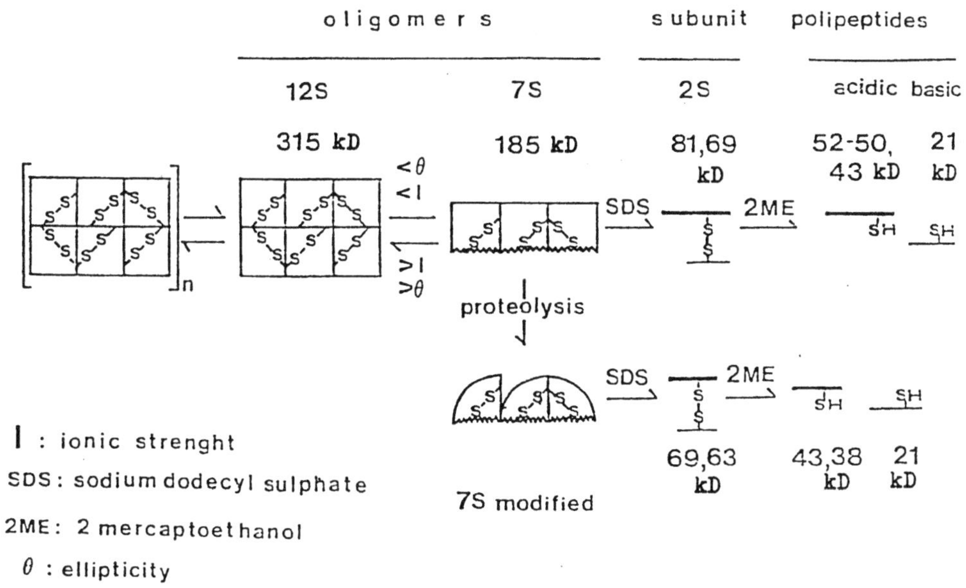


FIG. 4. Molecular Interactions and assembly of the legumin molecule.

**Activation**

As already stated autolysis of globulin 8 becomes apparent after 36 hours or more at 37°C. Also both proteinases require preincubation before their activity on the native globulin is evident.

For proteinase **1** the preincubation period is 30-40 hours at 37°C. On the other hand when the substrate is the isolated carboxymethylated $\alpha$-III subunit of pea legumin (9) or BAPA (8) activity is apparent at once: very likely the small molecule and the unfolded polypeptide have easy access to the active site, what does not happen with the native protein.

With proteinase **2** activity on globulin 8 becomes manifest after at least 24 hours incubation at 4°C in the presence of $Ca^{2+}$, also omitting the substrate: this suggests that the native enzyme is inactive on structural grounds that disappear in the presence of water due to conformational changes and/or autolysis. Interestingly $Ca^{2+}$ ions activate the proteolytic action of the enzyme.

**Effectors**

Autolysis is inhibited by 1.3 mM EDTA, 7.6 mM $NaN_3$ (1) and 3.0 mM $Zn^{++}$. EDTA (1.3 mM), sodium azide (7.6 mM) and $Zn^{++}$ (0.3 mM) (9) inhibit also proteinase **2**. Inhibition of proteinase **1** has been studied using BAPA as substrate: 2.5 mM EDTA does not inhibit (8).

Other inhibitors tested only on one proteolytic system are listed in Table 2 and serve to qualify proteinases **1** and **2** as a cysteine-protease and a metallo-protease, respectively.

**TABLE 2**

INHIBITORS OF PROTEASE ACTIVITY

| PROTEINASE **1** | | | PROTEINASE **2** | | |
|---|---|---|---|---|---|
| Inhibitor | mM | BAPAse act. Inhibition % | Inhibitor | mM | Proteolytic act. Inhibition % |
| EDTA | 2.5 | 3 | EDTA | 1.3 | +++ |
| NEM | 0.1 | 74 | $NaN_3$ | 7.6 | ++ |
| 2-mercapto--ethanol | 5.0 | 0 | dithio-threitol**(DTT)** | 2.0 | ++ |
| TLCK | 0.05 | 87 | $Zn^{++}$ | 0.3 | +++ |
| $HgCl_2$ | 0.26 | 100 | $Mn^{++}$ | 3.0 | + |
| Leupeptin | 0.002-0.25 | 46-100 | $Co^{++}$ | 3.0 | +++ |
| Salmin | 0.005 | 90 | $Mg^{++}$ | 3.0 | 0 |
| GLOBULIN 8 (Self-digestion) | | | | | |
| EDTA | 1.3 | +++ | | | |
| $NaN_3$ | 1.0,3.0,7.6 | +,++,+++ | | | |
| DTT | 2.0 | 0 | | | |
| $Zn^{++}$ | 3.0 | +++ | | | |

BAPAse activity was followed at 405 nm and 37°C in 50 mM Pi pH 8.0, 0.22 M NaCl on 0.33 mM BAPA. Proteinase **1** was 5 µg/ml.
Proteolytic activities were assayed in 50 mM Pi, 0.15 M NaCl. Globulin 8 was 0.5 mg/ml, proteinase **2**, where present, was 35 µg/mg globulin 8; divalent cations were assayed in 50 mM Tris-HCL, pH 8.0 containing 0.22 M NaCl.
The inhibitor was present from the beginning of incubation with the exception of DTT: this was incubated with the enzyme for 1 hour at 4°C in the conditions mentioned and, before adding substrate, it was removed by gel filtration on Sephadex G25 Fine.

If proteinase **2** is incubated with dithiothreitol (DTT) which is then removed, the protease activity decreases: this finding qualifies further the enzyme as a metalloendopeptidase (7). On the other hand DTT protects the BAPAse activity of proteinase **1**. Self-degradation of globulin 8 is enhanced in the presence of DTT. This however can be related with loss of structure due to reduction of the disulfide bridge that joins acidic and basic chains in the subunits.

<u>Endopeptidases and proteolysis in the dormant seed</u>

Proteinase **1** candidates as the agent of the limited proteolysis that brings the 12S oligomer to a 7S molecule. Proteinase **2** may act on both these oligomers and cleaves them somewhat more extensively. The action of both proteinases seems to be regulated by activation of the enzyme and, at least for what proteinase **2** is concerned, by the structural integrity, including conformation, of the substrate molecule. The specificity of both proteinases for acidic polypeptides may depend on lack of a proper sequence for cleavage in the basic polypeptide: however, at last for what concerns proteinase **1** which requires arginine residues close to the bond split, this aminoacid is present in both polypeptides (Table 1). An additional cause of specificity may be affinity for hydrophylic domains, as is the case for proteinase **1** (9): the basic polypeptide has namely highest average hydrophobicity.

We suggest that: a) both protease have a limited access or none at all to the sites of cleavage in the native 12S oligomer. Some sites become available after the transconformation associated with dissociation of the 12S oligomer to 7S; b) the two proteases are present in the quiescent seed and act sequentially: proteinase **1** acts on the 12S$\rightleftharpoons$7S form of the legumin and transforms it irreversibly into the modified 7S oligomer. The 12S oligomer and the 7S forms are cleaved by proteinase **2** and this opens the way to complete breakdown by proteases at germination.

The sequency of events, with conditions that affect the equilibria, are summarized in FIG. 4.

In germinating vetch seeds protease **1**, an acid thiol endopeptidase, acts on legumin and vicilin and on the modified proteins whereas protease **2**, a neutral thiol endopeptidase, only degrades globulins that have already been modified during the initial days of germination (10). Final breakdown to aminoacids is carried out by carboxypeptidases (11) and possibly arylamidases (12). Proteases **1** and **2** act on the acidic polypeptides of the legumin while basic chains are more resistant (10). A similar mode of action has been described in germinating pumpkin seeds (13) and for glycinin, the soybean legumin, (14) and seems quite general for legumes. The sequential action of proteases **1** and **2** is analogous to what we found for lupin: however protease **1** and **2** of vetch can only be detected some days after onset of germination (14) similarly to other enzymes active at germination in most legumes. In lupin, a plant that grows on dry soils, our endopeptidases are already present in the dry seed though their action is kept at a standstill on conformational grounds.

**Acknowledgements.** The research work was supported by CNR, Italy, Special Grant I.P.R.A. Sub-project 3.

## REFERENCES

[1] Duranti, M., Guerrieri, N., Takahashi, T. and Cerletti, P.: Phytochemistry, 27, 15-23, (1988)
[2] Guerrieri, N., Duranti, M., Giani, D. and Cerletti, P.: in Proteine 88, Società Italiana di Biochimica, p. 158-159 (1988)
[3] Plietz, P. and Damaschun, G.: Studia Biophysica, 116, 153-173 (1986)
[4] Sripad, G. and Narasinga Rao, M.S.: J. Agric. Food Chem., 35, 668-672 (1987)
[5] Cerletti, P., Duranti, M. and Bonomi, F.: in R.I. Zalewski, J.J. Skolik (eds.) Natural Product Chemistry 1984, Elsevier Sci. Publ. B.V. Amsterdam, p. 613-628 (1985)
[6] Bigelow, C.C.: J. Theoret. Biol., 116, 187-221 (1987)
[7] Giani, D., Duranti, M., Guerrieri, N. and Cerletti, P.: in Proteine 88, Società Italiana di Biochimica, p. 156-157 (1988)
[8] Duranti, M. and Cerletti, P.: in preparation
[9] Duranti, M., Gatehouse, J.A., Boulter, D. and Cerletti, P.: Phytochemistry 26, 627-631 (1987)
[10] Shutov, A.D., Bulmaja, V.P., Boldt, E.K. and Vaintraub, I.A.: Biokhimiya 46, 841-848 (1981)
[11] Shutov, A.D., Koroleva, T.N. and Vaintraub, I.A.: Fisiol. Rast. 25, 735-742 (1978)
[12] Zemchik, E.I., Fan Min Than, Shutov, T.N. and Vaintraub, I.A.: Biokhimiya, 40, 746-751 (1975)
[13] Hara, I. and Masubara, H.: Plant Physiol., 65, 103S (1980)
[14] Tan-Wilson, A.L. and Wilson, K.A. unpublished data, (1983)

**VARIATION OF SURFACE HYDROPHOBICITY OF WHEAT CLIADINS AND PEA GLOBULINS RELATED TO THEIR CONFORMATIONAL CHANGES**

Gueguen, J and Y. Popineau[1]

Surface hdrophobicity has to be considered as an important physicochemical characteristic of proteins as related to their functional properties [1, 2, 3]. It has been evaluated by many methods such as hydrophobic interaction chromatography, reversed phase high performance liquid chromatography [4, 5, 6], phase partition [7, 8, 9] and hydrophobic probe binding [10, 11].

The chromatography conditions are not sufficiently flexible to allow the study of the proteins in various conformation states depending on the solvent. On the other hand the ligand binding method could be used in various experimental conditions and permit moreover the determination of the number of sites and of the binding constants. In the present study, such a method was applied to the investigation of the hydrophobicity of wheat gliadins (γ, ω) and pea globulins (legumin, vicilin) in function of conformation changes induced by modifications of pH and salt concentration in the solvent. A special interest was devoted to the influence of dissociation and/or unfolding on the accessibility of the hydrophobic areas of these proteins.

## Materials and methods

### Materials

Pea (Variety AMINO) globulins were purified by ion exchange chromatography on DEAE Sepharose (Pharmacia) and purified by gel filtration on ACA34 ultragel (IBF Pharmindustrie) as described elsewhere [12, 13].

Purification procedure of gliadins was reported previously [14, 15]. It combined ion-exchange chromatography on SP-Trisacryl M, gel permeation chromatography on Sephadex G100 and hydrophobic interaction chromatography on Phenyl-Sepharose CL-4B.

[1]Ministère de la Recherche et de l'Enseignement Supérieur, I.N.R.A., Laboratoire de Biochimie et technologie des Protéines, Centre de Recherches Agroalimentaires, Rue de la Géraudière, 44072 Nantes, Cedex 03, France

## Methods

### Characterisation of the conformations

The conformational modifications depending on pH and ionic strengths were obtained for the pea globulins by solubilizing these proteins in the following 0.1M buffer systems: citrate-NaOH buffers pH $\leq$ 3 - 4; phosphate-NaOH buffers pH 7; glycine-NaOH buffers pH $\geq$ 9. They were investigated by ultracentrifugatin using a Beckman L565B centrifuge with a SW 40 Ti rotor [16].

Gliadin conformation changes were characterised by gel permeation chromatography on Sephacryl S-300, according to COLE et al [17]. Three solvents were used : $5 \cdot 10^{-2}$ M $CH_3$ COOH pH 3.0; $5 \cdot 10^{-2}$ M $CH_3$ COOH $10^{-2}$ M NaCL pH 3.0 and $10^{-3}$ M $CH_3$ COOH $10^{-2}$ M NaCL pH 5.0. Previous work showed that they promoted large conformation changes of a gliadin [17, 18]. 6M GuCL was also used to estimate the Stoke's radii of gliadins under unfolded conformation.

### Apolar ligand binding

Hydrophobicity was evaluated by the binding capacity of the protein for an apolar ligand 2 p-Toluidinylnaphtalene sulfonate (TNS) from Sigma Chemical Co [10]. Ultrafiltration was used for measuring the rate of TNS binding to the protein as suggested by SOPHIANOPOULOS et al. [19]. The complete experimental procedure were described recently [5, 20]. Binding isotherms and Scatchard plots were drawn to calculate the number of binding sites and binding constants. The experiments of binding were carried out in the various solvents used for inducing conformational changes except GuCl medium.

## Results and Discussion

### Conformational changes

The sedimentation coefficients of legumin were much more affected by pH variations than in the case of vicilin (Fig. 1, 2). Legumin sedimented only around 12.3S in the range pH 7 - 9, whereas vicilin adopted a native form (8S) between pH 6 and 10. Both proteins dissociated mainly into 3 - 4 S sedimenting components in extreme pH conditions. At pH 11.5, 45 % of legumin and 20 to 25 % of vicilin were still in their associated (12S and 8S) state considering the areas under the various sedimentation peaks. At pH 2.4 legumin is completely dissociated into subunits sedimenting around 3.5S. The native form has completely disappeared and it was previously shown [16] that the low sedimenting polypeptides corresponded to the AB subunits, assuming an hexameric structure 6(AB) for the native legumin. On the other hand, the 8S conformation of vicilin was still present at pH 2.4 whereas 2.7S sedimenting components were the major ones.

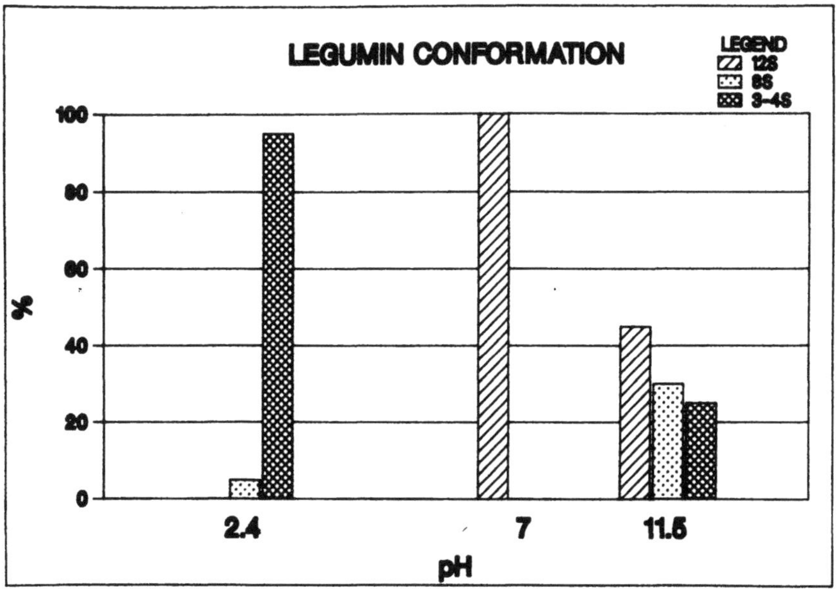


Figure 1: Influence of pH on legumin sedimentation coefficients

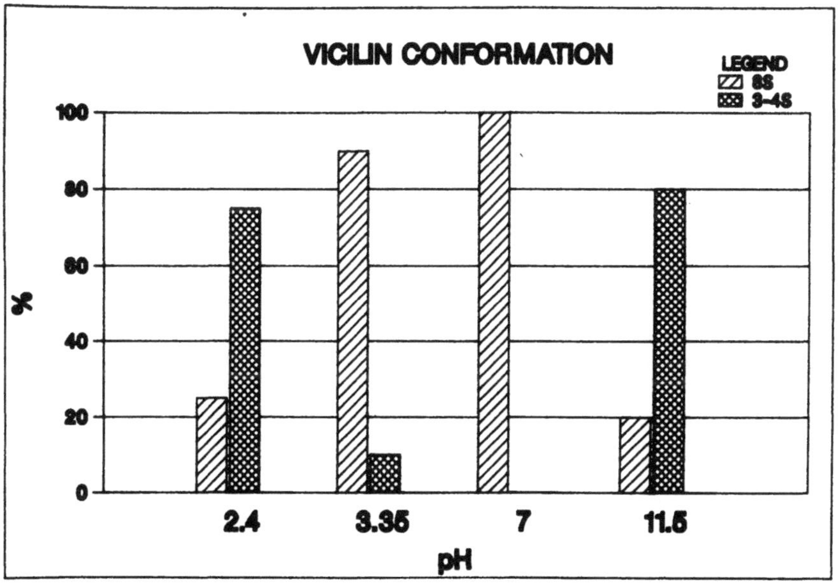


Figure 2: Influence of pH on vicilin sedimentation coefficients

Table 1: Influence of solvent conditions on the Stoke's radii of gliadins

| GLIADINS | | | LEGUMIN | | |
|---|---|---|---|---|---|
| | GAMMA 44 Re (nm) | OMEGA 17 Re (nm) | pH | $S_{20,w}$ | Re (nm) |
| $CH_3COOH$ 0.05M | 7.9 | 7.9 | 10.5 | 12.5 | 6.9 |
| pH3 | | | | 3.7 | n.d |
| $CH_3COOH$ 0.05M | 3.3 | 4.2 | 8.0 | 12.7 | 6.1 |
| NaCl 0.01M pH3 | | | | | |
| | | | 7.0 | 12.3 | 6.5 |
| $CH_3COOH$ 0.001M | 3.4 | n.d | | | |
| NaCl 0.01M pH5 | | | 2.5 | 3.5 | 8.3 |
| | | | | 2.2 | 6.8 |
| GuCl 6M pH 7 | 6.6 | 7.5 | | | |

Re: Stoke's radius

When gliadins were analysed in $5 \cdot 10^{-2}$ M $CH_3$ COOH pH 3.0, their Stoke's radii were higher than in 6 M GuCl even after reduction of the disulfides bridges (Table 1). However no aggregation was detected. The higher Stoke's radii in acetic acid were not due to protein association. It came most probably from an expanded conformation of the molecules, but resulting in a shape differing from randon coil. The smaller differences observed for gliadin Stoke's radii suggest that this particular shape may be due to the large proline-rich domain of gliadins.

The addition of NaCl to $5 \cdot 10^{-2}$ M $CH_3$ COOH resulted in a very large decrease of the Stoke's radii of both gliadins (Table 1). Their conformation were thus more compact than in the absence of salt, but no aggregation was observed, no turbidity was detected in samples and no peak was excluded from gel. Nevertheless, when gliadin Stoke's radii are compared to those of globular standard proteins of similar molecular weights, and they are significantly higher. Even under folded conformation gliadins are not globular. It may be related to the size of glutamine and proline rich domain and to its structure, because the largest discrepancy was observed with ω-gliadins. Solubility of gliadins in $10^{-3}$ M $CH_3$ COOH, $10^{-2}$ M NaCl pH 5.0 was only partial. So samples were first solubilised in $10^{-3}$ M $CH_3$ COOH, then salt concentration and pH were adjusted. However it resulted in turbid solutions indication that aggregation occured. ω17 was not analysed because of rapid precipitation of sample. No peak was observed at the column void volumes, but protein recovery was low. It was verified that some insoluble aggregates are retained into the gel, explaining why peaks corresponding to aggregated gliadins were never observed. Nevertheless, the Stoke's radius of the soluble aggregates eluting from the column could be determined for ω44-gliadin. It was found to be very close to the previous one in $5 \cdot 10^{-2}$ M $CH_3COOH$, $10^{-2}$ M NaCl pH 3. It might indicate that in these conditions gliadins aggregates were constituted by the association of compactly folded monomers.

## Apolar ligand binding

The number of accessible binding sites and binding constants were modified by the conformation changes (Table 2) for gliadins as well as for pea globulins.

Table 2: TNS binding parameters for gamma and omega gliadins

| | GAMMA 44 | | OMEGA 17 | |
|---|---|---|---|---|
| | **Number of sites** | **Binding Constant ($M^{-1}$)** | **Number of sites** | **Binding Constant ($M^{-1}$)** |
| **$CH_3COOH$ 0.05M pH3** | 20 | $5.4\ 10^4$ | 12 | $0.8\ 10^4$ |
| **$CH_3COOH$ 0.05M NaCl 0.01M pH3** | 14 | $4.8\ 10^4$ | 12 | $0.4\ 10^4$ |
| **$CH_3COOH$ 0.001M NaCl 0.01M pH5** | 7 | $2.3\ 10^4$ | 1 | n.d |

In the case of gliadins, passing from aggregates to folded monomers and to expanded chains resulted in the large increase of the number of accessible hydrophobic sites. This evolution is clearly observed with γ44-gliadin. 7 sites were measured under aggregating conditions ($10^{-3}$ M $CH_3$ COOH, $10^{-2}$ M NaCl, pH 5.0), 14 sites under folded conformation ($5 \cdot 10^{-2}$ M $CH_3$ COOH, $10^{-2}$ M NaCl, pH 4.0) and 20 when the polypeptide chain was completely expanded ($5 \cdot 10^{-2}$ M $CH_3$ COOH). Larger variations were observed for ω-gliadins. 1 or 2 sites were determined when aggregated. Unfolding led to more than 12 sites. Furthermore the shape of Scatchard plots was modified. In $10^{-3}$ M $CH_3$ COOH, $10^{-2}$ M NaCl pH 5.0, γ44-gliadin Scatchard plot was linear as seen on figure 3 a and corresponded to the presence of only one class of sites [21]. This was a major difference with other solvent conditions where upward curvature of Scatchard plots at lowest TNS concentrations indicated cooperative binding [22]. In the case of ω-gliadin, the Scatchard plot tends also to be linear under aggregating conditions but adopts a peculiar profile in $5 \cdot 10^{-2}$ M $CH_3$ COOH with a relatively constant

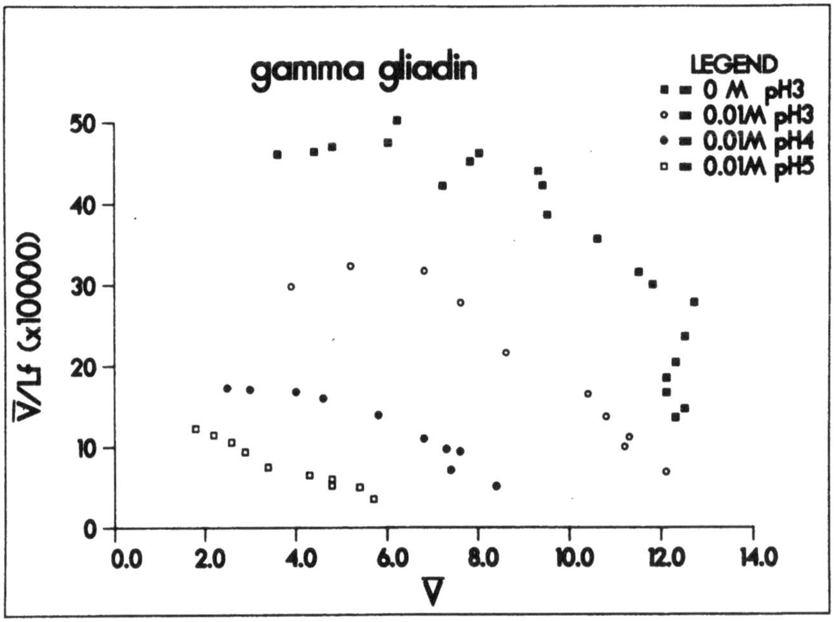


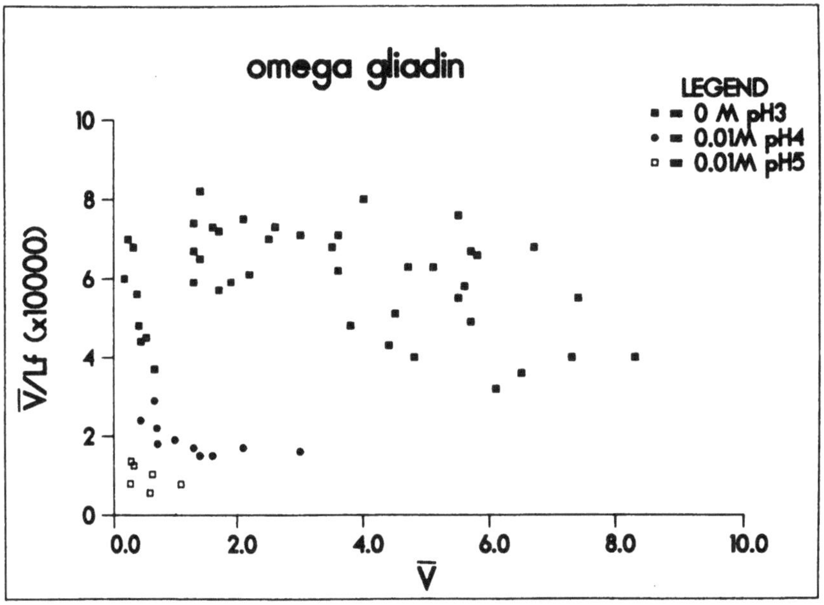


Figure 3: Scatchard plots of TNS binding by gamma gliadin (3 a above) and by omega gliadin (3 b below) solubilised in various solvents. $5 \cdot 10^{-2}$ M $CH_3$ COOH pH 3.0; $5 \cdot 10^{-2}$ M $CH_3$ COOH, $10^{-2}$ M NaCl pH 3.0; $5 \cdot 10^{-2}$ M $CH_3$ COOH, $10^{-2}$ M NaCl pH 4.0; $10^{-3}$ M $CH_3$ COOH $10^{-2}$ M NaCl pH 5.0

value of V/Lf wathever was the TNS concentration (Fig. 3 b). It signifies a large number of sites but the absolute value of which is experimentally difficult to determine.

The dissociation of the pea globulins and the unfolding of the resulting subunits in the acidic pH led also to the binding of a larger amount of hydrophobic ligand (Table 3).

Table 3: TNS binding parameters for legumin and vicilin

| | LEGUMIN | | VICILIN | |
|---|---|---|---|---|
| | Number of sites (n) | Binding Constant ( $M^{-1}$) | Number of sites (n) | Binding Constant ( $M^{-1}$) |
| pH 7 | $n_1$ 8<br>$n_2$ 11 | 4.5 $10^4$<br>3.5 $10^3$ | 2-3 | 1.7 $10^4$ |
| pH 11.5 | 16-18 | 3.9 $10^2$ | - | - |
| pH 2.4 | 895 | 5.7 $10^2$ | 244 | 1.5 $10^3$ |

$n_1$ Number of sites of strong affinity
$n_2$ Number of sites of weak affinity

The binding affinity constants are however decreased. In alkaline condition the binding parameters of legumin are only few modified. For vicilin at pH 11.5 the number of binding sites cannot be graphically determined but remained lower than at pH 2.4 on the basis of binding isotherms (Fig. 4).

These effects are consistent with our former results on the conformation changes, especially in the case of legumin for which it was shown that complete dissociation only occured in acidic pH range. Moreover, it was demonstrated in a previous study [16] that the unfolding of the dissociated legumin subunits at pH 2.4 led to the exposure of all the aromatic residues, indicating that most of the hydrophobic areas are exposed outwards. Taking into account the similar oligomeric forms of vicilin in extrem basic and acid conditions, the higher level of TNS binding by vicilin at pH 2.4 compared to pH 11.5 can olny be explained by the unfolding of the dissociated polypeptides, as happende for legumin in the same conditions.

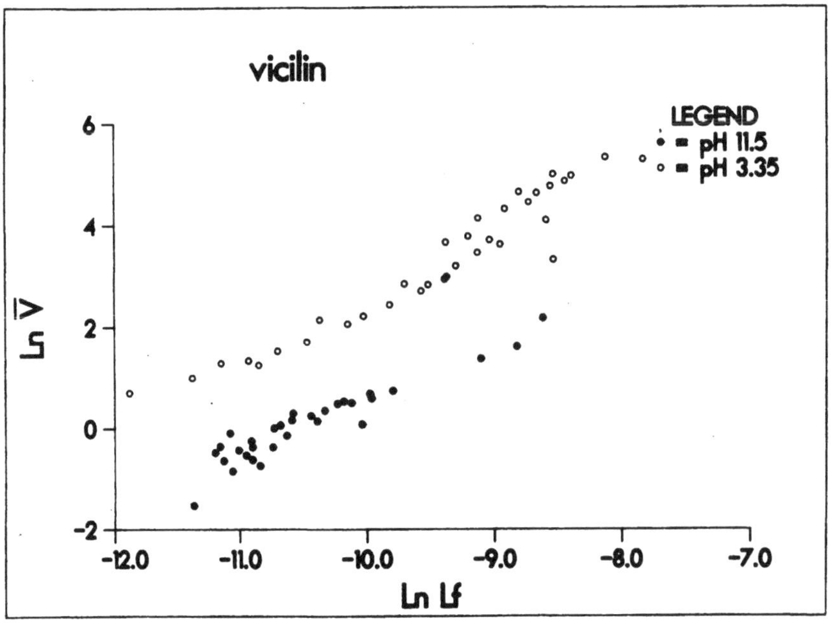


Figure 4: TNS binding isotherms of vicilin at pH 3.35 and 11.5.
V: number of moles of TNS bound/mole of protein.
Lf: concentration of free ligand.

The profiles of the Scatchard plots were also drastically modified by the conformation changes. At pH 7, native legumin (pH 7, 0.1 M) exhibited a Scatchard profile characteristic of two classes of sites. On the other hand, in acidic and alkaline conditions the binding of TNS by legumin was cooperative as shown by the profile of the Scatchard plots (Fig. 5). However, in alkaline condition, V/Lf values remained constant instead of decreasing for the higher ligand concentrations. The same variations of the Scatchard profiles were observed for vicilin. As native, this protein exhibit a linear Scatchard plot characteristic of one class of sites whereas a cooperative profile was obtained at pH 2.4 (Fig. 6). At pH 11.5 plateau value of V/Lf was also reached for the higher concentration of TNS. Thus, the binding of TNS by globulins was ruled by cooperative phenomena when they were dissociated or unfolded.

## Discussion

For gliadins as well as for pea globulins the folding and the aggregation was accompanied by surface hydrophobicity modifications. Expanded conformations corresponded to highest numbers of hydrophobic sites measured. In the case of gliadins folding reduced the number of accessible sites and in conditions promoting aggregation, the derease was very large.

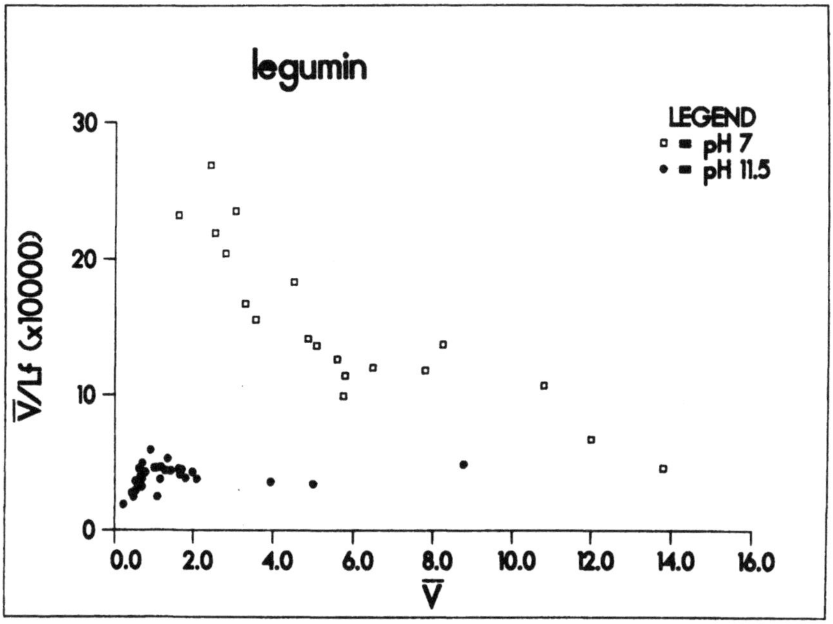


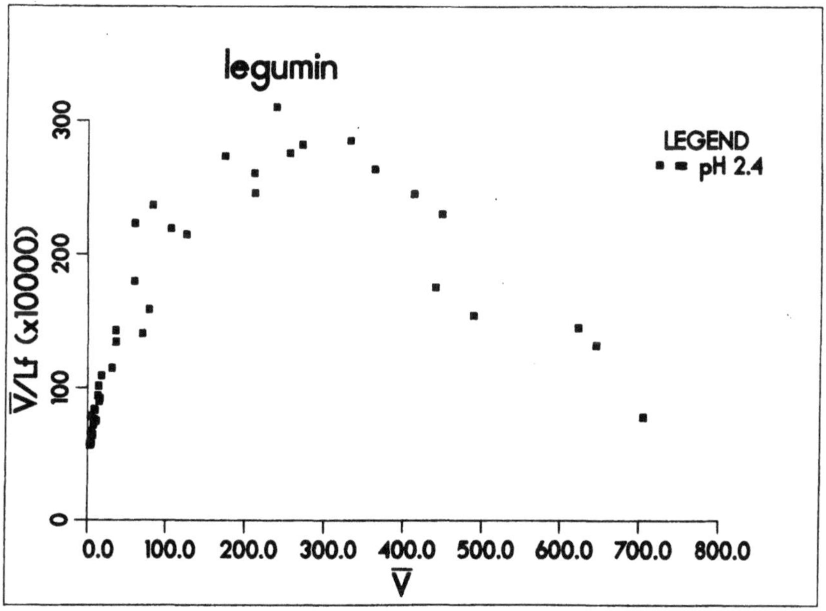


Figure 5: Scastchard plots of TNS binding by legumin.
(5 a, above) in neutral and alkaline pH range.
(5 b, below) in acidic pH range.
V: number of moles of TNS bound/mole of protein.
Lf: concentration of free ligand.

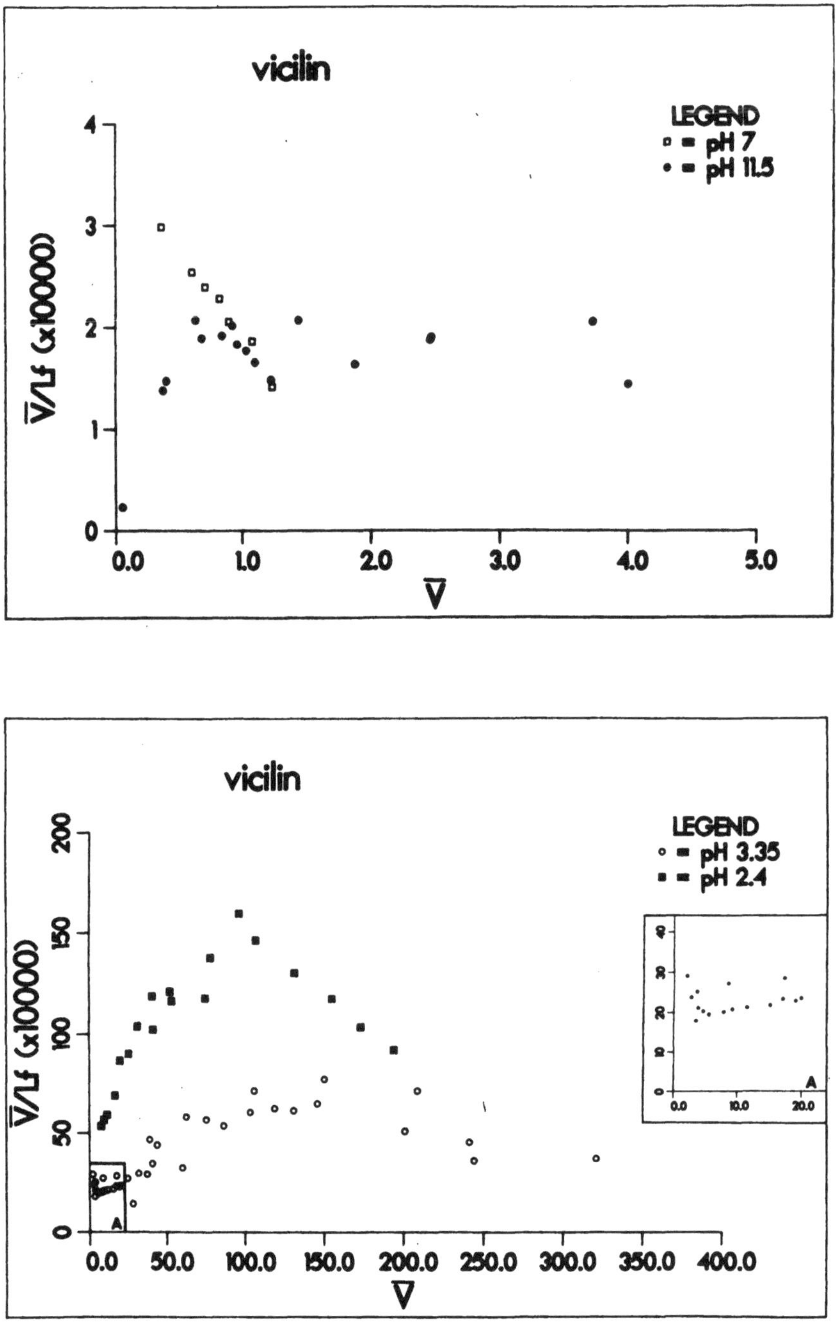


Figure 6: Scatchard plots of TNS binding by vicilin.
(6 a, above) in neutral and alkaline plH range.
(6 b, below) in acidic pH range. (6 bA) detail of the first part of the curve obtained for pH 3.35.
V: number of moles of TNS bound/mole of protein.
Lf: concentration of free ligand.

The number of sites is also unexpectedly large when pea globulins are dissociated and unfolded at pH 2.4. In opposite, their surface hydrophobicity is very low when they are under their closely packed structure. Those results show that only few hydrophobic sites are accessible when gliadins and globulin subunits are under folded and associated conformations. A large part of total sites was then probably buried inside the proteins, most of them being involved in the stabilization of the folded structure.

Moreover, the very high number of binding sites obtained for pea globulins at pH 2.4 and ω-gliadins in $5 \cdot 10^{-2}$ M $CH_3$ COOH could be due to the binding of successive layers of TNS stacked by electron Pi interactions to each others. It can be induced by a great density of the former TNS molecules bound along the completely accessible polypeptide chains. This hypothesis is supported by the aromatic amino acid composition of ω-gliadins and their behaviours in hydrophobic chromatography. They are less strongly adsorbed on hydrohpobic aliphatic columns than other gliadins althoungh they display high affinity for aromatic phase [5], bound larger amounts of TNS and have high content of phenylalanine.

The cooperativity which was observed for wheat gliadins as well as for pea globulins has to be discussed. It happened when proteins were unfolded or when the solvent conditions induced a weakening of the structure stabilizing forces (γ-gliadins in $5 \cdot 10^{-2}$ M $CH_3$ COOH, $10^{-2}$ M NaCl, pH 3 - pea globulins in extreme pH conditions). It can be easily imagined that the binding of new TNS molecules is easier due to the binding of the former ones as much as the structure stabilizing forces are weak.

The Scatchard plots adopted a peculiar profile when pea globulines are partially dissociated in alkaline conditions. Upward curvature of the Scatchard plots were observed for the lower TNS concentration whereas constant value of V/Lf were obtained for the higher ones. Taking into account the first part of the curve at pH 11.5 the number of binding sites could be graphically determined around 8 and 3, respectively, for legumin and vicilin. These values are very close to those obtained for native forms. Thus, the partial dissociation which occurs in alkaline pH range did not increase very much the number of binding sites, but high concentration of TNS seemed however to be able to open the proteins structure favourizing the accessibility of new hydrophobic areas. It should be due to modifications of the hydrophobic interactions which stabilize the oligomeric strucutre of these proteins.

A similar procedure of binding should occur for vicilin at pH 3.35. In this condition, this protein is only few dissociated. Here the first part of the Scatchard plots ($V < 10$) is linear and lead graphically to 6 binding sites. This value is not so far from the number of binding sites obtained at pH 7. For ω-gliadin solubilised in $5 \cdot 10^{-2}$ M $CH_3$ COOH, a linear part can also be distinguished in the Scatchard plots for the lower TNS concentrtion ($V < 1$). Taking into account this part only, around one site was obtained as for the protein under aggregating conditions.

In some cases the number of ligand bound molecules is exessively high in comparison with the size of the protein. Near horizontal Scatchard plots were observed indication a continuous binding with increasing free ligand concentrations.

It suggested that in those conditions the results did not measure the actual number of hydrophobic sites of these proteins but reflects the formation of ligand-protein complexes able to associate still larger amounts of ligand. Additionnal experiments are needed to elucidate these phenomena. However, such binding behaviours could have a bearing in the functional properties of proteins in terms of interactions with non-polar small molecules as in emulsions. It emphasizes also the importance of a systematic investigation of the binding isotherms when functional properties are concerned.

**References**

[1] Nakai, S.; J. Agric. Food Chem. **31**, 676 (1983)

[2] Nakai, S., E. Li Chan and S. Hayakawa; Nahrung **30**, 327 (1986)

[3] Li Chan, E., S. Nakai and D.F. Wood; J. Food Sci. **49**, 2, 345 (1984)

[4] Bietz, J.A. and T. Burnouf; Theoretical and Applied Genetics **70**, 599 (1985)

[5] Popineau, Y, and F. Pineau; J. Cereal Sci. **5**, 215 (1987)

[6] Fausnaugh, J.L., L.A. Kennedy and F.E. Regnier; J. Chrom. **317**, 141 (1984)

[7] Zaslavski, B. Yu., N.M. Mestechkina and S.V. Rogozhin; J. Chrom. **260**, 329 (1983)

[8] Axelsson, C.G.; Biochim. Biophys. Acta **533**, 34 (1978)

[9] Albertsson, P.A.; Endeavour (New Series) **1**, 2, 69 (1977)

[10] McClure, W.O. and G.M Edelman; Biochem. **5**, 1908 (1966)

[11] Kato, A., T. Matsuda, N Matsudomi and K. Kobayashi; J. Agric. Food Chem. **32**, 2, 284 (1984)

[12] Gueguen, J., A.T. Vu and F. Schaeffer; J. Sci. Food Agric. **35**, 1024 (1984)

[13] Larre, C. and Gueguen; J. Chrom. **361**, 169 (1986)

[14] Popineau, Y., J.L. le Guerroue and F. Pineau; Lebensm. Wiss. Techn. **19**, 266 (1986)

[15] Popineau, Y. and F. Pineau; J. Cereal Sci. **3**, 363 (1985)

[16] Gueguen, J., M. Chevalier, J. Barbot and J. Schaeffer; J. Sci. Food Agric. In press.

[17] Cole, E.W., J.V. Torres and D.D. Kasarda; Cereal Chem. **60**, 306 (1983)

[18] Cole, E.W., D.D. Kasarda and D. Lafiandra; Biochim. Biophys. Acta, **787**, 244 (1984)

[19] Sophianopoulos, J.A., J.S. Durham, A.J. Sophianopoulos, H.L. Ragsdale and W.P. Cropper; Arch. Biochem. Biphys. **187**, 132 (1978)

[20] Gueguen, J.; J. Agric. Food Chem., submitted for publication

[21] Cantor, A.C. and P.R. Schimmel; "Biophysical Chemistry Part III: the Behaviour of Biological Macromolecules", San Francisco: W.H. Freeman, p 844, (1980)

[22] Thakur, A.K., M.L. Jaffe and D. Rodbard; Anal. Biochemm. **107**, 279 (1980)

# NAPIN, THE 2S PROTEIN IN RAPESEED
# - CONFORMATIONAL STABILITY AND RELATIONSHIP TO OTHER 2S PLANT PROTEINS

K.D. Schwenke[1], B. Raab[1], W. Pähtz[1], and D. Zirwer[2]

## Abstract

The low molecular mass basic rapeseed protein fraction (napin) represents helical proteins (40 - 45 % helix) the secondary structure of which is stabilized by interchain and intrachain disulfide bridges. Succinylation or acetylation did not change significantly the secondary or tertiary structure which was investigated by means of far and near ultraviolet CD and by fluorescence spectroscopy. Both the formerly predicted secondary structure and exposed and flexible regions (Schwenke, Drescher, Zirwer, Raab, Biochem. Physiol. Pflanzen, 183, 219 (1988)) were used for a first approximation of a structural model which corresponds to the physico-chemical and functional properties of napin.

The comparison of the napin with other low-molecular mass plant proteins revealed a relationship (and certain homology) to other 2S storage proteins and some enzyme inhibitors.

## Introduction

The low molecular mass 2S protein fraction represents a closely related group of water soluble storage proteins in rapeseed (*Brassica napus L.*) [1 - 4]. Owing to its high content in rapeseed, the napin fraction contributes significantly to the functional properties of the total rapeseed proteins. The last years have thrown new light on the structure and biosynthesis of this protein fraction by elucidating the amino acid sequence from the coding DNA base sequence [5] and direct sequence analysis [6]. This fraction wich has been called "napins" by CROUCH [5] comprises homologous proteins with molecular masses of 12 000 - 14 000 g/mol and isoelectric points > 10. The latter are composed of two polypeptide chains which are connected by disulfide bridges. In the present paper the peculiarities of the napin structure and their relationship to other low molecular mass storage proteins and enzyme inhibitors are discussed. It is shown that the structural stability of napins follows from the presence of disulfide bridges in the molecule.

1) Central Institute of Nutrition in Potsdam-Rehbrücke, Academy of Sciences of the GDR, DDR-1505 Bergholz-Rehbrücke, Arthur-Scheunert-Allee 114 - 116

2) Central Institute of Molecular Biology, Academy of Sciences of the GDR, DDR-1115 Berlin-Buch, Robert-Rössle-Str. 10

## Napins as helical proteins

The low molecular mass and the high isoelectric point of napins may point to a relationship to other highly basic protein families as ribosomal proteins or histones. There are however peculiarities in the napin composition and structure which allow us to exclude such a relationship: The napins contain a relatively high amount of cysteins lacking in those proteins and they are rich in helical conformation, which is poor in the other ones.

The far ultraviolet circular dichroism spectrum of napins is characterized by two negative maxima at 208 and 222 nm which are typical for helical proteins [4]. The evaluation of the spectrum gave 40 - 45 % helix and 16 - 20 % ß-sheet structure for the native proteins. Differences in the helix content of napins from various rapeseed varieties could not be found.

## Predicted napin structure

The secondary structure has been predicted from the amino acid sequence published by CROUCH [5] using a modified version of the methods CHOU and FASMAN [7] and GARNIER et al. [8]. That results in 37 % helix and 16 % ß-sheet content in good correspondence which the experimental data [9]. Figure 1 shows the location of helices and ß-strands in an arrangement which allows the interaction of helices and the formation of interchain disulfide bridges.

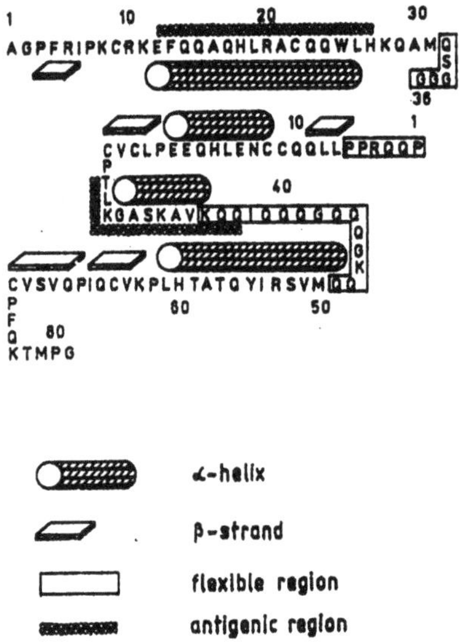


Fig. 1: Predicted secondary structure and regions of high flexibility and antigenic determinants of a napin, according to [9].

The small polypeptide chain contains one helix, while three helices are located in the large polypeptide chain. The two half cystine residues in the short polypeptide chain take part in the formation of two interchain disulfide bridges (Fig. 2), one of which is at a helix. Their half cystine counterparts in the large chain are still unknown.

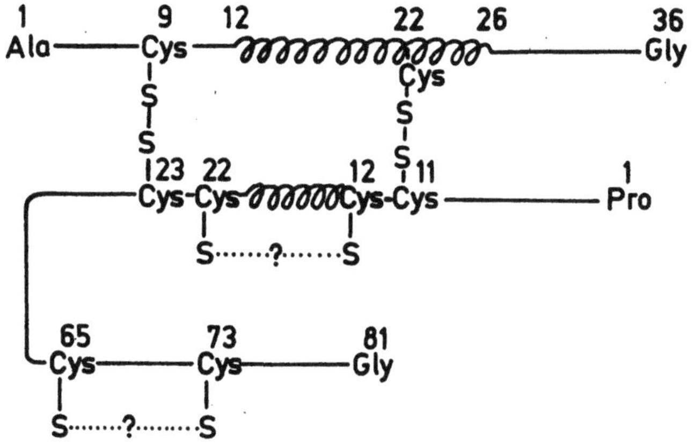


Hypothetical location of disulfide bridges in napin

Fig. 2: Hypothetical location of disulfide bridges in napin

Some region of high flexibility were predicted according to KARPLUS and SCHULTZ [10]. They are in the C-terminal sequence of the large one. At both terminal sites the splitting of a sequence comprising 20 amino acids has taken place in the precursor polypeptide [5].
The largest flexible sequence is located between the second and the third helix of the large chain (Fig. 1).

Two antigen determinants were predicted according to WELLING et al. [11]. Both the flexible parts of the chains and the antigen determinants exposed on the molecular surface are considered to be involved in the formation of protein foams. Napins exhibit a high foam capacity and stability [12].

Moreover, there are two regions of high positive charge density in the protein. The first one is the sequence 5 - 11 of the small chain with two lysine and two arginine residues at the beginning of the large exposed region. The second one comprising three lysines lies within the antigen determinant in the large chain (positions 28, 32, 35). Both are believed to be preferred sites for electrostatic interactions. The predominance of a dimeric protein-phytic acid complex [13] may point to a favoured site of interaction. The cumulation of basic amino acid residues, especially of lysine, in both regions favours a nucleophilic attack by splitting products of thioglycosinolates or other reagents.

**Relationship and homology between 2 S storage proteins and enzyme inhibitors**

The napins belong to a group of similarly structured 2S storage proteins which are widely distributed in oilseeds and legumes. They were found in the seeds of sunflower [3], safflor [14], sesame [15], poppy [16], lupin [17], in castor bean [18, 19], linseed [20] and Brazil nut [21 - 24]. So far as the secondary structure of these proteins was investigated, a high content of helix conformation was found, reaching from 30 % in the safflor protein to 60 % in the protein from Brazil nut (Tab. 1).

Table 1: Secondary structure (helix content) in 2S storage proteins

| Origin | Secondary structure Method | evaluation % helix | author |
|---|---|---|---|
| Rape (*Brassica napus*) | CD | 40 - 45 | Schwenke et al. [4] |
| Sunflower (*Helianthus anuus*) | CD | +++ | Raab [25] |
| Safflor (*Carthamus tinct.*) | CD | 30 | Sridhara/Prakash [14] |
| Sesame (*Sesamum ind.*) | CD | 30 | Rajendra/ Prakash [15] |
| Linseed (*Linum usit.*) | CD | +++ | Madhusudhan [20] |
| Lupin (*Lupinus angust.*) | ORD/CD | 38 | Lilley [17] |
| Brazil nut (*Bertholletia excelsa*) | Prediction | 60 | Drescher [26] |

This structural relationship was underlined by a certain homology of the amino acid sequences. Thus, the Brazil nut protein shows 33 % homology with that of the castor bean and 25 % with that of napin [21]. Moreover, their relationship becomes evident when the relative positions of cysteine residues are considered (Fig. 3).
The cysteine positions in the 2S storage proteins are highly conservative. We found them in a similar arragement in some proteinase inhibitors of the BOWMAN-BIRK type [27, 28] and in the sweet plant protein thaumatin from the fruit of *Thaumatococcus daniellii* [19]. SHARIEF and LI found a high homology between the large subunit of the castor bean protein and the BOWMAN-BIRK inhibitor. In the case of the Bowman-Birk inhibitor sequence, the Lys-Ser in position 26-27 is the active site of the trypsin inhibitor [29, 30]. The Arg-Ser at position 3-4 of the lare subunit might also be involved in a similar function, since this native protein seems to be resistant to digestion by trypsin, chymotrypsin and thermolysin [19]. The Arg-Ile sequence at position 53-54 in the sequence of the large chain of napin (Fig. 1) may be involved in such a function, too. The question arises, whether the large

subunit of the 2S storage proteins may function as an endogenous proteinase inhibitor. A comparison of the sequences of three proteins, napin, castor bean 2S protein, and trypsin inhibitor from barley gave a high alignment scores in a computer analysis [6]. The inhibitor active sequence in position 33-34 of the barley inhibitor lacks, however, in the napin sequence.

```
                                             small chain

Rapeseed    -Lys- Cys-Arg -Lys - - - - - Ala- Cys-Gln -
Brazil nut  -Gln- Cys-Arg -Asp - - - - - His- Cys-Arg -
Castor bean -Gly- Cys-Arg -Gly - - - - - Cys- Cys-Gln -

                                             large chain

Rapeseed    -Gln- Cys-Cys -Asn - - - - - Leu- Cys-Val-Cys-Pro -
Brazil nut  -Glu- Cys-Cys -Glu - - - - - Glu- Cys-Arg-Cys-Glu -
Castor bean -Gly- Cys-Cys -Asp - - - - - Gln- Cys-Arg-Cys-Glu -

Rapeseed    - Cys -Gln-Ile-Pro-Gln-Val-Ser-Val- Cys-Pro -
Brazil nut  - Cys -Asn-Leu-Ser-Pro - Met - Arg- Cys-Pro -
Castor bean - Cys -Gly-Val-Ser-Pro - Thr - Gln- Cys-Arg -
```

Figure 3: Relative positions of cysteine residues in amino acid sequences of 2S proteins from rapeseed [5] Brazil nut [21] and castor bean [19]

**Chemical modification and structural stability of the napin fraction**

The ε-amino groups of the lysine residues in the napins are quickly blocked by acetylation or succinylation [12, 31]. More slowly, the hydroxyl groups of the serine and threeine residues and the phenolic group of the tyrosine are esterfied by this reaction. The surface hydrophobicity, estimated by the ANS probe technique, increases continuously with the total number of acetyl groups connected with both the amino and hydroxyl groups [31]. Nevertheless, an alteration of the functional surface properties could not be observed [32]. Moreover, the secondary structure of the protein did not change after acylation (Tab. 2).

Table 2: Results of secondary structure evaluation of the native and acylated napin fraction, according to [9]

| Protein sample | % α-helix | % ß-sheet | % remainder |
|---|---|---|---|
| native[1] | 41 ± 1 | 16 ± 2 | 43 ± 1 |
| native[2] | 45 ± 1 | 20 ± 1 | 35 ± 1 |
| 30 % succinyl.[3] | 38 ± 2 | 20 ± 2 | 42 ± 1 |
| 87 % succinyl.[3] | 44 ± 1 | 17 ± 1 | 39 ± 1 |
| 98 % acetyl.[3] | 44 ± 4 | | |

[1] according to [4]; protein isolated from the rapeseed variety "Großlüsewitzer Spätsaatverträgliche"; secondary struture evaluation according to [33]
[2] protein isolated from the rapeseed variety "Sollux"; secondary structure evaluation according to [34]
[3] protein isolated from the rapeseed variety "Marinus"; secondary structure (α-helix) evaluation using the $[\theta]_{222\ nm}$-method

The lack of a shift of the maximum in the fluorescence emission spectrum and the lack of significant changes of the positions of the main maxima in the near UV CD spectrum (Fig. 4) [31] after acetylation are a proof for the stability of the tertiary structure, too. There are, however, three facts which point to a certain chain flexibility in the tertiary structure. These are the quenching of tryptophan fluorescence, the changes of the cysteine absorption in the near UV DC spectrum (250-270 nm) and the changes of intrinsic viscosity depending on the degree of modification [31].

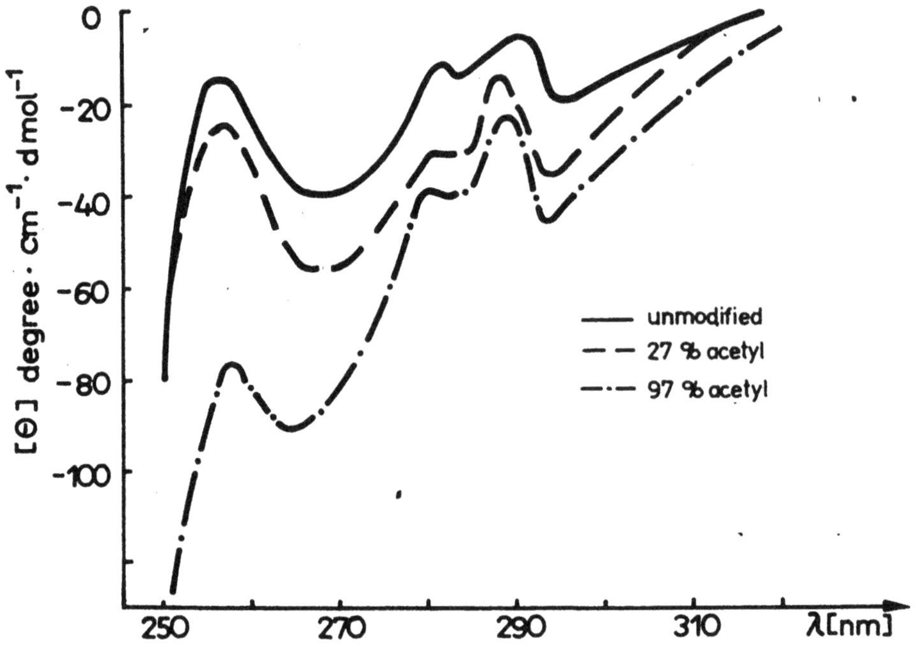


Fig. 4: Near ultraviolet circular dichroism spectra of a native and two acetylated napin samples, according to [31].

The relatively high conformational stability of the napin has been shown by measuring the CD after heating the protein solution (Tab. 3). The helix content remained unchanged after heating the acidic, neutral and weak alkaline solutions, respectively, for 10 min at 80°C. Higher temperatures or pH values were necessary to induce a significant decrease of helix content.

Splitting of the disulfide bridges by reduction using sulfhydryl reagents decreases the helix content, too. The reduced, alkylated and chromatographically separated small and large polypeptide chains show a helix content of only 8 and 6 % (Tab. 3). The disulfide bonds, responsible for the stability of the structure, must be available to the reagent, because they were reduced in the absence of a denaturant.

In the absence of a reducing agent the helix content was decreased by urea, but the secondary structure could be restored to a high degree after removing the denaturant (Tab. 3).

Table 3: Secondary structure evaluation of heat-treated and reduced napin and napin subunits, according to [9]

| Protein sample | modification | secondary structure (%) | | |
|---|---|---|---|---|
| | | α-helix | β-sheet | remainder |
| napin | pH 9.1 80°C | 40 | 14 | 46 |
| | pH 11.8 80°C | 30 | 17 | 53 |
| | pH 9.1 100°C | 20 | 19 | 61 |
| | pH 11.8 100°C | 14 | 22 | 64 |
| napin | 8 M urea | 20 | 15 | 65 |
| | 6 M urea; renaturation | 30 | | |
| napin | reduction; without urea (DTE) | <10 | | |
| large subunit | reduction | 6 | | |
| small subunit | SH-alkylation | 8 | | |

These results underline clearly the role of disulfide bridges in stabilizing the napin structure. Moreover, the conserved relative positions of the cysteine residues in the 2S storage proteins suggest that disulfide bridges constitute a major structural element in this protein group. The structural homology of those proteins points to their evolution from a common ancestral gene which might be regarded as an ancestor of enzyme inhibitor genes, too.

## References

[1] Bhatty, R.S., S.L. McKenzie and A.J. Finlayson, Can. J. Biochem. **46**, 1191 (1969)

[2] Lönnerdal, B. and J.C. Janson, Biochim. Biophys. Acta **278**, 175 (1972)

[3] Schwenke, K.D., B. Raab, J. Uhlig, H. Tkocz, J. Behlke, M. Böttger and U. Freimuth, Nahrung **17**, 791 (1973)

[4] Schwenke, K.D., B. Raab and M. Schultz, Studia biophysica **51**, 161 (1975)

[5] Crouch, M.L., K.M. Tenbarge, A.E. Simon and R. Ferl, J. molec. appl. genetics **2**, 273 (1983)

[6] Ericson, M.L., J. Rödin, M. Lenman, K. Glimelius, L.-G. Josefsson and L. Rask, J. Biol. Chem. **261**, 14576 (1986)

[7] Chou, P.J., and G.D. Fasman, Advances in Enzymology **47**, 45 (1978)

[8] Garnier, J., D.J. Osguthorpe and B. Robson, J. Mol. Biol. **130**, 97 (1978)

[9] Schwenke, K.D., B. Drescher, D. Zirwer and B. Raab, Biochem. Physiol. Pflanzen **183**, 219 (1988)

[10] Karplus, P.A., and G.E. Schultz, Naturwissenschaften **72**, 212 (1985)

[11] Welling, G.W., W.J. Weijer, W.J. van der Zee and S. Welling-Wister, FEBS Letters 188, 215 (1985)

[12] Nitecka, E., B. Raab and K.D. Schwenke, Nahrung 30, 975 (1986)

[13] Schwenke, K.D., R. Mothes, K. Gast and D. Zirwer, these proceedings, p.

[14] Sridhara, S. and V. Prakash, J. Agric. Food Chem. 35, 676 (1987)

[15] Rajendran, S. and V. Prakash, J. Agric. Food Chem. 36, 269 (1988)

[16] Srinivas, H., Ph. D. Thesis, Univ. Mysore 1985, quoted in [14]

[17] Lilley, G.G., J. Sci. Food Agric. 37, 895 (1986)

[18] Youle, R.J. and A.H.C. Huang, Plant Physiol. 61, 13 (1978)

[19] Sharief, F.S. and St.S.-L. Li, J. Biol. Chem. 257, 14753 (1982)

[20] Madhusudhan, K.T. and N. Singh, Phytochemistry 24, 2507 (1985)

[21] Ampe, Ch., J. van Damme, L.A.B. de Castro, M.J.A.M. Sampaio, M. van Montagu and J. Vandekerckhove, Eur. J. Biochem. 159, 597 (1986)

[22] Sun, S.S.M., F.W. Leung and J.C. Tomic, J. Agric. Food Chem. 35, 232 (1987)

[23] Sun, S.M., S.B. Altenback and F.W. Leung, Eur. J. Biochem. 162, 477 (1987)

[24] Altenback, S.B., K.W. Pearson, F.W. Leung and S.S.M. Sun, Plant Molecular Biol. 8, 239 (1987)

[25] Raab, B., Thesis, TU Dresden 1974

[26] Drescher, B., personal communication

[27] Krahn, J., and F.C. Stevens, Biochemistry 9, 2646 (1970)

[28] Tan, C.G.L., and F.C. Stevens, Eur. J. Biochem. 18, 515 (1971)

[29] Iyengar, R.B., P. Smits, F van der Quaderaa, H. van der Wel, J. van Browershaven, R. Ravestein, G. Richters and P.D. van Wassenaar, Eur. J. Biochem. 96, 193 (1979)

[30] Odani, S. and T. Ikenaka, J. Biochem. 71, 839 (1972)

[31] Schwenke, K.D., B. Raab, W. Pähtz, D. Zirwer and Kim Yung Hak, J. Food Biochem. in preparation

[32] Schwenke, K.D., Kim Yung Hak, B. Raab, W. Pähtz, A. Krajewski, D. Zirwer, E. Lange and G. Mieth, Proceedings of the 7th Internat. Rapeseed Congress, Poznan 11 - 14 May 1988, Poland

[33] Saxena, V.P. and D. Wetlaufer, Proc. Natl. Acad. Sci. USA 68, 969 (1971)

[34] Provencher, S.W. and J. Gloeckner, Biochemistry 20, 33 (1981)

# IS THERE A STRUCTURAL SIMILARITY AMONGST THE LOW MOLECULAR WEIGHT PROTEIN FRACTIONS ALSO FROM VARIOUS OISLEEDS ?

V. Prakash[1]

The presence of several protein components in the oilseed is based probably for their function in the seed either during formation, dormancy or germination. With an extensive research still going on in this area, it is not very clear what role has each one of these different protein components are playing in the seed.

The existing literature on the physico-chemical properties of the various protein fractions from peanut, soybean, sesame seed, mustard seed rapeseed, sunflower seed, safflower seed, cottonseed, poppyseed and linseed is fairly extensive [1]. The analysis of data of the high molecular weight protein fraction (HMW) in terms of their structural similarities has been attempted by Prakash and Narasinga Rao [2]. The analysis indicated that in the HMW protein fractions of oilseeds of peanut, soybean, sesame seed, mustard seed, rapeseed, sunflower seed, safflower seed and cotton seed, there is structural similarity in terms of their amino acid composition, size and shape, molecular weight, secondary structure, subunit composition, association-dissociation at high and low pH, stability towards proteolysis by proteases and quaternary structure. Based on these similarities a working model has been proposed for the association, dissociation, denaturation and reassociation of proteins of oilseeds [2].

Similar to the high molecular weight proteins, there is considerable amount of literature available on the low molecular weight protein fractions from sesame seed, mustard seed, rapeseed, sunflower seed, safflower seed, cotton seed, poppyseed and linseed [1]. Eventhough there is an extensive literature on several of the fractions of soybean and peanut no single fraction can represent the total low molecular weight protein fraction like other oilseeds and hence is not included for the purpose of comparison and discussion in the present paper.

Most of the oilseeds predominantly had four protein fractions namely 2S, 7S, 11S and 15 - 18S (polymer). For the purpose of present discussion the low molecular weight protein fraction is designated as LMW protein. It generally sediments as a $2 \pm 0.3$S component in most of the oilseeds. It is observed that substances such as trypsin inhibitor, hemaglutinins, polyphenols, glucosinolates, color, bitter principles and other antinutritional factors which are inherents in some of the oilseeds are generally found to a higher extent in the 2S or the LMW protein.

[1] Biophysical Chemistry Unit, Food Chemistry Department,
Central Food Technological Research Institute, Mysore-570 013, India

In the present paper the similarity in amino acid composition, hydrophobicity and related parameters, molecular weight secondary structure, size and shape, partial specific volume and stability towards denaturants will be discussed.

## LMW proteins

Table 1 summarises the percent composition of the 1.3 to 2.4S protein fractions present in the total protein of sesame seed, mustard seed, rapeseed, sunflower seed, safflower seed, cottonseed, poppyseed and linseed.

In the literature these proteins are usually referred to as 2S proteins. This has resulted in a tremendous confusion with regard to specific identification of protein. To avoid confusion names based on botanical species and in relation to HMW protein fraction is suggested (Table 1). New names are suggested for the LMW proteins of sesame seed, sunflower seed, mustard seed, rapeseed, poppyseed and linseed, except the conbrassins, most of the LMW proteins are present to the extent of 20 - 30 percent.

## 1. Amino acid composition

The amino acid composition of LMW proteins from eight different seeds are given in Table 2. All the amino acids in LMW proteins are normalised to the total number of residues present for molecular weight of 16 000 (Please see discussion on molecular weight). A striking similarity is very apparent in the amino acid composition in that nearly 35 % of the amino acids is represented by glutamic acid in all the LMW proteins. They are also having a high content of sulfur amino acids, lysine, arginine and glycine as compared to HMW proteins. The large variation one sees in Table 2 could be due to the heterogenity of LMW proteins and also different methods being utilised to determine amino acids and acid hydrolysis values not being extrapolated to zero time and other experimental variations. It is very essential that amino acid analysis under identical conditions of highly purified LMW protein is performed to understand the intrinsic homology in the amino acid compositions of the proteins. It may also indicate whether there is a homology in the length of the polypeptide chain also. In the absence of these data we have analysed the existing amino acid data in terms of hydrophobicity and other indices.

## 2. Hydrophobicity and related indices

It has become customary to evaluate hydrophobicity index, HQ [3], Fisher's P or the ratio of the volume occupied by polar residues to the volume occupied by nonpolar residues, [4] the fractional charge value, C and Waugh's NPS or frequency of nonpolar side chains based on

Table 1: Low Molecular Weight Protein fraction from various oilseeds

(*Superscripts indicate the source of information)

| Oilseeds | Botanical name | Existing name | Suggested name | $S_{20,w}$* | % in total protein |
|---|---|---|---|---|---|
| Sesame seed | *Sesamum indicum* | β-globulin | Consesamin | 2.0[11] | 20 |
| Mustard seed | *Brassica species* | 2S protein | Conbrassin (M) | 1.3[12] | 70 |
| Rapeseed | *Brassica species* | Albumin | Conbrassin (R) | 2.0[18] | 40 - 60 |
| Sunflower seed | *Helianthus annus* | Albumin | Conhelianthin | 2.0[12] | 20 |
| Safflower seed | *Carthamus tinctorius* | LMW protein | Concarmin | 1.5[13] | 25 |
| Cottonseed | *Gossypium species* | Albumin | Congossypin | 2.0[14] | 30 |
| Poppyseed | *Papaver somniferum* | LMW protein | Conpoppyverin | 0.8[15] | 20 |
| Linseed | *Linum usitatissium* | LMW protein | Conlinin | 1.6[16] | 20 |

Table 2: Content of aminoacids of LMW protein from various oilseeds (residues/16 000 gm protein)

| AMINO ACID | Consesamin[11] (M) | Conbrassin[12] (M) | Conbrassin[12,18] (R) | Conheli-anthin[12] | Concarmin[13] | Congossypin[14] | Conpoppy-verin[15] | Conlinin[16] |
|---|---|---|---|---|---|---|---|---|
| Aspartic acid | 6 | 4 | 2 | 11 | 9 | 12 | 7 | 8 |
| Threonine | 2 | 5 | 2 | 7 | 4 | 5 | 5 | 4 |
| Serine | 6 | 8 | 7 | 9 | 5 | 8 | 7 | 8 |
| Glutamic acid | 48 | 39 | 33 | 32 | 48 | 34 | 50 | 42 |
| Proline | 4 | - | 15 | 8 | 3 | 5 | 7 | 5 |
| Glycine | 9 | 13 | 10 | 15 | 21 | 24 | 10 | 24 |
| Alanine | 5 | 8 | 9 | 11 | 7 | 10 | 5 | 5 |
| Valine | 4 | 11 | 8 | 8 | 6 | 3 | 2 | 4 |
| Methionine | 3 | 7 | 2 | 3 | 2 | 2 | 5 | 3 |
| Half-cysteine | 4 | - | 9 | 9 | 5 | 12 | 5 | 1 |
| Isoleucine | 4 | 7 | 5 | 6 | 3 | 2 | 2 | 4 |
| Leucine | 6 | 11 | 10 | 9 | 7 | 4 | 5 | 8 |
| Tyrosine | 3 | 2 | 1 | 1 | 3 | 3 | 2 | 1 |
| Phenylalanine | 2 | 3 | 4 | 2 | 3 | 2 | 1 | 3 |
| Lysine | 2 | 9 | 10 | 7 | 5 | 9 | 2 | 7 |
| Histidine | 2 | 5 | 5 | 2 | 3 | 3 | 1 | 2 |
| Arginine | 15 | - | 7 | 8 | 12 | 11 | 17 | 13 |
| Tryptophan | 2 | - | 1 | - | - | 1 | - | 2 |

Table 3: Calculated values of hydrophobicity and related parameters of the LMW proteins from various oilseeds

| PROTEIN | $HQ^a$ | $NFS^b$ | $P^c$ | $C^d$ | Total number of amino acid per 16 000 g of protein |
|---|---|---|---|---|---|
| Consesamin[11] | 545 | 0.40 | 2.86 | 0.60 | 127 |
| Conbrassin (M)[12] | 680 | 0.55 | 1.80 | 0.45 | 132 |
| Conbrassin (R)[12] | 622 | 0.56 | 2.05 | 0.40 | 149 |
| Conhelianthin[12] | 663 | 0.59 | 2.03 | 0.41 | 148 |
| Concarmin[13] | 478 | 0.45 | 3.13 | 0.55 | 146 |
| Congossypin[14] | 554 | 0.52 | 3.70 | 0.48 | 150 |
| Conpoppyverin[15] | 439 | 0.41 | 4.44 | 0.59 | 133 |
| Conlinin[16] | 535 | 0.49 | 2.69 | 0.51 | 144 |
| Ovalbumin | 1110 | 0.34 | 0.92 | – | – |
| HMW protein in oilseeds | 860 | 0.28 | 1.31 | – | $865 \pm 61^e$ |

a: Average hydrophobicity [3]. b: Frequency of nonpolar side chains [5, 3]. c: Ratio of the volume occupied by polar residues to that occupied by nonpolar residues [4, 3]. d: Frequency of polar sidechains [5, 3]. e: Amino acids per 1 000 000 g of protein.

Table 4: Secondary structure, intrinsic viscosity, molecular weight, fluorescence emission maximum and carbohaydrate conent of the LMW proteins from various oilseeds (nd: not detectable)

| PROTEIN | % Secondary structure | | | Viscosity | Molecular | Fluorescence | % Carbohydrate |
|---|---|---|---|---|---|---|---|
| | α-Helix | β-structure | Aperiodic | (ν) ml/g | weight | emission maximum (nm) | |
| Consesamin[11] | 35 | 45 | 20 | 4.10 | 15 000 | 336 | nd |
| Conbrassin (M)[12] | 31 | 44 | 25 | 5.40 | 15 000 | 334 | 1.8 |
| Conbrassin (R)[12] | 45 | 16 | 39 | 7.27 | 14 900 | 335 | – |
| Conhelianthin[12,17] | 36 | 40 | 24 | 7.28 | 14 600 | 333 | – |
| Concarmin[13] | 30 | 47 | 23 | 6.50 | 15 000 | 338 | 1.6 |
| Congossypin[14] | 32 | 41 | 23 | – | 16 600 | 334 | – |
| Conpoppyverin[15] | 35 | 56 | 09 | – | 16 000 | 332 | 3.1 |
| Conlinin[16] | 30 | 51 | 19 | – | 17 000 | 340 | 0.5 |

Tanford's free energy of transfer of amino acid side chain from an organic environment to an aqueous environment. In Table 3 is shown the average hydrophobicity, NPS, P and C values of LMW protein. For the purpose of comparison the data on ovalbumin, a typical globular animal protein, and the average value of HMW protein of oilseeds are also shown. These values were calculated as described in the above cited papers.

The analysis of hydrophobicity and other parameters indicate that except for conbrassin (M) most of the other LMW proteins have hydrophobicity index in the range of 550 calories/residue. This value is much lower compared to hydrophobicity value of 860 ± 50 calories/residue for the HMW proteins of various seed proteins as shown by Prakash and Narasinga Rao [2]. Also very similar to the HMW proteins the values of hydrophobicity index do not fit any portion of Biglow's plot of average hydrophobicity versus molecular weight [3]. The hydrophobicity index for the LMW protein indicates the general trend and may be related to the high content of α-helix and ß-structure in these proteins.

## 3. Secondary structure

The circular dichroic (CD) spectra of LMW protein in the far ultraviolet region are generally characterized by a minimum at 208 - 210 nm with a pronounced shoulder at 222 nm [1]. This empirically indicates rather high content of α-helix in the protein. Table 4 summarises the secondary structure of LMW proteins as calculated from CD curves. They all have nearly 35 % α-helix, and 40 % ß-structure; the rest being aperiodic structure. However attempts have not been made to calculate the number of ß-turns from the CD data. This highlights another important generality among the LMW protein that they all have very high α-helical content compared to very low α-helical content of HMW protein.

These LMW proteins have very low amount of proline in them, on an average nearly 5 residues per mole of the protein (for 16 000 molecular weight). Blake and Johnson [6] have classified most proteins into five classes based on their secondary structure. The MLW proteins fit into class three defined by them, that is α + ß proteins. On the contrary the HMW proteins has been shown not to fit into any of the Blake and Johnson classes of proteins as they are peculiarly rich in ß-sheet and aperiodic structure.

## 4. Intrinsic viscosity

The intrinsic viscosity values of LMW proteins in Table 4. The data is not available for all the proteins. However, with the available data it is seen that the intrinsic viscosity is between 4 and 7 ml/g indicating an extended structure based on Tanford's criterion for globular proteins and its relation to intrinsic viscosity. These data indicate that there is a general trend in the shape of the LMW proteins. On the other hand the HMW proteins are shown to be highly globular in shape [1].

## 5. Molecular weight

The determination of molecular weight of LMW proteins by several methods such as sedimentation-diffusion method, approach to equilibrium method and other routine techniques such as SDS-polyacrylamide gel electrophoresis, might be the main reason why one sees variation in the value of molecular weight from as low a value of 14 900 to as high a value of 17 000, (Table 4) eventhough the precision of these methods cover this range of values. With this background one can empirically conclude that these LMW proteins have a molecular weight of 16 000 ± 1 000. This analysis demands a more precise and thermodynamically sound method such as sedimentation equilibrium for the determination of molelcular weight for all the LMW proteins. The observation also indicates that the length of the polypeptide chain appears to be conserved as one sees from the average molecular weight point of view indication a structural similarity amongst LMW proteins.

## 6. Fluorescence

Fluorescence emission maxima of LMW protein is around 333 - 340 nm as shown in Table 4. The origin of fluorescence is very well established to be due to tryptophan residues in the protein, on an average nearly two tryptophan residues are present per mole of the protein assuming a molecular weight of 16 000. Eventhough on an average nearly 3 tyrosine residues are present per mole of the protein the fluorescence is predominantly due to tryptophan residues. It is well established that tryptophanyl fluorescence dominantes over the tyrosinyl fluorescence especially if they are present in equimolar quantities in a protein [7, 8]. Also it is shown that tryptophan or its amide in water has a fluorescence emission maximum around 340 nm [8]. The fluorescence emission maximum of LMW protein at 337 ± 3 nm indicates that most of the tryptophanyl residues are exposed to the bulk solvent. This is in conformity with intrinsic viscosity results of LMW protein which shows extended shape for the protein. The above results indicate that there is similarity in the location of the tryptophanyl groups in the LMW proteins.

## 7. Carbohydrate content

Compared to HMW proteins these LMW proteins contain higher content of carbohydrate in them (Table 4). It is not clear whether these are glycoproteins. It is quite possible that the carbohydrate moiety might be assisting in folding of the LMW protein [9, 10].

More work is needed in identifying the nature of carbohydrate residue and its precise function in the LMW proteins.

It is necessary to emphasise the need for more data of LMW proteins in terms of their behaviour towards specific proteases, effect of detergents and denaturants, subunit if any and the forces holding them. Only then one can conclude the existence of structural similarity amongst LMW proteins. It also needs to be emphasised that there is necessity for developing simpler and faster isolating techniques for LMW proteins in larger quantities to carry out indepth studies with regard to biophysical, biochemical and chemical properties of the protein. Such work is in progress in the authors laboratory.


References

[1] Prakash, V. and Narasinga Rao, M.S.; CRC Crit. Rev. in Biochem., **20**, (1986) 265 - 364

[2] Prakash, V. and Narasinga Rao, M.S.; J. Bioscience, 1988 in press

[3] Bigelow, C.C.; J. Theor, Biol., **16** (1967) 187 - 211

[4] Fisher, H.F.; Proc. Natl. Acad. Sci., USA, **51** (1964) 1285 - 1291

[5] Waugh, D.F.; Advances in Protein Chemistry, (Anson, M.L., Edsall, J.T. and Bailey, K., Eds.) Academic Press, New York, **9** (1954) 326

[6] Blake, C.C.F. and Johnson, L.N.; Trends in Biochem. Sci., **9** (1984) 147 - 151

[7] Shiffrin, S., Luborsky, S.W. and Grochowski, B.I.; J. Biol. Chem., **246** (1971) 7708 - 7714

[8] Teale, F.W.J.; Biochem. J., **76** (1960) 381 - 388

[9] Sharon, N. and Lis, H.; Chem. Eng. News. **59**, (1981) 21 - 25

[10] Sharon, N.; Trends in Biochem. Sci., **9** (1984) 198 - 201

[11] Rajendran, S. and Prakash, V.; J. Agric. Fd. Chem., **36** (1988) 269 - 275

[12] Schwenke, K.D., Raab, B., Uhlig, J., Tkocz, H., Behlke M., and Freimuth, V.; Die Nahrung, **17** (1973), 791 - 809

[13] Sridhara, S. and Prakash, V.; J. Agric. Fd. Chem., **35** (1987) 676 - 679

[14] Youle, R.J. and Huang, A.H.L.; J. Agric Fd. Chem. **27** (1979) 500 - 503

[15] Srinivas, H. and Rao, M.S.N.; J. Agric. Fd. Chem., **35** (1987) 12 - 14, ibid **29** (1981) 1235 - 1239

[16] Madhusudhan, K.T. and Narendra, Singh; Phytochemistry **24** (1985) 2507 - 2509

[17] Prakash, V.; Unpublished results

DYNAMIC LIGHT SCATTERING FROM HUMAN $\alpha$-LACTALBUMIN: COMPARISON OF MOLECULAR DIMENSIONS IN NATIVE AND DENATURED STATES

K. Gast[1)], D. Zirwer[1)], H. Welfle[1)], V.E. Bychkova[2)] and O. B. Ptitsyn[2)]

## 1. Introduction

The experiments which are reported here are part of extensive investigations with different methods directed to the problem of protein folding. The relevance of our results with respect to this general problem should therefore be discussed first.

The formation of a biologically active protein molecule comprises two important steps: the biosynthesis of the polypeptide chain and the folding of the chain into the native three-dimensional structure. It is an interesting feature of the folding process that the protein finds its native structure very quickly compared to the time necessary for a random walk search starting from the unfolded chain. This points to the existence of a particular folding pathway. Protein folding does not demand in general the presence of special biological factors and can thus be studied under in-vitro conditions. For in-vitro folding and unfolding experiments the reversibility of this process is an important demand.

Until now little is known about the pathway of folding. Some hypotheses and models exist from which we discuss the sequential folding model of Ptitsyn /7/. According to the sequential model, folding occurs in an unique and defined sequence of steps. At least three steps are to be considered:

(1) formation of a fluctuating secondary structure,
(2) merging of preexisting blocks with a secondary structure to an intermediate globular structure, and
(3) adjustment of this intermediate structure into the final specific native tertiary structure.

We consider here only the folding of small globular proteins.

To demonstrate sequential folding, it is essential to detect and to characterize intermediate states in the folding pathway. However, the intermediates must be stable enough and sufficiently populated compared to the unfolded and native states to be detectable. Furthermore, as most

---

1) Zentralinstitut für Molekularbiologie der Akademie der Wissenschaften der DDR, 1115 Berlin-Buch, Robert-Rössle-Str. 10

2) Institute of Protein Research, USSR Academy of Sciences, 142292 Poustchino, Moscow Region, USSR

of the physical methods which give structural information are time-consuming, especially equilibrium intermediates existing for a long time under defined conditions are needed. According to the present knowledge these requirements are fulfilled in folding experiments with some of the globular proteins, e.g. human and bovine α-lactalbumin (HαLA, BαLA), bovine carbonic anhydrase B (BCAB), ribonuclease A, and penicillinase. Essential characteristics of intermediates are: the amount of secondary and tertiary structure, the compactness, the conditions under which such a state exists, and how they can be transformed either to the native or the unfolded states and vice versa.
The aim of our work was the estimation of the compactness of an intermediate state called the 'molten globule' state which occurs in the folding and unfolding processes of HαLA. Reversibility was guaranteed under our conditions. The native state was chosen as an reference point. The investigations were done by measuring the hydrodynamic Stokes' radii of the protein molecules in the native, intermediate, and unfolded states using dynamic light scattering (DLS). Highly disordered and unfolded states are mainly found at high concentrations of strong denaturants such as guanidine hydrochloride (GuHCl) or urea, while other denaturating influences as high temperature, extreme pH, etc. leave some features of protein structure. The conditions used in our experiments are discussed later on.

## 2. Features of the intermediate state of α-lactalbumin molecules

First experimental evidence of the existence of an intermediate state was given for BαLA and HαLA by Kuwajima and co-workers in 1976 /3/ and 1978 /4/.They found by CD-measurements a three state unfolding transition upon GuHCl denaturation. The stable intermediate state at approximately 2M GuHCl is similar to the denatured state at low pH, called the acid or A-form. Further extensive investigations were performed by Ptitsyn and co-workers /2/. According to the experimental findings denatured states produced by acid pH (A-form), 2M GuHCl, and also thermal melting are very similar. They exhibit qualitatively the same properties: no specific tertiary structure but a secondary structure, which is similar to that of the native protein.
This behaviour is well demonstrated by the CD spectra shown in fig. 1 (data from Dolgikh et al /2/)for the native (——), the acid (---), the temperature denatured (-·-·-), and unfolded (— —) forms. In the spectral range between 200 nm and 230 nm (fig. 1a) which reflects the secondary structure, the CD spectra of the A-form and the temperature denatured form are similar to the spectrum of the native form. In contrast, in the aromatic region (fig. 1b) the CD spectra of both the acid and temperature denatured forms are drastically reduced similar to the spectrum of the

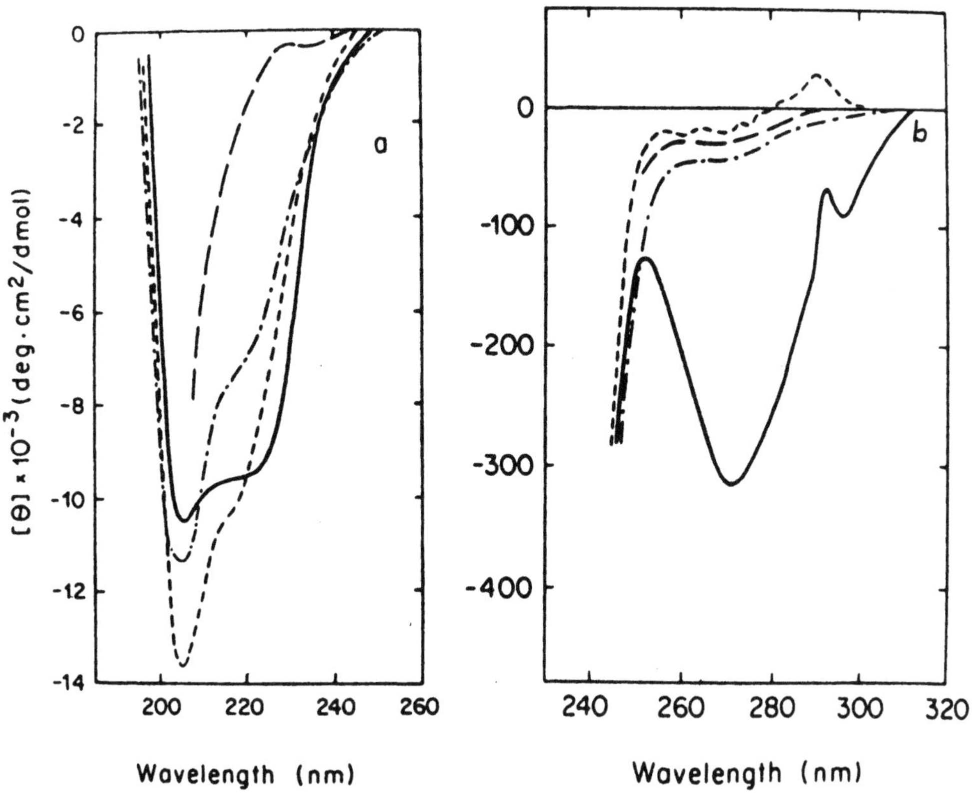


Fig. 1 CD spectra in the far UV region (a) and the near UV region (b) for the native (————), the acid (----), the temperature denatured (-·-·-) and the unfolded (— — —) forms.

unfolded form, pointing to a loss of the specific tertiary structure. The latter fact led initially to the assumption of a rather expanded intermediate state (Kuwajima 1976 /3/). This was not confirmed later on. Measurements of the dimensions and the compactness are therefore essential to the understanding of the physical nature of this intermediate state.

A further important feature of the A-form is the absence of any cooperative transition upon heating in scanning calorimetry. This was shown by Pfeil et al. /5/ in comparison with the melting of native HαLA. These results and the fact that the temperature denatured form of HαLA belongs to the same intermediate state allows the conclusion that the cooperative temperature melting of small globular proteins is not due to the unfolding of the chain but due to the destruction of the specific tertiary structure.

### 3. Estimation of the dimensions by DLS

The DLS measurements were done using a laboratory-built apparatus consisting of an argon laser operating at a wavelength $\lambda$ = 514.5 nm and a single clipped correlator, which calculates the time-autocorrelation function of the scattered light intensity, measured at a scattering angle of 90 deg.. The translational diffusion coefficients and the corresponding Stokes' radii of the protein molecules were derived from the autocorrelation functions performing an inverse Laplace transformation with the program CONTIN of Provencher /6/.
Depending on the conditions specified in table 1, different states of

Table 1: Human $\alpha$-lactalbumin: buffer conditions

| Form | Buffer |
|---|---|
| Native | 20 mM Tris-HCl, pH 7.5, 1 mM $CaCl_2$ |
| $Ca^{2+}$-free | 20 mM Tris-HCl, pH 7.5, 10 mM EDTA |
| Acid | 50 mM KCl-HCl, pH 2.0 |
| Unfolded | 20 mM Tris-HCl, pH 7.5, 6 M guanidine hydrochloride |

H$\alpha$LA were obtained. The acid form was investigated at pH 2 and the unfolded form in 6M GuHCl. $\alpha$-lactalbumin is a Ca-binding protein. The native form was therefore studied in the presence of $CaCl_2$. The removal of Ca by EDTA does not lead to a conformational change but decreases the stability of the protein shifting the midpoint of melting from 65°C to 30°C. For technical convenience the DLS studies of the temperature denaturation were performed with the Ca-free apo-protein. The results of the DLS measurements are summarized in fig. 2. The native and the unfolded forms were investigated at 20°C, whereas for the acid and the Ca-free forms a temperature dependence between 4°C and 50°C was recorded. The value of the Stokes' radius of the native protein is 1.77 nm. This is in rather good agreement with earlier data from the literature. The Stokes' radius of the Ca-free protein at 4°C is practically the same as that of the native protein. The change of the Stokes' radius between 10°C and 40°C reflects the thermal melting of the protein molecule. The temperature dependence of the Stokes' radius of the acid form is negligible within the experimental error.
The main result of our investigations is that both acid and temperature denaturation lead to an increase in the hydrodynamic effective dimensions of the molecules of only about 10% which is much smaller than the increase of about 40% at its unfolding by 6M GuHCl. The similarities

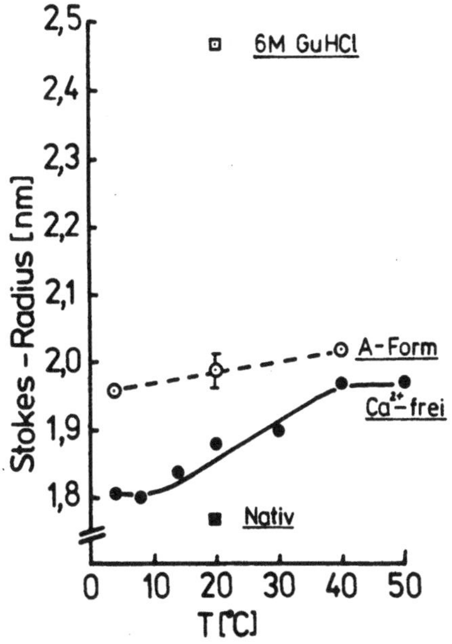


| Form | T[°C] | Stokes Radius R[nm] | $Q=\frac{R}{R_{Nat.}}$ |
|---|---|---|---|
| Nativ | 20 | 1,77 | 1,00 |
| $Ca^{2+}$-frei | 4 | 1,81 | 1,02 |
| " | 20 | 1,88 | 1,06 |
| " | 50 | 1,97 | 1,11 |
| A-Form | 20 | 1,99 | 1,12 |
| 6M GuHCl | 20 | 2,47 | 1,40 |

Fig. 2 Stokes' radii of different forms of H$\alpha$LA measured by DLS (the conditions are listed in table 1).

between the acid and the temperature denatured forms are also confirmed by our experiments. Hence, it is reasonable to consider these states as a special type of a folding intermediate, which was called the 'molten globule' state.

## 4. Discussion and summary

The results of the DLS experiments demonstrate that the 'molten globule' state found in the folding pathway of H$\alpha$LA is nearly as compact as the native state. It has no specific tertiary structure and, as revealed by NMR and deuterium exchange experiments, the intramolecular fluctuations are increased compared to the native structure. The state has a considerable secondary structure but exhibits no cooperative melting transition in scanning calorimetry. Evidence that a protein in the 'molten globule' state is essentially compact is also demonstrated by wide-angle X-ray scattering experiments of Damaschun et al /1/ who showed that the density of side goup packing in the 'molten globule' state (A-form) does not differ very much from that in the native state. The transition from the native to the 'molten globule' state can be considered as a first order phase transition. The important conclusion can be drawn that the cooperative melting transition found in protein denaturation is the destruction of the specific tertiary structure rather than the destruction of the secondary structure and the unfolding of the chain.

References


/1/ Damaschun, G., Ch. Gernat, H. Damschun, V.E. Bychkova and O.B. Ptitsyn: Comparison of intramolecular packing of a protein in native and "molten globule" states. Int. J. Biol. Macromol. 8 (1986), 226 - 230.

/2/ Dolgikh, D.A., R.I. Gilmanshin, E.V. Brazhnikov, V.E. Bychkova, G.V. Semisotnov, S.Yu. Venyaminov and O.B. Ptitsyn: α-lactalbumin: compact state with fluctuating tertiary structure? FEBS Lett. 136 (1981), 311 - 315.

/3/ Kuwajima, K., K. Nitta, M. Yoneyama and S. Sugai: Three-state denaturation of α-lactalbumin by guanidine hydrochloride. J. Mol. Biol. 106 (1976), 359-373.

/4/ Nozaka, M., K. Kuwajima, K. Nitta and S. Sugai: Detection and characterization of the intermediate on the folding pathway of human α-lactalbumin. Biochemistry 17 (1978), 3753-3758.

/5/ Pfeil, W., V.E. Bychkova and O.B. Ptitsyn: Physical nature of the phase transition in globular porteins. FEBS Lett. 198 (1986)2, 287-291.

/6/ Provencher, S.W.: CONTIN: A general purpose constrained regularization program for inverting noisy linear algebraic and integral equations. Comput. Phys. Commun. 27 (1982), 229-242.

/7/ Ptitsyn, O.B.: Stepwise mechanism of self-organization of protein molecules: Dokl. Akad. Nauk SSSR 210 (1973), 1213-1215.

# USE OF FLUORESCENT TECHNIQUES TO FOLLOW THE DENATURATION OF VICILIN, A STORAGE PROTEIN FROM VICIA FABA

S.D. Arntfield, M.A.H. Ismond and E.D. Murray[1]

## Introduction

In working with food proteins, especially plant storage proteins, there are problems associated with the assessment of conformational change. This is due to a lack of biological activity and difficulties in terms of solubilization. One technique which has been valuable in this respect is differential scanning calorimetry (DSC) as evidenced by the number of papers and review articles written on the subject. [1,2,3] However, a reduced $\Delta H$ value for the denaturation endotherm produced with this technique does not necessarily reflect a change in the conformation of the protein. Vital wheat gluten, for example, gives very small or no endotherms with DSC analysis. [1,4,5] This has been explained by a balance of exothermic and endothermic reactions [1] or a lack of long range order in the native gluten [5]. The presence of non proteinaceous components such as hulls, starch or oil can also influence the thermal properties without significantly altering the conformation of the protein. [6] For this reason, it is desirable to have a complementary approach for the assessment of conformational changes in food proteins.

There are several reasons for considering the use of fluorescent techniques and in particular, intrinsic fluorescence for this purpose. First, the technique itself should have minimal influence on protein conformation as all that is required for sample preparation is the addition of water or a suitable buffer. Secondly, the sensitivity of the technique is such that very low concentrations of protein are required, and solubility problems are minimized.

The use of intrinsic fluorescence with proteins is based on the fact that those amino acids which absorb light also emit that absorbed light at a longer wavelength. The fluorescence emission spectra of these amino acids consist of single bands with maxima at 282 nm for phenylalanine, 303 nm for tyrosine and 348 nm for tryptophan. [7] The fluorescence characteristics when incorporated into a protein, however, are not identical to those of the neutral solutions of free amino acids. In general, when a protein contains only one of these three amino acids, the emission spectrum is characteristic of that amino acid. Quantum yield values (quanta emitted / quanta absorbed), however, tend to be lower due to the quenching effects of the other amino acid residues in the proteins. If only phenylalanine and tyrosine are present (e.g. ribonuclease), a characteristic tyrosine emission spectrum results. This is in part related to the low quantum yield for phenylalanine (0.04) in comparison to tyrosine (0.21). When all three amino acids are present, a characteristic tryptophan emission results. It is generally accepted that there is either quenching by the environment around the tyrosine residue or a transfer of energy from tyrosine to tryptophan so that tyrosine fluorescence is not observed. [7] This behavior has been noted in the presence of even a single tryptophan residue (e.g. human serum albumin). [8] The contribution that tryptophan actually makes to the observed spectrum, and hence the degree of energy transfer from tyrosine to tryptophan, can be determined by using an excitation wavelength of 295 nm where only the tryptophan residue will absorb light.

---

1). Food Science Department, University of Manitoba, Winnipeg, Manitoba, CANADA R3T 2N2

Interestingly, upon denaturation, this energy transfer relationship is altered such that the emission spectrum contains two distinct peaks at 306 and 353 nm, corresponding to tyrosine and tryptophan fluorescence, respectively. It has been observed that the wavelength of maximum emission for tryptophan shifts from 342 in a nonpolar environment (such as buried in the hydrophobic core of a protein) to 353 nm in a polar solvent such as water. As a result, there are several parameters associated with intrinsic fluorescence which can be used to assess protein denaturation. These include a) the appearance of an emission peak representing tyrosine, b) a shift in the emission peak for tryptophan from 348 to 353 nm and c) an increase in the quantum yield values. For practical purposes, quantum values are determined by comparing the absorbance and relative fluorescence values of a protein to those for the pure amino acids, for which quantum yield values. In this way, the values obtained will be corrected for variations due to different light sources.

One further variation on intrinsic fluorescence measurements is an assessment of the degree of polarization. This involves the use of a polarizing attachment which utilizes polarizing filters to adjust both excitation and emission light independently into either vertical or horizontal planes. The degree of polarization (P) can then by calculated using the following formula:

$$P = \frac{I_{vv} - GI_{vh}}{I_{vv} + GI_{vh}}$$

where I = relative fluorescence intensity, G is the grating conversion factor given by $G = I_{vh} / I_{hh}$, and the first and second subscripts refer to the vertical (v) and horizontal (h) positions for the excitation and emission polarization filters, respectively. This reflects the rotational freedom of the fluorescing group, which should be low in the native protein and increase as the protein unfolds. Increased rotational freedom is measured as a decrease in the degree of polarization.

**Fluorescent Properties of Native Vicilin**

Examination of the amino acid composition of vicilin reveals that it contains all three fluorescing amino acids at the following concentrations: phenylalanine - 5.82 g / 100 g protein [9]; tyrosine - 1.09 g / 100 g protein [9]; and tryptophan - 0.16 g / 100 protein [10]. Due to discrepancies in the literature as to the tryptophan content in vicilin, a value obtained using amino acid analysis following alkaline hydrolysis rather than a spectrophotometric technique has been adopted. Interestingly, the emission spectrum for vicilin obtained with an excitation wavelength of 274 nm is characteristic of tyrosine fluorescence (Fig. 1). This response would suggest a lack of tryptophan in the vicilin molecule. The emission spectrum resulting from excitation at 295 nm, however, contains two peaks, the first at 331 nm representing the Raman band of water and the second at 347 nm, typical of tryptophan fluorescence. It would appear that due to a combination of the relatively large size of vicilin (molecular weight = 158,000) and its low tryptophan content, there is no transfer of energy from tyrosine to tryptophan residues. Furthermore, the low quantum yield for tryptophan in this environment (0.034) compared to tyrosine (0.24) may account for the lack of a tryptophan peak when using an excitation wavelength of 274 nm. This dominance of tyrosine fluorescence in the native protein removes one of the parameters (appearance of a tyrosine emission peak) suggested as an indicator for conformational change. The lack of energy transfer, however, makes it possible to examine the behavior of the tyrosine and tryptophan residues independently simply be selecting the appropriate excitation wavelength (274 nm for tyrosine and 295 nm for tryptophan).

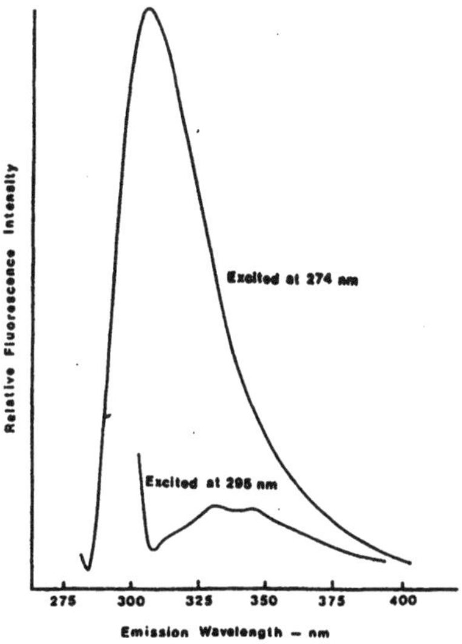


**Figure 1.** Fluorescence emission spectra of native vicilin obtained using excitation wavelengths of 274 and 295 nm. [10]

**Fluorescence Characteristics of the Tyrosine Residues in Vicilin in the Presence of Denaturants**

The addition of urea to vicilin results in a change in both the size and shape of the emission spectrum obtained using an excitation wavelength of 274 nm (Fig. 2). From these representative curves, it is clear that as urea concentration is increased, the relative fluorescence intensity for tyrosine emissions at 306 nm decreases and a second peak appears at 356 nm corresponding to the emission expected for tryptophan. The same trend has been observed for guanidine hydrochloride (GdnHCl), although the shoulder at 356 nm is much less pronounced. [10]

The decrease in relative fluorescence intensity in both denaturants reflects a decrease in the absorption of the sample analyzed due to protein dilution upon the addition of the denaturant rather than changes in quantum yield. In fact, the quantum yield values in urea are basically unchanged over the entire concentration range except for a slight decrease at 5.0 M (Fig. 3). With GdnHCl, the quantum yield values remain unchanged up to a denaturant concentration of 4.0 M, after which a slight increase is observed. It is possible that the expected increase in quantum yield has been counteracted by the quenching effect of the solvent. As a result, this parameter has little value in following protein denaturation.

Changes in the degree of polarization for tyrosine fluorescence are more informative. For both urea and GdnHCl, the effect of denaturant concentration on the degree of polarization divides these values into two distinctively different groups. For urea, values at concentrations greater than 4.0 M are significantly different from those below and with GdnHCl a similar change is noted at a concentration of 2.0 M. Due to the large degree of error in polarization measurements, only these general distinctions can be made. The change, however, does provide a measure as to when vicilin goes from a native state into a denatured state.

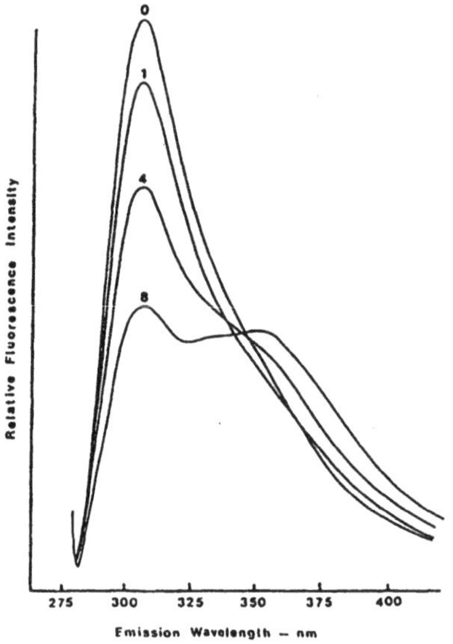


**Figure 2.** Effect of urea on the fluorescence emission spectrum of vicilin at an excitation wavelength of 274 nm. Numbers on the figure refer to the molarity of urea. [10]

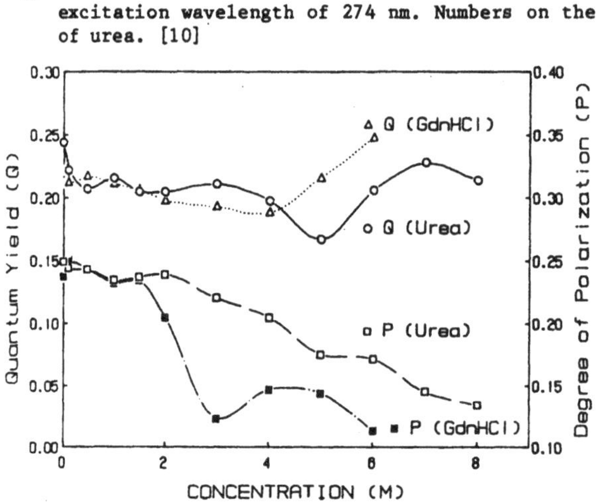


**Figure 3.** Effect of urea and GdnHCl on the fluorescence quantum yield (Q) and degree of polarization (P) of the tyrosine residue in vicilin.

**Fluorescence Characteristics of the Tryptophan Residues in Vicilin in the Presence of Denaturants**

The response of the tryptophan emission spectrum for vicilin excited at 295 nm, to the addition of urea is substantially different from that obtained by exciting at 274 nm (Fig. 4). In this situation, the relative fluorescence intensity increases with increasing urea concentration despite a decrease in absorption; as a result the Raman band for water is masked at higher urea concentrations. A shift in the wavelength of maximum emission is also evident.

Upon closer examination of these parameters, it can be seen that at urea concentration greater than 2.0 M, there is a gradual increase in quantum yield values

(Fig 5). At this same concentration, there is a shift in the wavelength of maximum emission from 345 to 353 nm. Moreover, there is no change in the degree of polarization for tryptophan until a urea concentration of 4.0 M; this is the same concentration at which there is a change in the degree of polarization for tyrosine.

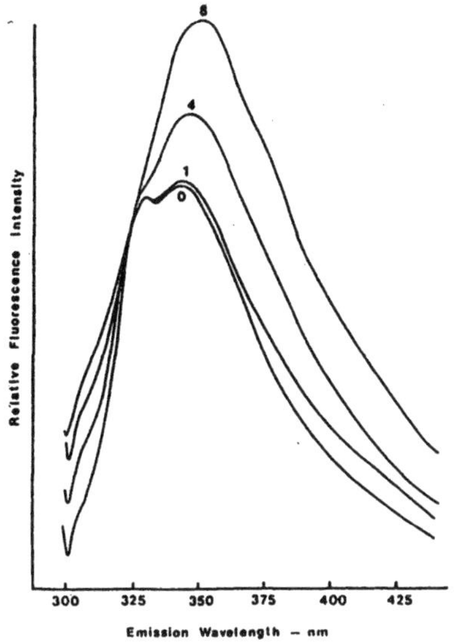


**Figure 4.** Effect of urea on the fluorescence emission spectrum of vicilin using an excitation wavelength of 295 nm. Numbers on figure refer to the molarity of urea. [10]

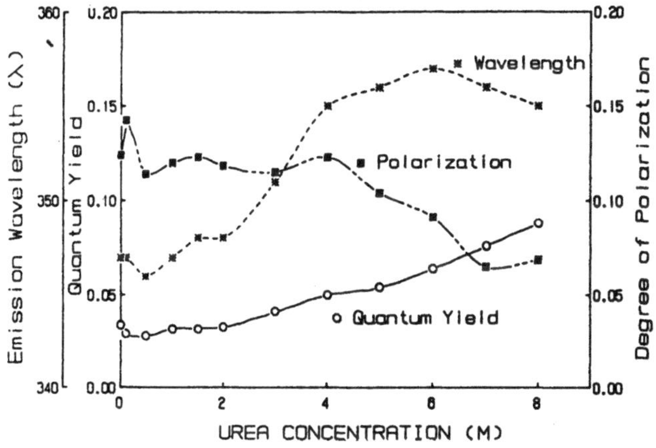


**Figure 5.** Effect of urea on the intrinsic fluorescent properties of the tryptophan residues in vicilin.

The effects of GdnHCl are similar, except the concentration required for changes of any given parameter are generally lower, suggesting GdnHCl is a more effective denaturation (Fig. 6). The increase in quantum yield is only slight with concentrations of 5.0 and 6.0 M GdnHCl required to give a significant change. At concentrations greater than 1.5 M, there is a significant increase in the wavelength of maximum emission, while concentrations greater than 2.0 M are required for changes in the degree of polarization.

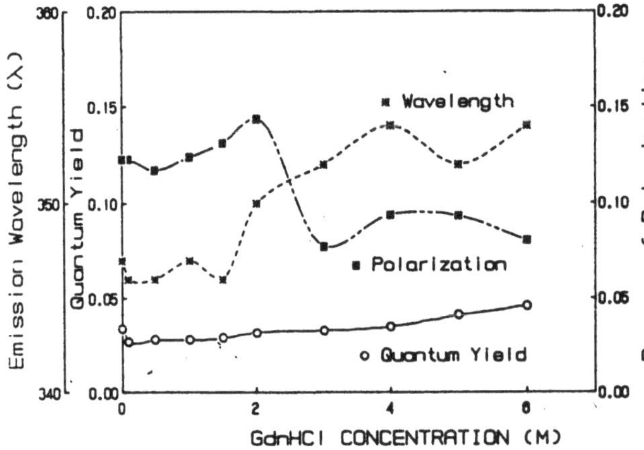


**Figure 6.** Effect of GdnHCl on the intrinsic fluorescence properties of the tryptophan residues in vicilin.

One noticeable difference between the effects of the two denaturants is the quantum yield response, where the increase with urea was considerably higher than that for GdnHCl. This exaltation of tryptophan fluorescence by urea has also been reported for the pure amino acid [8] and makes it questionable as to whether changes in quantum yield would be of value in assessing conformational changes in other environments. Changes in the wavelength of maximum emission as well as degree of polarization make it possible to detect major conformational changes for vicilin in both urea and GdnHCl. Interestingly, for both denaturants, the change in wavelength occurred at a concentration slightly lower that at which a change in the degree of polarization was observed. This observation, in conjunction with the gradual change in quantum yield values, supported the idea that vicilin denaturation is a progressive process reflecting the multisubunit nature of the vicilin molecule.

Overall, despite the low levels of tryptophan in vicilin, it is the fluorescence of this amino acid residue which makes it possible to use intrinsic fluorescence techniques to monitor conformational changes. Vicilin denaturation is characterized by an increase in the wavelength of maximum emission for trpytophan and a decrease in the degree of polarization; changes in quantum yield values are not as useful in this respect. It should be noted that changes in the degree of polarization for tyrosine are comparable to those for tryptophan when used to assess concentrations associated with major conformational change. The sensitivity of fluorescent techniques, which makes the use of low protein concentrations possible, can also be a cause of concern. The influence of solvent on the quantum yield values in this study was evident for both tyrosine and tryptophan fluorescence. The influence of temperature on fluorescence can also be quite dramatic; higher temperatures increase the loss of energy through vibration and hence quantum yield values and relative fluorescence intensities are low. As a result, there are situations when the use of a fluorescent probe may be of more value in following protein denaturation.

**Changes in ANS Fluorescence during Temperature Denaturation of Vicilin**

There are a number of fluorescent probes available whose properties change when they bind to hydrophobic regions of a protein. Both ANS (1-anilino-naphthalene-8-sulfonate) and cis-parinaric acid have been used to measure protein surface hydrophobicity. [11] In addition, ANS fluorescence has been used to follow thermal transitions of myosin [12] based on the concept that as the protein unfolds, the hydrophobic residues are exposed, so that binding of ANS increases as does the relative fluorescence intensity. Using a similar approach with vicilin subjected to a controlled heating regime, ANS was added to the sample at the desired temperature and cooled to room temperature prior to assessment of relative fluorescence intensity thus eliminating any problems associated with temperature effects.

For vicilin in 0.1M NaCl at pH 5.0, ANS fluorescence begins to increase at temperatures greater than 80°C and continue to rise with increasing temperatures (Fig. 7). This correlates well with the DSC thermal curve in that the first increase in relative fluorescence intensity corresponds to the Td value for the denaturation endotherm. There is also an interesting relationship between protein unfolding and the development of structure as demonstrated by an increase in the G' value (elastic modulus) determined using small amplitude oscillatory testing with a Bohlin rheometer. The increase in G' corresponds to the initial change in ANS fluorescence; it then levels off and then increase sharply as protein unfolding is completed.

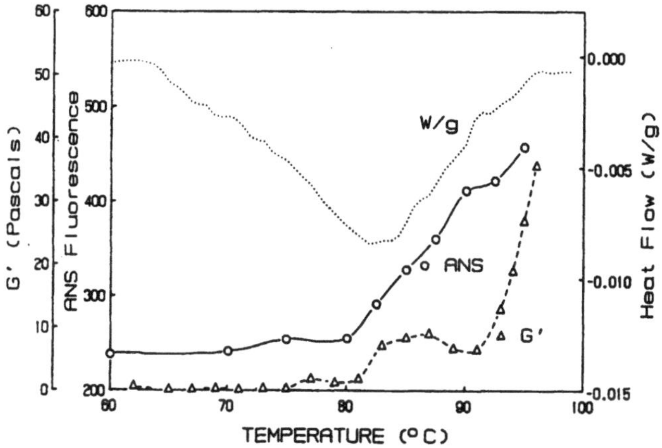


**Figure 7.** Relationship between DSC thermal curve (heat flow), ANS fluorescence, and structure development (G') as a function of temperature for vicilin at pH 5. Heating rate is 2°C/min.

An increase in the pH of the vicilin preparation to pH 9 changes the relationship between these parameters. Under these conditions, changes in ANS fluorescence correspond more to the onset temperature of the thermal curve rather than the peak temperature as was the case at pH 5. The ANS fluorescence appears to respond to the minor conformation changes at lower temperatures in this environment. Also, structure development was delayed relative to the conformational changes observed with ANS fluorescence and the DSC endotherm. A certain degree of protein unfolding appears to be required prior to structure development at this pH. The slight decrease in ANS fluorescence at temperatures greater than 90°C corresponds to the area of maximum structure development suggesting the hydrophobic residues necessary for ANS binding are buried during structure development.

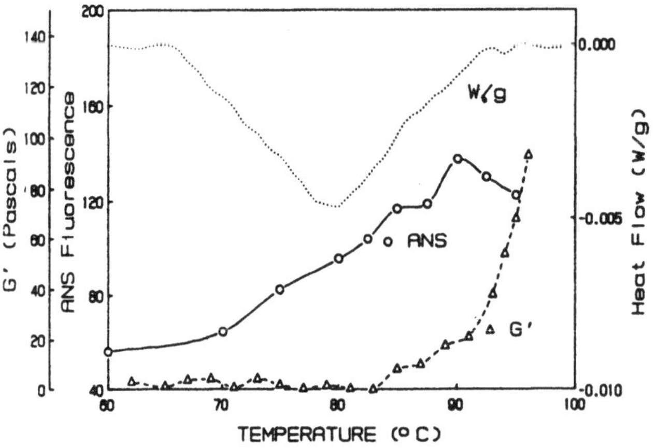


**Figure 8.** Relationship between DSC thermal curve (heat flow), ANS fluorescence and structure development (G') as a function of temperature for vicilin at pH 9. Heating rate is 2°C/min.

It can be seen, therefore, that the a fluorescent probe can be used to follow protein denaturation by monitoring the relative fluorescence intensity; this provides a good compliment to thermoanalytical techniques. When used in conjunction with other types of analysis, it can provide valuable information as to the relationship between protein denaturation and protein structure development.

**References**

[1] Arntfield, S.D. and E.D. Murray: The influence of processing parameters on food protein functionality I. Differential scanning calorimetry as an indicator of protein denaturation. Can. Inst. Food Sci. Technol. J. 14 (1981) 289-294.

[2] Biliaderis, C.G.: Differential scanning calorimetry in food research - A review. Food Chem. 10 (1983) 239-265.

[3] Wright, D.J.: Thermoanalytical methods in food research. Crit. Reports Applied Chem. 5 (1984) 1-36.

[4] Eliasson, A.C. and P.O. Hegg: Thermal stability of wheat gluten. Cereal Chem. 57 (1980) 436-437.

[5] Hoseney, R.C., K. Zeleznak and C.S. Lai: Wheat gluten; a glassy polymer. Cereal Chem. 63 (1986) 285-286.

[6] Murray, E.D., S.D. Arntfield and M.A.H. Ismond: The influence of processing parameters on food protein functionality II. Factors affecting thermal properties as analyzed by differential scanning calorimetry. Can. Inst. Food Sci. Technol. J. 18 (1985) 158-162.

[7] Brand, L. and B. Whitholt: Fluorescence measurements. Meth. Enz. 11 (1962) 776-856.

[8] Kronman, M.J. and L.G. Holmes: The fluorescence of native denatured and reduced-denatured proteins. Photochem. Photobiol. 14 (1971) 113-134.

[9] Ismond, M.A.H.: The role of noncovalent forces in food protein interactions - a study system using the legume storage protein vicilin. Ph.D. Thesis. University of Manitoba, Canada (1984).

[10] Arntfield, S.D., M.A.H. Ismond and E.D. Murray: Use of intrinsic fluorescence to follow the denaturation of vicilin, a storage protein from Vicia faba. Int J. Peptide Protein Res. 29 (1987) 9-20.

[11] Voutsinas, L.P., E. Cheung and S. Nakai: Relationships of hydrophobicity to emulsifying properties of heat denatured proteins. J. Food Sci. 48 (1983) 26-32.

[12] Wicker, L., R.C. Lanier, D.D. Hamann and T. Akahana: Thermal transitions in myosin-ANS fluorescence and gel rigidity. J. Food Sci. 51 (1986) 1540-1562.

# PROTEIN - PHYTIC ACID - METALLIC ION INTERACTIONS

Ljubomir Lásztity[1], Radomir Lásztity[2] and András Salgó[2]

**Abstract**

Similarily to some other polyphosphate compounds phytic acid bind strongly to proteins. The binding is electrostatic in nature and involves the anionic phosphate groups of phytate and the cationic groups of proteins such as arginyl, lysyl and histidyl groups. The ability of phytic acid to complex with proteins has been also the subject of investigations from several reasons but predominantly from chemical and nutritional point of view. In the presence both of polyvalent cations and phytic acid a formation of ternary phytic acid - cation - protein complexes is also possible. The formation of such complexes influence not only the nutritive value but also the functionality of protein systems, so it has also an importance from technological point of view.

Model systems containing proteins (glycinin, gluten proteins, sunflower seed globulin) phytic acid and polyvalent cations (Ca-, Mg- and Zn ions) were investigated. Formation of complexes and solubility of systems were investigated. The effect of pH was also controlled. All types of interactions (phytic acid - metallic ion, metallic ion - protein and protein - metallic ion - phytic acid) may be formed depending on the conditions and concentration levels.

Generally all the proteins to be investigated bind phytic acid at pH-values below the isoelectric point. The quantity of bound phytic acid is in good correlation with the number of cationic groups.

## Introduction

The ability of phytic acid to complex with proteins has been a subject of investigation for several reasons, but predominantly from chemical and nutritional point of view.

Recently the effect of phytates on the functional properties of protein concentrates and isolates were also studied. The phytate content of different legumes and cereals varies in a wide range. Some data measured in our laboratory are shown in Table 1. Depending on the conditions of processing the protein concentrates and isolates also contain phytates. In the Table 2 some data measured in our laboratory are collected.

[1]Department of Inorganic Chemistry, Eötvös Lóránd University, Budapest, Múzeum krt. 6 - 8., Hungary

[2]Department of Biochemistry and Food Technology, Technical University, Budapest, H-1502, Pf. 91., Hungary

Table 1: Phytic acid content of some cereals and legumes [g/100 g]

| Product | Phytic acid content* |
|---|---|
| Wheat [MV-4] | 0.85 |
| Wheat [Besostaya-1] | 0.93 |
| Wheat [durum, GK Basa] | 0.72 |
| Maize [yellow dent] | 1.02 |
| Maize [flint] | 0.90 |
| Maize [sweet] | 0.85 |
| Barley | 0.97 |
| Oats | 1.01 |
| Soybean | 1.43 |
| Cowpea | 0.42 |
| Common bean | 0.55 |
| Peas | 1.02 |

*Calculated phytic acid content assuming 28.20 % phosphorus in the molecule

Table 2: Phytic acid content of some protein preparations [g/100 g]

| Product | Phytic acid content* |
|---|---|
| Soy protein isolate | 0.82 |
| Soy protein concentrate | 1.81 |
| Wheat gluten [vital] | 1.90 |
| Sunflower seed protein isolate | 0.92 |

*Calculated phytic acid content assuming 28.20 % phosphorus in the molecule

Investigating from theoretical point of view the possible interactions of phytic acid and proteins first of all we must take in mind the structure of the phytic acid.

Having 12 dissociable hydrogens (protons) depending on the pH phytic acid has allways more or less negative charges. So in all cases if protein is also charged (pH below isoelectric point) a possibility of ionic interactions exists.

This is evident from several studies indicating involvement of lysyl, histidyl, arginyl and amino terminal groups in the formation of protein - phytic acid complexes. Formation of ternary complexes of phytic acid, bi- or multivalent cations and proteins is also possible. Finally an esterification of primary alcoholic groups (e.g. serine side chain) may not be excluded.

**Materials and methods**

Soy glycinin, gluten proteins, and sunflower seed globulin preparations were used in experiments. Phytic acid used in experiments was prepared according to the procedure described by Okubo et al. [1].

The binding of phytic acid controlled using gelchromatography on Sephadex G-75 columns or by turbidimetric titration using procedure of Okubo et al. [1]. $CaCl_2$, $MgCl_2$ and $ZnCl_2$ was used in experiments investigating effect of these cations in concentration range 0-20 mM. The quantity of ions coprecipitated or coeluated with protein was controlled using AAS technique.

**Results and discussion**

Glycinin binds phytic acid strongly below the isoelectric point of this protein (pH = 4.9). At pH values above the isoelectric point (pH = 6; pH = 8; pH = 12) no binding of phytic acid was observed. A decrease of solubility and precipitation was observed in the pH-range 2.0 - 5.5. The maximum quantity of bound phytate was 126 mol/$10^5$ g protein. This result is in good agreement with the number of cationic groups in the glycinin (calculated on the basis of amino acid composition) and also with data published by Okubo et al. [1].

Sunflower seed globulin showed very similar properties concerning the binding of phytic acid. This fact may be connected with the similar solubility of two proteins and some similarities in the amino acid composition.

The isoelectric point was found to be something lower (pH = 4.5) than that of glycinin. Phytic acid binding was observed in this case also only below the isoelectric point. The highest quantity bound by this protein was lower (90 equivalents of phytic acid per $10^5$ g protein).

Gluten proteins solubilized by AUC method were investigated only in acid pH region (pH = 2.0 - 4.0). The binding of phytic acid was much lower than in the case of two globulins. This fact may be connected with the lower quantity of cationic groups espcially in gliadin components. The maximum value of bound phytic acid was only 30 equivalents of phytic acid per $10^5$ g of protein.

All metallic ions $Ca^{++}$, $Mg^{++}$ and $Zn^{++}$ lowered the quantity of bound phytic acid at pH = 3. This fact may be explained with the observation that phytic acid forms chelates with metallic ions and so a direct competition between the ions and cationic groups of proteins occurs [1]. An other explanation may be that the ions form chelates with cationic groups of protein [2]. Both explanation are acceptable. The effect of $Zn^{++}$ is much greater probably because they form more stable complexes with phytic acid [3]. At lower metallic ion concentrations detection of both phytic acid and metallic ions in protein fractions separated at Sephadex G-75 column was possible. Isolation of phytic acid-metallic ion-protein complexes will be the next step of investigation.

**Literature**


[1] Okubo, K., D.V. Myers and G.A. Jacobucci; Cereal Chem. **53** (1976) 4, 513 - 524

[2] Barré, R., J. E. Courtois and G. Wormser; Ann. Sci. Fenn. Serie A2, **60** (1953) 104 - 112

[3] Láztity, Lj. and R. Lásztity; Periodica Polytechnica Chem. Eng. **32** (1988) (in press)

# INTERACTION OF PHYTIC ACID WITH α-GLOBULIN FROM SESAME SEED (*Sesamum indicum L.*)

Rajendran, S., and V. Prakash[1]

One of the major undesirable constitutent in sesame seed is phytic acid. It is generally present as its calcium or magnesium salt in the embroyonic tissue. It also plays an important role in influencing the properties of protein mainly due to electrostatic interaction [1, 2]. It also forms a stable insoluble complex with the protein. In sesame seed proteins which are heat labile, it is not clear whether the presence of phytic acid has any role in the coagulation process [3]. Hence it is necessary to study the influence of phytic acid on the properties of major protein fraction, α-globulin. This has been investigated in detail.

Several studies are available on interaction of phytic acid with proteins of rapeseed, soyabean, mustard and other oilseed proteins [4-12]. Also the interaction of proteins with polyphosphates has resulted in development of newer procedures for extraction of proteins from cottonseed, rapeseed and sunflower seed proteins [13 - 16].

The homogeneous protein α-globulin has been isolated and very well characterised for its physical, physico-chemical and biophysical properties under various solution conditions both from the hydrodynamic as well as spectral properties of the protein [17].

The present paper focuses a study of interaction of phytic acid with α-globulin, (phytic acid free), the major protein fraction of sesame seed. The investigation is ultimately aimed at developing rational methods for removing or lessening of phytic acid from edible protein meals such that they can be used for food purposes with better functional properties.

## Materials and Methods

Sesame seeds (*Sesamum indicum L.*) were obtained from local market. They are processed by the method of Prakash and Nandi [18] to yield a flour containing nearly 1 % fat and 50 % protein in it. All the chemicals used were of analytical reagent grade.

Sesame α-globulin was isolated by the method of Prakash and Nandi [18] using the above prepared flour. The final precipitate was dissolved in 0.15 M Glycine-HCl buffer of pH 2.3 and used for all the experiments.

[1]Biophysical Chemistry Unit, Food Chemistry Department,
Central Food Technological Research Institute, Mysore-570 013, India

Protein concentration was determined spectrophotometrically by using an absorption coefficient $E^{280nm}_{1\%, 1cm}$ of 10.8 [18]. Phytate was hydrolyzed by using 10 N $H_2SO_4$ and the inorganic phosphorus was estimated by the method of Taussky and Shorr [19]. Phytate concentration is expressed as phytic phosphorus.

The percentage of protein precipitation was determined at various phytate to protein concentrations by obtaining the $A_{280}$ reading of the protein solution with and without phytate. The $A_{280}$ reading of the supernatant after removal of the precipitate was used in calculating the percentages.

Sedimentation velocity experiments were carried out at 27°C in a Spinco Model E analytical ultracentrifuge at various concentrations of phytic acid in glycine-HCl buffer of 0.15 M, pH 2.3, at 59780 rpm in a Kel F cell at 27°C. $S_{20,w}$ values were calculated by the method of Schachman [20].

Fluorescence emission measurements were performed in an Aminco-Bowman spectrofluorimeter at 27°C with 0.01 % protein solution at 279 nm in presence of different concentrations of phytic acid.

## Results and Discussions

From. Fig. 1 it can be seen that the protein phytic acid complex precipitates. From pH 2.3 to pH 7.0 the precipitation was decreasing linearly with increase in pH. This is confirmed by the amount of phosphorus in the supernatant estimated as a function of pH as shown in Fig. 1 inset.

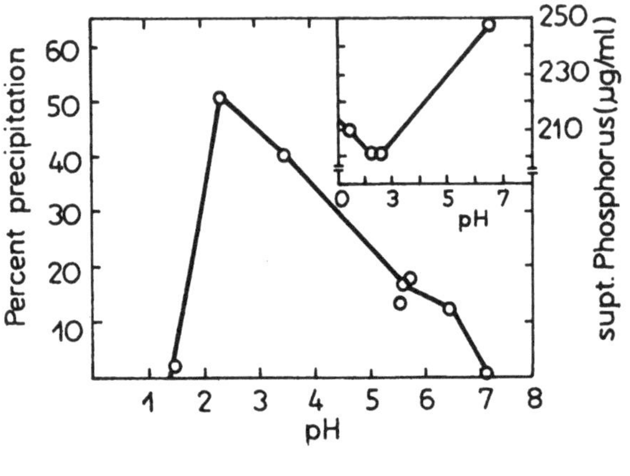


Figure 1: Effect of pH on percent precipitation of α-globulin at $1.8 \cdot 10^{-3}$M phytate concentration. (In set) Supernatant phosphorus in the precipitation mixture as a function of pH at $1.8 \cdot 10^{-3}$M phytate concentration.

The results indicate that between pH 2 and 3 there is minimum phosphorus in the supernatant indicating that most of it was bound to the protein. Unlike in mustard-phytic acid complex [12], the protein precipitate did not solubilize even at a very low pH.

These results may be explained in the light of observations made by Prakash and Nandi [21] of the effect of low pH on α-globulin. It has been observed that the dissociation and denaturation of α-globulin occurs at pH value around 3 [21]. At this pH value since the protein has got large excess of positive charge and the various binding sites are fully exposed, the binding of phytate at pH 2.3 would represent the total binding and can be correlated to the total number of basic amino acid residues present in the system. From Fig. 2 it is apparent that the curve can be divided into two regions, one up to a phytate to protein ratio of approximately 200 and rest of the curve above this concentration. As the phytate concentration increases it can be seen from the figure that the precipitation increases up to 30 % above which the amount of precipitate is constant with increase in phytate concentration. Above the phytate to protein concentration of 200 there is an increase in precipitation with increase in phytate concentration. From this result it can be concluded that the first phase of precipitation is mainly acountable by

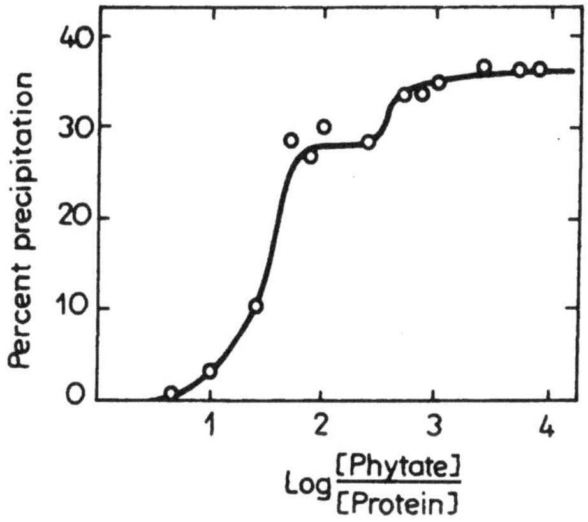


Figure 2: Effect of variation of total phytate concentration at constant protein concentration on the percent precipitation of α-globulin at pH 2.3

binding with nearly 200 basic groups in the protein. Above which not much significant precipitation is seen with increase in phytate concentration. This marginal increase in precipitation could be due to dissociation of protein leading to denaturation which might expose the remaining charged groups which might have been otherwise buried inside the protein.

In Fig. 3 is shown the effect of ionic strength on the percent precipitation of α-globulin at a phytic acid concentration of $10^{-2}$M and protein concentration of 10 mg/ml. From the figure it can be seen that wilth decrease in ionic strength the precipitation increases. This enormous difference could be possibly due to the competition of buffer ions with phytic acid. Also the interactions of buffer ions with amide dipole will be favoured at higher ionic strength making less of them available for the phytic acid to interact.

The effect of phytate concentration on the sedimentation velocity profile has been shown in Fig. 4. α-globulin which sediments as a single 11S component at pH 7.5 dissociates at pH 2.3 as shown in Fig. 4a. With the addition of phytic acid at $5 \cdot 10^{-5}$ M at constant protein concentration not much effect is seen in the sedimentation velocity pattern (Fig. 4b). Above this concentration, the protein dissociates and is entirely present as 2S component with concomittant binding of phytic acid as shown by earlier results. Above this concentration of phytic acid the sedimentation coefficient decreases further possibly due to conformational changes of the protein.

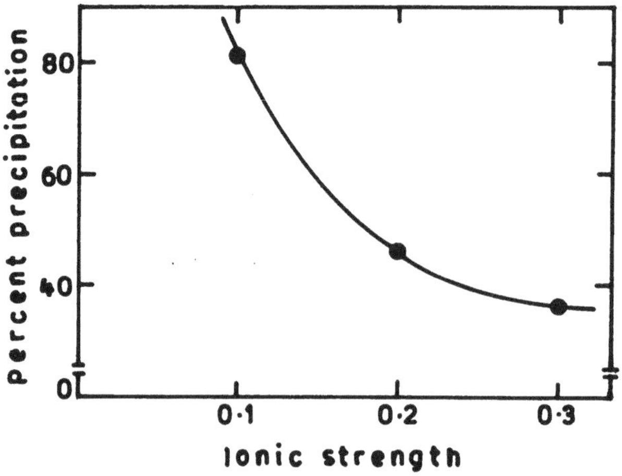


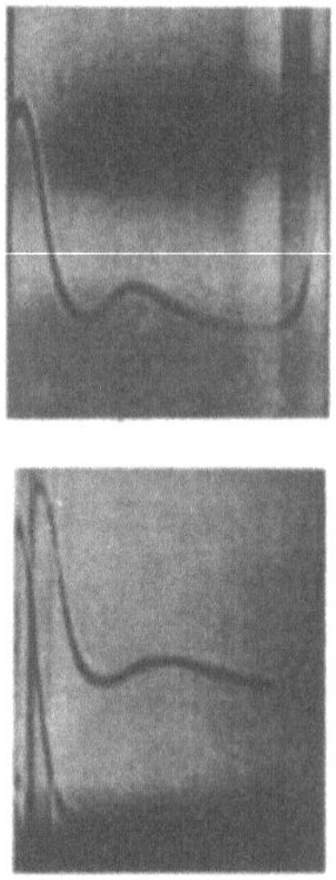


Figure 3: Effect of ionic strength on the percent precipitation of α-globulin at pH 2.3 and $1 \cdot 10^{-2}$ M phytate and $3.6 \cdot 10^{-6}$ M protein concentration.

Figure 4: Sedimentation velocity pattern of α-globulin (a) at pH 2.3 - control (b) upper - $5 \cdot 10^{-5}$ M free phytic acid concentration, lower - $5 \cdot 10^{-4}$ M free phytic acid concentration. Photographs were taken at 42 minutes after reaching two thirds of maximum speed.

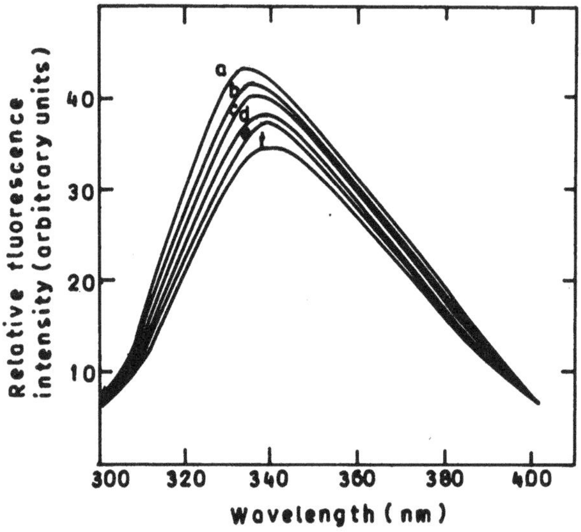


Figure 5: Fluorescence emission spectra of α-globulin (a) at pH 2.3 (b) $5 \cdot 10^{-5}$ M (c) $1 \cdot 10^{-3}$ M (d) $5 \cdot 10^{-3}$ M (e) $7.5 \cdot 10^{-3}$ M (f) $1 \cdot 10^{-2}$ M phytate concentration. The excitation was at 279 nm.

In order to follow the conformational changes in the protein as a function of phytate concentration, the fluorescence spectra of protein is followed and is shown in Fig. 5. With increase in phytate concentration two things are observed: (a) the decrease in fluorescence intensity and (b) a red shift in the emission maxima. These results indicate that the conformational status of the protein is changed due to binding of phytic acid to the protein resulting in the exposure of tryptophanyl groups to the bulk solvent which changes the fluorescence characteristics of the protein [21].

The above results indicate that the protein has an optimum binding below its isoelectric pH as a function of phytate and protein concentration resulting in dissociation of the protein to a 2S component. At higher phytate concentrations the binding induces conformational changes resulting in the exposure of chromophores.

Work is in progress with respect to monitoring the structural changes, binding isotherm, spectral properties and characterization of phytic acid facilitated dissociation, denaturation and aggregation of α-globulin.

## References


[1] Maga, J.A.; J. Agric Food Chem., **30**, (1982) 1-9 .

[2] Cheriyan, M.; CRC Crit. Rev. Food Sci. Nutrit. **13**, (1980) 297-335

[3] Lakshmi, T.S., Nandi, P.K., and Prakash, V.; Ind. J. Biochem. Biophys. **22**, (1985) 274-280

[4] Schwenke, K.D., Mothes, R., Marzilga, K., Borowska, J., and Kozlowska, H.; Die Nahrung, **31**, (1987) 1001-1014

[5] Gillberg, L., and Tornell, B.; J. Food Sci., **41**, (1976) 1063-1069

[6] Schwenke, K.D., Elkowicz, K., and Kozlowska, H.; Die Nahrung, **23**, (1979) 967-970

[7] Saio, K., Koyama, E., and Watanabe, T.; Agr. Biol. Chem., **31**, 819679 1195-1200, ibid 32, (1968) 448-452

[8] Saio, K., Koyama, E., Yamazaki, B., and Watanabe, T.; Agric. Biol. Chem., **33**, (1969) 36-42

[9] Okubo, K., Myers, K.B., and Iucobucci, G.A.; Cereal Chem., **53** (1976) 513-524

[10] De Rham, O. and Jost, T.; J. Food Sci., **44**, (1979) 596-600

[11] O'Dell, B.L., and De Boland, A.; J. Agric. Food Chem., **24**, (1976) 804-808

[12] Kishore Kumar Murthy, N.V., and Narasinga Rao, M.S.; J. Agric. Food Chem. **32**, (1984) 493-498

[13] Shemer, M., Mizrahi, S., Berk, Z., and Moady, S.; J. Agric. Food Chem., **21**, (1973) 460-462

[14] Thompson, L.U., Allum-Poon, P., and Procope, C.; J. Can. Inst. Food Sci. Tech., **9**, (1976) 15-19

[15] Schwenke, K.D., Raab, B., and Ender, B.; Die Nahrung, **19**, (1975) 935-939

[16] Gillberg, L., and Tornell, B.; J. Food Sci., **41**, (1976) 1070-1075

[17] Prakash, V., and Narasinga Rao, M.S.; CRC Critical Reviews in Biochemistry, **20**, (1986) 264-363

[18] Prakash, V., and Nandi, P.K.; J. Agric. Food Chem., **26**, (1978) 320-323

[19] Tausky, H.H., and Shorr, E.; J. Biol. Chem., **202**, (1953) 675-685

[20] Schachman, H.K.; Ultracentrifugation in Biochemistry, Academic Press, New York, (1959)

[21] Prakash, V., and Nandi, P.K.; Int. J. Peptide and Protein Res., **9**, (1977) 319-328

# INTERACTIONS BETWEEN SOYBEAN PROTEINS AND ANTHOCYANINS

A.S. Muntyan and I.A. Vaintraub

Soybean proteins being increasingly used for the fortification of fruit beverages and pastes, it is of certain interest to study their interaction with anthocyanins.

Soybean globulins are insoluble in water in the pH interval from 4 to 6. Under these conditions they bind the grape juice anthocyanins (Fig. 1). The latter are not extracted by acidified ethanol from the insoluble complex formed.

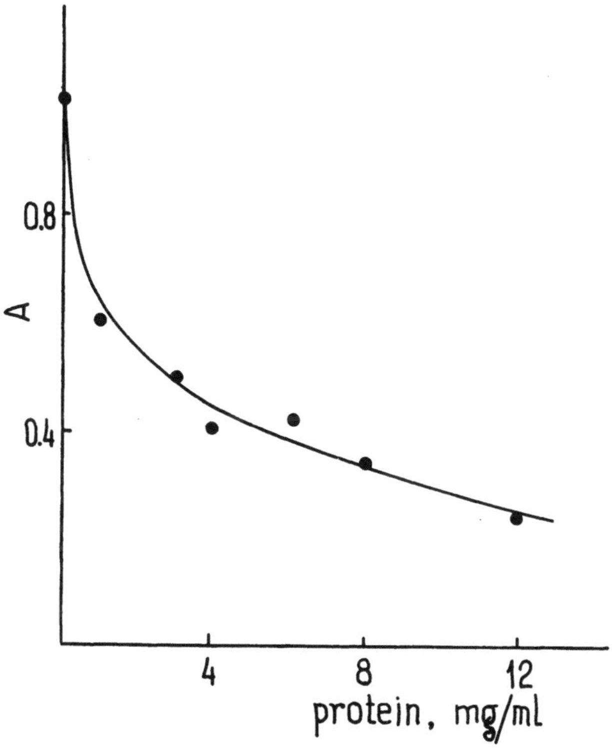


Fig. 1. Binding of grape juice anthocyanins to soybean globulins (decrease in anthocyanins absorption by added protein); pH 4.5

---

Laboratory of Protein Chemistry, V.I. Lenin State University of Kishinev, Kishinev 277014, U.S.S.R.

The interaction of the total preparation of anthocyanins extracted from the grape skin and purified by adsorption on talc /1/ with soybean 11S protein isolated according to /4/ was studied further at pH 2.0 where the 11S protein is soluble and the anthocyanins are mainly in cationic form. The protein-anthocyanin complex was separated from the excess of free anthocyanin by gel filtration on Sephadex G-25. The absorption maximum of the bound anthocyanin is flattened and shifted from 517 to 540 nm which is characteristic of quinoidal pseudobase form (Fig. 2). Probably the 11S protein which is positively charged at pH 2.0 binds only the neutral form and shifts the flavylium cation - pseudobase equilibrium. If it is true, the association constants determined below are apparent ones including the equilibrium constant between the cationic and neutral forms of the anthocyanins.

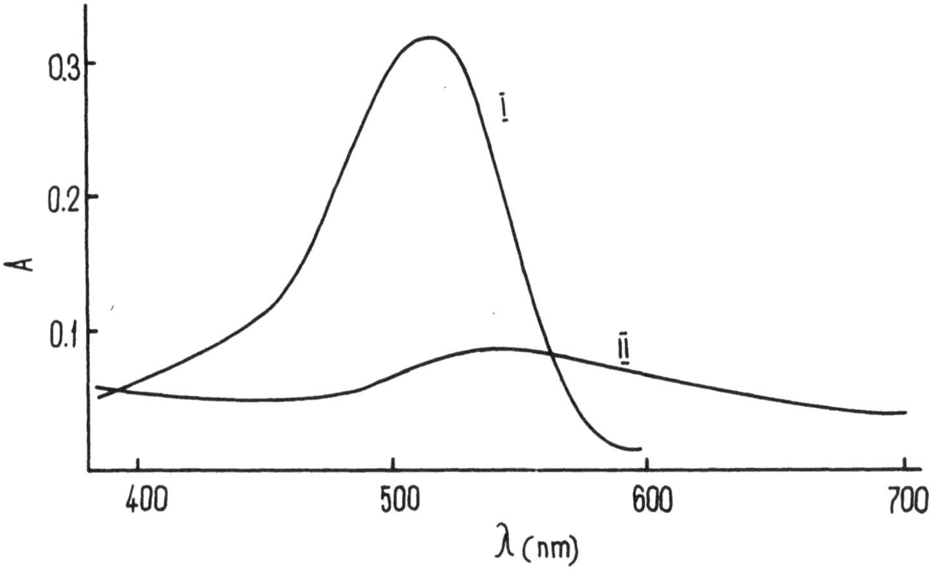


Fig. 2. Absorption spectra of free (I) and protein-bound (II) anthocyanins.

Association constants of the complex were determined by equilibrium dialysis method. 4-40 μM solutions of anthocyanins in 0.02 M KCl-HCl pH 2.0 were used. The protein concentration was 0.5 mg/ml. The three temperatures used in the experiment were 20, 30 and 40° C. The anthocyanin concentration was determined spectrophotometrically after acidification taking the value of molar extinction $E_{517}=5\cdot10^4$ /3/.

All the Scatchard plots obtained are linear (Fig. 3). Apparently the association constants of at least the main anthocyanins of grape differ but unsignificantly. This is supported by the coincidence of the Scatchard plots obtained at 30° C by the total anthocyanin preparation and individual anthocyanin (Fig. 3). The latter was isolated by repeated column chromatography on cellulose powder.

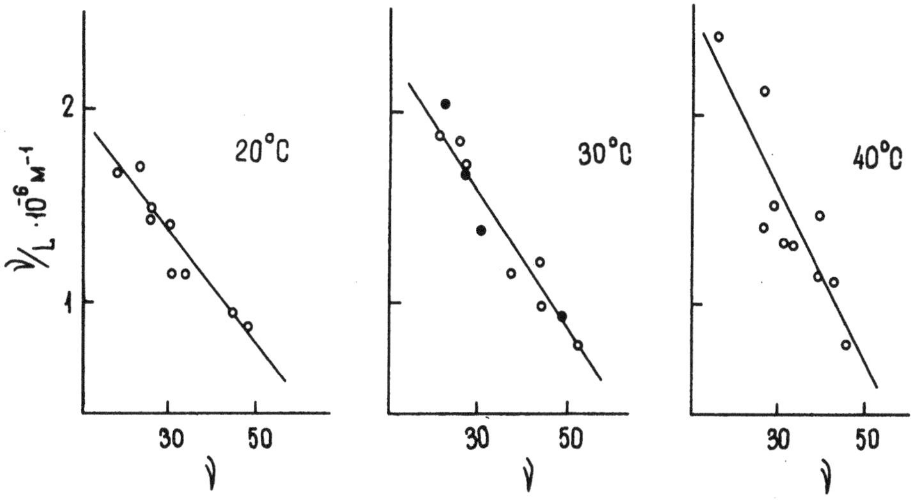


Fig. 3. Scatchard plots of soybean 11S protein - grape anthocyanins interaction.
o - total anthocyanin preparation; • - individual anthocyanin.

The number of binding sites calculated from the Scatchard plots is equal to 66-77. At pH 2.0 the soybean 11S protein is dissociated to six subunits /5/. Each subunit posseses, therefore 11-13 binding sites.

The association constants at 20, 30 and 40° C are equal to 31000± 4000, 38000±3000, 48000±9000 $M^{-1}$, respectively.

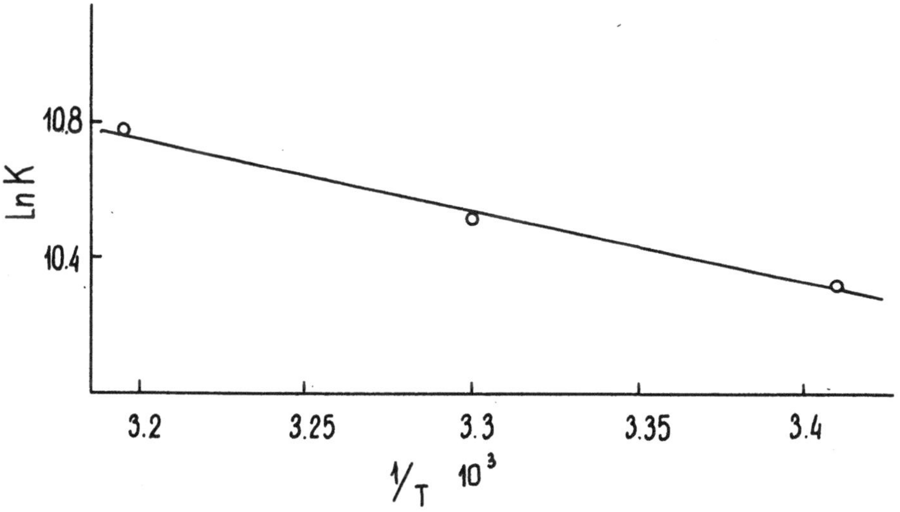


Fig. 4. Temperature dependence of association constants of soybean 11S protein and grape anthocyanins at pH 2.0 according to the Van't Hoff equation.

From the temperature dependence of the association constants according to the Van't Hoff equation (Fig. 4) the thermodynamic parameters of 11S protein-anthocyanins interaction were calculated. At pH 2.0 they were as follows: $\Delta G=-6.3$ kcal/mol, $\Delta H=4.2$ kcal/mol, $\Delta S=35$ eu.

The positive values of enthalpy and entropy changes indicate a process which is entropy driven, i.e. the hydrophobic binding of anthocyanins to soybean 11S protein.

## References


1. Bokuchava M.A., G.G. Valuiko and A.M. Filippov: Isolation of anthocyans from grapes and their study by means of IR-spectroscopy. Fiziol. Biochim. Kult. Rast.. 3 (1971) 2, 210-214.
2. Britton, G.: The biochemistry of natural pigments. Cambridge University Press, Cambridge 1983.
3. Fuleki, T. and F.J. Francis: Quantitative methods for anthocyanins. 1. Extraction and determination of total anthocyanins in cranberries. J. Food Sci.. 33 (1968) 1, 72-77.
4. Thanh, V.H. and K. Shibasaki: Major proteins of soybean seeds. A straightforward fractionation and their characterization. J. Agric. Food Chem.. 24 (1976) 6, 1117-1121.
5. Wolf, W.J., J.J. Rackis, A.K. Smith, H.A. Sasame and G.E. Babcock: Behavior of the 11S protein of soybeans in acid solutions. 1. Effect of pH, ionic strength and time on ultracentrifugal and optical rotatory properties. J. Amer. Chem. Soc.. 80 (1958) 21, 5730.

LEAF PROTEIN - CALCIUM ION INTERACTIONS

S.Gwiazda[1/] and K.Saio[2/]

## Introduction

In the preparation of leaf protein concentrates intended for human use, it is desirable to separate the soluble white proteins (cytoplasmic fraction) from the pigmented chloroplast membranes (chloroplastic fraction). The different methods suggested for separation of green and soluble leaf proteins from expressed green juice include ultracentrifugation, ultrafiltration, selective heat coagulation, the use of organic solvents or polyanionic flocculants followed by centrifugation.

In our previous work (Gwiazda and Saio, 1981) we sought the combination of calcium salts and mild heat pretreatment to improve the separation of chloroplastic fraction and increase the yield of white leaf protein concentrate (WLPC). It resulted in almost threefold increase of the yield of WLPC from Italian ryegrass. The present study deals with the influence of calcium salts on agglomeration of chloroplastic fraction and coprecipitation of cytoplasmic fraction as well as on the functional properties of Ca-treated WLPC.

## Materials and methods

Italian ryegrass and alfalfa were pressed with a screw press to provide green juice and press cake. From the green juice chloroplastic fraction was separated by: ultracentrifugation (160.000xg, 1 hr),heat treatment (to 60$^{o}$C) and centrifugation (10.000xg, 5 min.) or mild heating (39-43$^{o}$C) of calcium treated green juice |1.6 - 3.2 g Ca/dm$^{3}$| followed by centrifugation (10.000xg, 5 min.). From the chloroplast free juice the cytoplasmic fraction was precipitated by heating to 85$^{o}$C then washed and freeze dried.

Fraction I protein from alfalfa was isolated by the method of Jones and Mangan (1976). SDS polyacrylamide gel electrophoresis (SDS-PAGE) was performed according to Weber and Osborn (1969).

Water absorption capacity (WAC) and fat absorption capacity (FAC) were determined by centrifugation method (Gwiazda and Kocoń, 1979). Foam expansion (FE) and foam stability (FS) were measured according to Muschiolik et al., (1986).

1/ Agricultural University of Warsaw, Poland
2/ National Food Research Institute, Tsukuba, Japan

Results and discussion

The thermal precipitation of chloroplastic material from green juice in order to get edible cytoplasmic fraction (WLPC) is not highly specific. Heating of green juice at 56-60$^{o}$C - the temperature necessary to agglomerate chloroplastic fraction, results in precipitation of 20-40% of alfalfa soluble white proteins (Knuckles et al., 1980). Fractionation of Italian ryegrass green juice under these conditions has shown that more than 60% of soluble proteins are coagulated and separated as a part of chloroplastic fraction (Fig.1). Therefore, to obtain higher yield, suitable

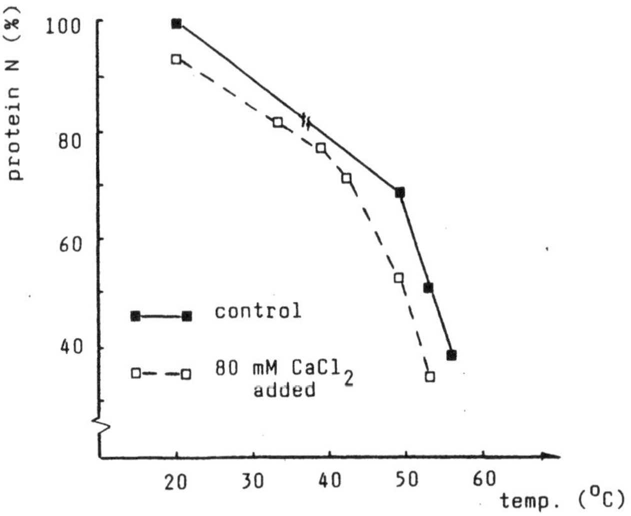


Fig.1. The influence of heating of Italian ryegrass green juice on the losses of cytoplasmic fraction. The chloroplastic fraction was removed by ultracentrifugation

conditions of the fractionation which allow to remove chloroplastic fraction at temperature lower than 60$^{o}$C have to be assured. This may be achieved for example by the addition of calcium chloride to green juice (Gwiazda and Saio, 1981). Although heating of Ca treated green juice caused higher losses of soluble proteins than untreated samples (Fig.1) the separation of chloroplastic materials from these samples was conducted already at 39-43$^{o}$C when 3.2 or 1.6 g Ca/dm$^3$ were added. The presented results indicate that under applied conditions soluble proteins are less Ca sensitive than chloroplastic fraction. This may come from different chemical characteristic of both fractions. Contrary to cytoplasmic fraction, chloroplastic fraction contains about 10% of fat and most of them (80%) is in form of polar lipids (Hudson and Karis, 1973). The result reported by Stifel et al., (1968) have shown that polar lipids actively compete with leaf proteins for Ca binding. Therefore addition of $CaCl_2$ to green juice may enhance aggregation through formation of intermolecular salt-bridging and as a result of this destabilization of the colloidal structure of chloroplastic particles would take place.

Interaction of $CaCl_2$ with soluble proteins of the chloroplast free juice allowed to decrease the coagulation temperature of cytoplasmic fraction from 85°C to 70°C at the same yield of the final product. Moreover, the results presented in Fig.2

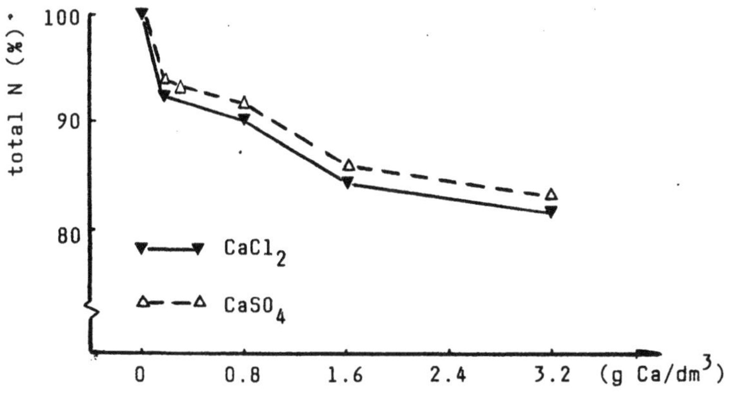


Fig.2. The effect of calcium salts on N substances remaining in whey during fractionation of Italian ryegrass

suggest that during the coagulation of cytoplasmic fraction, $CaCl_2$ remaining in the chloroplast free juice coprecipitates the low molecular weight nitrogenous substances. It was found that addition of calcium salts to green juice in the amount of 1.6 g Ca/dm$^3$ could additionally increase, due to coprecipitation, the recovery of N substances by 15%. This effect was not observed when lactone (GDL) was used (0.1 - 4.0%, pH=3.5) and there was virtually no difference in the amount of the N substances remaining in the resulted whey (heat soluble) of control and lactone treated samples.

Interaction of Ca ions with leaf proteins has improved not only the yield of WLPC but also contributes to its functional properties (Tab.1). The excellent foaming properties of Italian ryegrass WLPC, superior to

Table 1. Some functional properties of WLPC

| Raw material | Method | WAC ($g\ H_2O/g$) | FAC (g oil/g) | FE (%) | FS (%) |
|---|---|---|---|---|---|
| alfalfa | control | $5.1 \pm 0.2$ | $2.4 \pm 0.2$ | $225 \pm 10$ | $11 \pm 4$ |
| Italian ryegrass | control | $2.7 \pm 0.2$ | $1.0 \pm 0.1$ | $390 \pm 14$ | $83 \pm 8$ |
| | $CaCl_2$ | $3.3 \pm 0.2$ | $1.5 \pm 0.2$ | $341 \pm 8$ | $82 \pm 6$ |

alfalfa WLPC, may reflect higher content of low molecular weight proteins. On the other hand better water and fat absorption capacity that alfalfa WLPC possessed, are related to high molecular weight fraction I protein (Sheen and Sheen, 1985). Therefore, as a result of relatively high ratio of fraction I in Italian ryegrass WLPC prepared from $CaCl_2$ treated green juice (Fig.3) its superior absorption properties can be explained.

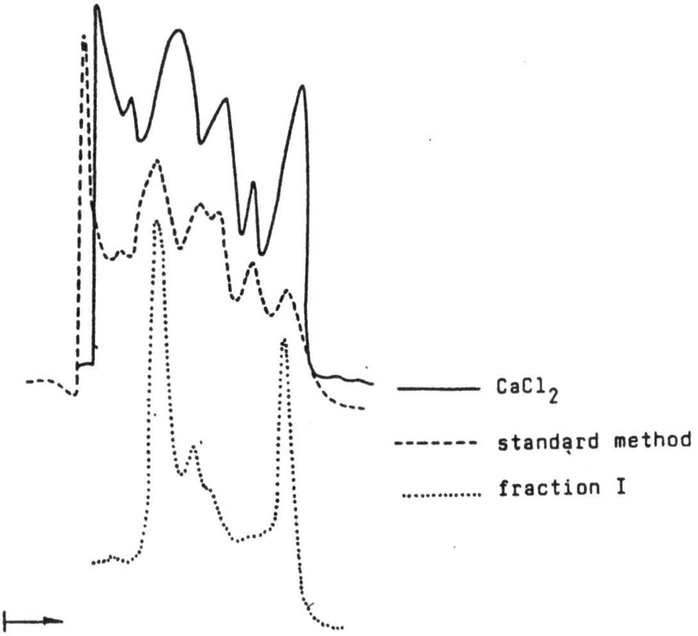


Fig.3. Densitograms of SDS-PAGE of WLPC prepared by standard method and with $CaCl_2$ as compared to fraction I protein

Literature


1. Gwiazda, S., and J.Kocoń: Acta Alim. Pol. 5 (1979), 71-80.
2. Gwiazda, S., and K.Saio: Agric. Biol. Chem. 45 (1981), 2659-2660.
3. Hudson, B.J.F., and I.G.Karis: J. Sci. Food Agric. 24 (1973), 1541-1550.
4. Jones, W.T., and J.L.Mangan: J. Agric. Sci. 86 (1976), 495-501.
5. Knuckles, B.E., R.H.Edwards, G.O.Kohler, and L.F.Whitney: J. Agric. Food Chem. 28 (1980), 32-36.
6. Muschiolik, G., H.Hörske, Ch.Schneider, M.Schultz, and H.Schmandtke: Nahrung 30 (1986), 431-434.
7. Sheen, S.J., and V.L.Sheen: J. Agric. Food Chem. 33 (1985), 79-83.
8. Stifel, F.B., R.L.Vetter, and R.S.Allen: J. Agric. Food Chem. 16 (1968), 500-505.
9. Weber, K., and M.Osborn: J.Biol.Chem. 244 (1969), 4406-4412.

# PROTEIN-METAL COMPLEXES AND THEIR DETERMINATION

E. Gábor[1)]

The homogeneous enrichement of different foodstuffs and fodders with micro elements is a very difficult problem because of the very small quantity of the enriching component. There is a possibility to diminish this problem by using organic metal compounds for this purpose. Their metal content can be regulated through the complex-producing process.

Our aim was to produce protein-copper complex compounds.

Milk proteins were reacted with a special copper-containing reagent.

The copper content of the protein-copper complex depends on the ratio of the milk and copper reagent.

These compounds have blue colours of different intensities. The complexes can be dissolved in various organic and inorganic acids and also in alkali solutions.

## 1. Production of the protein-copper complexes

The copper reagent consisted of 12,5 g of $Cu(NO_3)_2$ dissolved in 200 $cm^3$ of acetone.

Skimmed milk was used as protein source.

Various complexes were produced with different copper contents in the following way:

1. 50.00 $cm^3$ of milk were reacted with 0.50 $cm^3$ of reagent diluted with 1.50 $cm^3$ of acetone. 50.00 $cm^3$ of ethanol (96 v/v %) were used to complete the precipitation of the complex. It was filtered off and washed with aqueous ethanol (50 v/v %).
2. The reaction was carried out in the same way except for the quantity of the reagent: 1.00 $cm^3$ of copper solution and 1.00 $cm^3$ of acetone were used in this case.
3. 1.50 $cm^3$ reagent were diluted with 0.50 $cm^3$ of acetone.
4. 2.00 $cm^3$ of copper solution were reacted with milk.

## 2. Analysis of protein-copper compound

### 2.1 Protein content determination

This was carried out by UV-spectrophotometry (1., 2., 3., 4., 5.). 0.0500 g of the sample was weighed into a glass-stoppered test tube and

1)University of Horticulture and Food Industry
C.Faculty of Food Industry, Szeged

5.00 $cm^3$ of formic acid (98 v/v %) were then added to it. The reaction mixture was heated at 90 °C for 2 minutes. In this way a colloid solution was produced, wich was cooled and then diluted with 2.50 $cm^3$ of methylene chloride and 2.50 $cm^3$ of absolute ethanol. The light absorption of the resulting clear solution was measured at the absorption maximum, 277 nm. The spectrum of the solution can be seen in Fig.1.

Calibration measurements were necessary for the protein content calculations. Four samples with different protein contents were produced from the protein-copper (made by method 1./, and mixed with starch in different ratios. These samples were also analysed by the above-mentioned spectrophotometric method and by the Kjeldahl technique, too.

A calibration line was plotted (or a regression equation could be calculated) from the data.

The average protein content of the samples ranged between 48 % and 80 %, depending on the water content.

2.2 <u>Copper-ion determination</u>

The copper-ion of the complex was determined by spectrophotometry. 0.500 g of the protein-copper complex was weighed and transferred into a glass-stoppered test tube. It was heated with 4.00 $cm^3$ of formic acid (98 v/v %) in a boiling water bath for twenty minutes. After cooling 4.00 $cm^3$ of methylene chloride was added to it. The light absorption of the clear solution was measured at the maximum of the spectrum, 257 nm (Fig.2).

Calibration measurements had to be carried out for the calculation of copper content from the measured absorbance values. The protein-copper complexes were analysed in the following way. 0.500 g of the samples (with different copper content) were ashed. The ash was reacted with 5.00 $cm^3$ of $H_2SO_4$ solution (30 %) in a water bath for 10 minutes. The solution was filtered out in a 25 $cm^3$ of volumetric flask and the clear solution was filled up with $H_2SO_4$ solution (5 %).An aliquot quantity was determined iodometrically.

A calibration line can be plotted or a regression equation can be calculated from the data got by the analysis of the two methods.

The copper content of the samples produced by prescriptions 1.-4.moved from 0.20 % to 0.94 %.

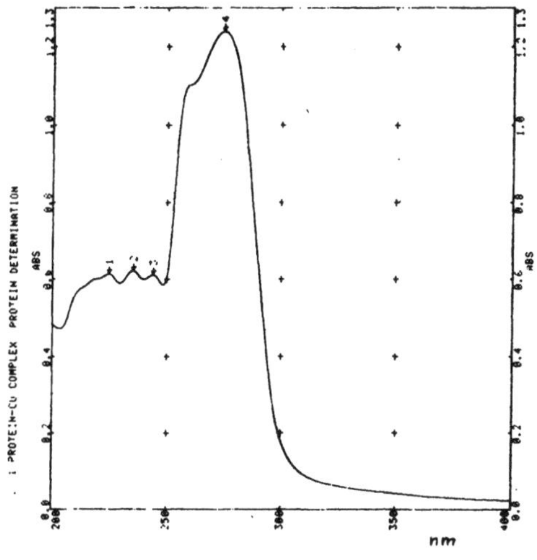


Fig.1. Protein content determination of protein-copper compound

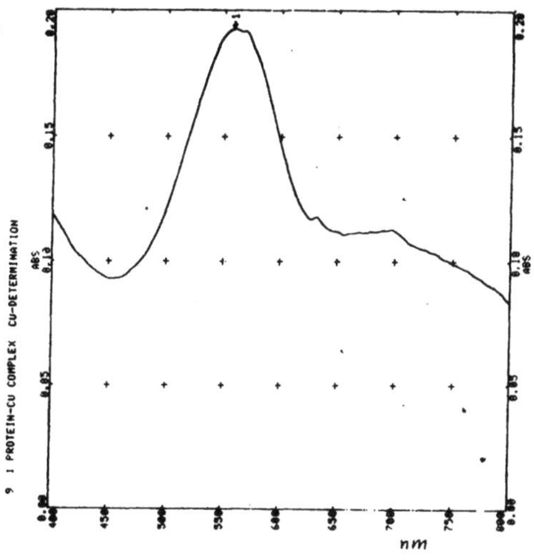


Fig.2. Copper content determination of protein-copper compound

## 3. Literature


(1) Kiermeyer, F.: Handbuch d. Lebensmittelchemie III/2, 989-998, Springer Verlag, Berlin-Heidelberg-New York, 1968.

(2) Wrigley, C.W. - Webster, H.L.: Spectrophotomteric estimation of protein in presence of ultraviolet absorbing impurities; J.Chromatogr., 33 (1968) 534.

(3) Gábor, E.: Determination of the protein content of certain meat products by ultraviolet absorption spectrophotometry; Acta Alimentaria 8 (1979) 157-167.

(4) Gábor, E.: Bestimmung des Eiweissgehaltes von Fleisch und Fleischwaren mittels Spectrophotometrie in ultravioletten Bereich; Fleisch, 37 (1983) 194-198.

(5) Gábor, E.: Applicability and advantage of spectrophotometry in food quality control; First European Seminar of WOQC Food Section May 26-28. Budapest, Hungary, Proceedings, (1986) 180.

# INTERACTIONS BETWEEN SINAPINE AND RAPESEED ALBUMIN. PRELIMINARY STUDY

K.J.Dąbrowski[1/] and K.D.Schwenke[2/]

## Introduction

The potential uses of rapeseed proteins are limited by the high cost of the process, associated with low yield and poor organoleptic quality i.e. bitter taste and dark appearance of the product.

Sinapine, major phenolic compound of rapeseed has been found as a bitter and astringent that contributes to unpleasant taste of rapeseed flour, concentrates (ISMAIL et al., 1981). Typical processes for flour, concentrate and isolate preparation gave products containing still 17-40% of initial phenolics content (DABROWSKI and SOSULSKI, 1983). It may be associated with binding of phenolics to proteins under processing conditions as has been proved in the case of sunflower.

The objectives of the present study were to isolate pure substrates i.e. albumin and sinapine from rapeseed meal and evaluate in a model system interaction between these two compounds.

## Materials and methods

Both substrates, albumin and sinapine (in form of sinapine bisulfate), were isolated from defatted double improved rapeseed meal by the methods of RAAB and SCHWENKE, (1984) and CLANDININ, (1961), respectively. Purity of albumin and sinapine was tested by gel electrophoresis and melting temperature measurements, respectively. Albumin was tested for phenolics presence by alkaline hydrolysis and TLC/UV detection DABROWSKI and SOSULSKI, (1984).

Absorption spectra of albumin, sinapine and albumin-sinapine reaction mixtures at weight ratio of 50:1 in standard Theorell-Stenhagen buffer were recorded in the range of 240-500 nm with a Beckman DU-6 Spectrophotometer in 1 cm cuvette. Albumin conc. was 0.5 mg/ml.

Fluorescence emission spectra of albumin, sinapine and their mixtures at weight ratio from 60:1 to 5:1 in the standard buffer were recorded with a Perkin-Elmer LS-5 Luminescence Spectrometer. Excitation wavelenght was 280 nm, spectra range 300-560 nm, albumin conc. 0.5 mg/ml, max. sinapine 0.1 mg/ml.

Reaction mixtures of albumin-sinapine were prepared as follows: to 5 ml measuring flask 2.5 mg of albumin and varying amounts of sinapine were added so that weight ratio of albumin to sinapine was from 60:1 to 5:1,

[1/] Agricultural University of Warsaw, Poland
[2/] Central Institute of Nutrition, GDR

and flask made up with standard buffer at pH 6; 8; 10; 12. The samples were vigorously shaken, emission and absorption spectra were taken after one hour and 18 hrs of reaction at room temperature, respectively. Based on fluorescence emission spectra, binding curve - $\Delta$F (difference in flourescence intensity between albumin and albumin-sinapine) as a function of sinapine concentration (C), and a Scatchard plot of sinapine binding to albumin - $\Delta$F/(C) as a function of $\Delta$F were drawn according to MURTHY and RAO, (1979).

## Results and discussion

### Substrates evaluation

Purity of albumin fraction as determined by gel electrophoresis was satisfactory, similarly as obtained by RAAB and SCHWENKE, (1984). Isolated albumin was free of phenolics since in its alkaline hydrolysate neither sinapic acid nor sinapine was detected by TLC separation and UV visualization. Crystals of sinapine bisulfate had a melting point of $187^{o}C$ which is in a good agreement with data of CLANDININ, (1961). Prior to study albumin-sinapine interaction, absorption and fluorescence emission spectra of separate substrates were taken. The albumin dissolved in universal buffer had similar absorption and fluorescence emission in acidic and in mild alkali range with max. absorption and emission at 280 and 332-336 nm, respectively (Tab.1). At pH above 11, a red shift in both spectra occured, which reflects ionisation of hyd-

Table 1. Wavelenght of maximum absorption and fluorescence emission of albumin and sinapine in the pH range of 2-12

| pH | Absorption maximum (nm) | | Emission maximum (nm) | |
|---|---|---|---|---|
| | Albumin | Sinapine | Albumin | Sinapine |
| 2-7 | 280 | 326 | 332 | 465 |
| 8 | 280 | 327<br>380 | 333 | 480 |
| 9 | 280 | 388 | 335 | 480 |
| 10 | 280 | 389 | 335 | 500 |
| 12 | 282<br>290 | 353 | 345 | 475 |

roxyl group of tyrosine. Sinapine exhibits an absorption max. at 326 nm at acidic range while values of 388 and 353 nm at pH 10 and 12 were obtained, respectively (Tab.1). At pH 8 two peaks at 326 and 380 nm were observed that can be associated with ionisation of hydroxyl group of sinapine. Fluorescence spectra of sinapine showed an emission max. at 465 nm in the acidic and 475 to 500 nm in alkali range (Tab.1).

### Reaction mixtures of albumin-sinapine

Absorption spectra of the reaction mixtures at weight ratio of 50:1 in the pH range of 2- 9 showed separation of albumin peak into two peaks at 283 and 290 nm, while at pH 10-12 albumin shoulder only was observed (Fig.1). Albumin added to sinapine in reaction mixture caused a blue shift of sinapine at pH 9 (323 vs 328 nm) and a red shift at pH 12 (382 vs 388 nm). Absorbancies of both compounds were higher in

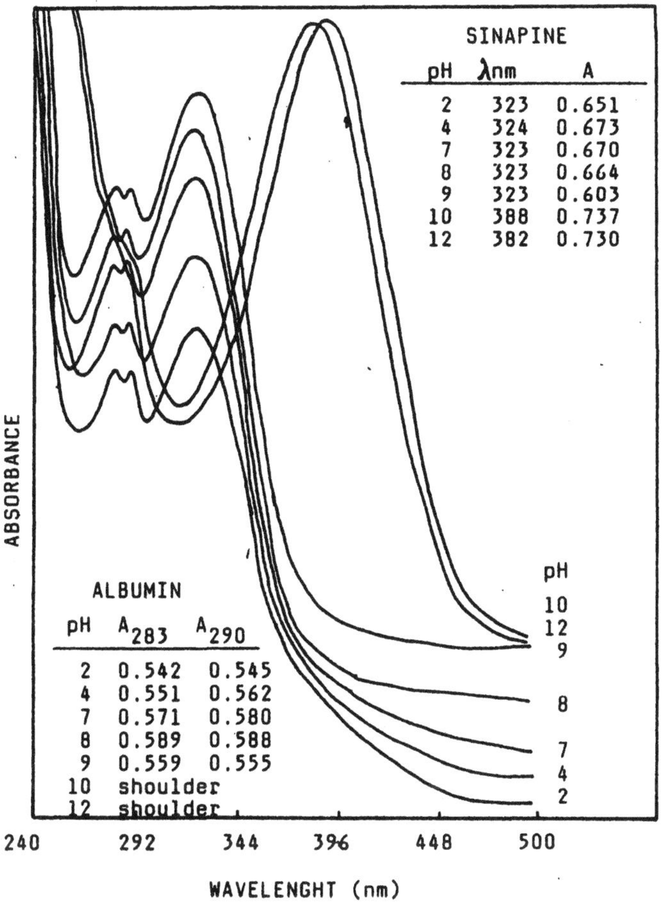


Fig.1. Absorption spectra of the albumin-sinapine reaction mixtures at weight ratio of 50:1 in the standard buffer solutions

reaction mixture than as measured separately at the same concentrations (Fig.1). Displacement of wavelenght of max. absorption of studied compounds in certain conditions may be attributed to interaction between them.

Fluorescence emission spectra of the albumin-sinapine reaction mixtures exhibited quenching effect, more stronger with increasing amounts of sinapine added to reaction mixture. First portions of sinapine added to albumin caused drastic decrease in fluorescence intensity of albumin while reaching albumin/sinapine ratio of 20:1 further quenching was low. Decreasing rate of quenching was in order of pH 6; 8; 12; 10 (Fig.2A). At the same time depending on pH a red (pH 6;8) or blue shift (pH 10; 12) was observed. A Scatchard plot of sinapine binding to albumin is shown in Fig.2B. Low slope value representing association constant indicate weak type of interaction between two examined compounds. Addition of 25 mM of sodium sulphite kept reducing environment thus rate of quenching was decreased while 1 M sodium chloride did not affect emission spectra.

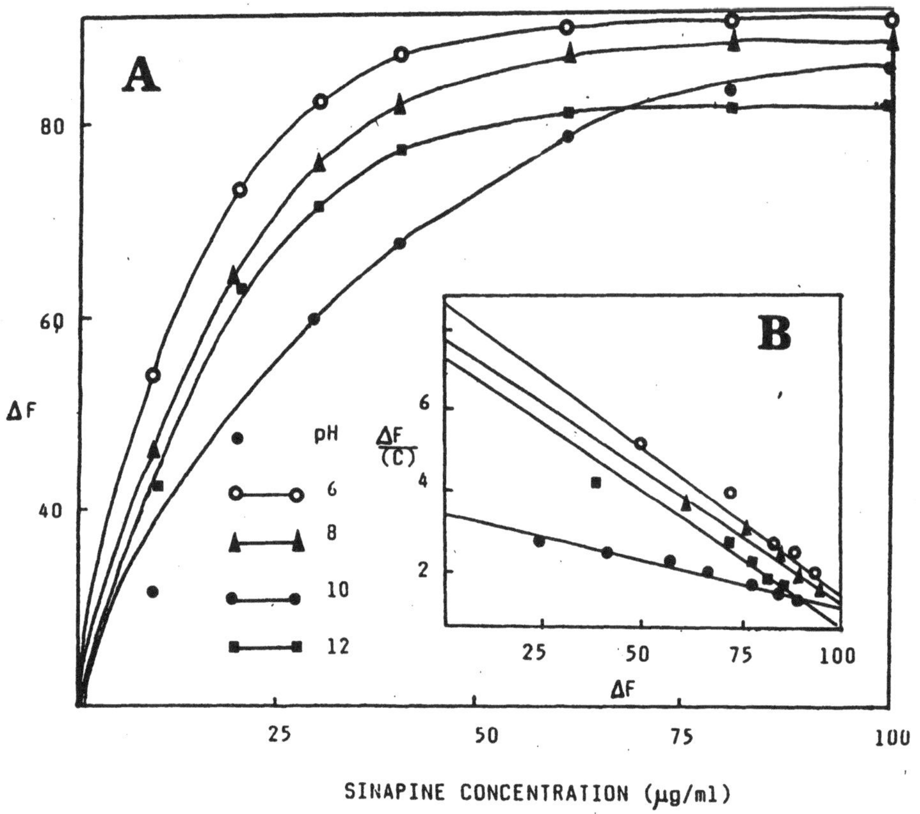


Fig.2. A. Albumin-sinapine binding curve
B. A Scatchard plot of the binding data

Using data obtained with fluorescence method, type of binding can not be established since free ligand is not separated and number of sinapine bound to albumin can not be determined. Classical method recommended for this kind of study is equilibrium dialysis (CREIGHTON, 1984), unavailable in this study. Further study is now underway using ultrafiltration for separation and quantitation of sinapine bound to albumin therefore described here data will be further discussed.

Literature


1. CLANDININ, D.R.: Poultry Science 40 (1961), 484-487.
2. CREIGHTON, T.E.: Proteins. W.H.Freeman and Company, New York 1983.
3. DABROWSKI, K. and F.SOSULSKI: Proc. 6th Rapeseed Conf., (1983), 1338-1342
4. DABROWSKI, K. and F.SOSULSKI: J.Agri.Food Chem., 32 (1983), 123-127.
5. ISMAIL, F., M.VAISEY-GENSER, and B.FYFE: J.Food Sci., 46 (1981), 1241-1244
6. MURTHY N.V.K.K., and M.S.N. RAO: J.Biosci., 1 (1979), 125-133.
7. RAAB, B., and SCHWENKE K.D.: Die Nahrung 28 (1984), 863-866.

# FLUORESCENCE STUDY OF SINAPIC ACID INTERACTION WITH PROTEIN IN MODEL SYSTEM

B. Smyk, R. Drebent

Academy of Agriculture and Technology
Institute of Physics and Food Chemistry,
Department of Physics
Olsztyn, Poland

Phenolic compounds present in the seeds of oleaginous plants lower the organoleptic quality of the protein concentrates produced from these seeds /1, 2/. So it is necessary to study the interaction between these phenolic compounds and proteins. The sinapic acid is one of the phenolic compounds, which exist in rapeseeds in high concentrration /3/.

The aim of this investigation was to determine the interaction of sinapic acid /SA/ with bovine serum albumin /BSA/ in a model system.

The absorption sepctra were measured using a spectrophotometer SPECORD M40 produced by Carl Zeiss Jena, and the fluorescence was measured using a typical apparatus of our own construction /4/.

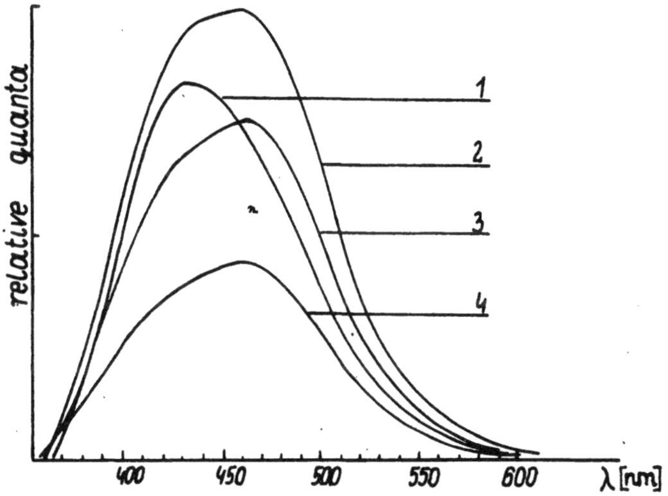


Fig. 1. The comparison of the fluorescence spectra of $SA^-$ /curve 1 - $C_{SA^-} = 10^{-3}M$/ with a few fluorescence spectra of SA + BSA /curves: 2 - $C_{SA^-} = 10^{-3}M$, 3 - $C_{SA^-} = 3 \cdot 10^{-4}M$, 4 - $C_{SA^-} = 10^{-4}M$/

Sinapic acid /SA/ produced by Fluka and bovine serum albumin /BSA/ purchased from the P.P.H. Polish Chemical Reagents in Gliwice, /albumin content ≥ 99%/ were used. The samples were prepared in the buffer of Britton-Robinson, pH 6.4. At this pH, SA occurs as a monovalent anion with carboxyl group totally dissociated /$pk_a$ = 4.47/ /4/.

The concentration of BSA in every solutions was $4 \cdot 10^{-5}$M, but the concentration of $SA^-$ in solutions with and without BSA varied from $8 \cdot 10^{-6}$M to $10^{-3}$M. The solutions were prepared by using dilution method /5/. The solutions of sinapic acid and protein with sinapic acid were excited with light at wavelength 333 nm /$\lambda_{max}$ of $SA^-$ absorption is 305 nm/ /4/. The corrected fluorescence spectra for 16 different concentrations of $SA^-$ in solutions with and without BSA were measured.

On the Fig. 1 the fluorescence spectrum of $SA^-$ /curve 1/ and a few fluorescence spectra of $SA^-$ + BSA solutions /curve 2 - 4/ are shown.

As it is seen from this figure the fluorescence spectra of $SA^-$ + BSA are changed with $SA^-$ concentration and a new fluorescence band appeares. This band is shifted toward longer wavelength and the fluorescence became more intensive compared with "free" $SA^-$. It indicates that monoanionic form of the sinapic acid interact with BSA. As a result of this interaction a fluorescent BSA-$SA^-$ complex is created.

REFERENCES

1. Sosulski, F., JAOCS 56, 711 /1979/
2. Kozłowska, H., Rotkiewicz, D.A., Zadernowski, R., JAOCS 60, 1119 /1983/
3. Zadernowski, R., and Kozłowska, H., Lebensm. - Wiss. u. - Technol. 16, 110 /1983/
4. Smyk, B., Drabent, R. "Spectroscopic investigations of the ionic forms of sinapic acid" /in preparation/.
5. Daniel, E., and Weber, G., Biochem. 5, 1893 /1966/

# THE DETERMINATION OF ELECTROSTATIC INTERACTION CONSTANTS OF PROTEINS IN SOLUTIONS

Vainerman E.S., Kurskaya E.A., Rogozhin S.V.[1)]

The study of electrostatic interactions between proteins is an important task in the isolation and purification of proteins and their conversion into food forms. The composition and a number of functional properties of protein electrostatic complexes can be changed in favourable direction by the variation of pH, ionic strength values, and molar ratio of interacting protein components. Due to the polyampholytic nature of proteins they can act as polycations or polyanions. Thus within the range of isoelectric points from 5 to 9 acid-process gelatin (A) and alkaline-process gelatin (B) possess opposite charges and can form electrostatic complexes of various composition and solubility. Unsoluble complexes were found to be neutral and soluble ones - to be charged [1]. Relatively low charge density of protein macromolecules results in low values of stability constants of protein electrostatic complexes. This hampers the use of nonequilibrium transport methods and also those methods, where high ionic strength and electrostatic potential are to be employed for quantitative analysis of electrostatic complex formation. For these purposes the equilibrium ion-exchange resin method can be applied. In case when the interaction process is described in terms of multiple equilibrium scheme [2], the association constants of complexes can be determined. This method was successfully used for the investigation of metal - ligands [3] as well as polyamine - nucleotide [4] interactions. The method is based on the following principle. The equilibrium of the ion-exchange resin with one of the two interacting protein components (acceptor) leads to its electrostatic adsorbtion. The distribution coefficient ($K_{d_o}$) is the ratio of acceptors' concentrations on the resin and in the solution. We shall call larger net charge density protein component an "acceptor". When oppositely charged second component (ligand) is added to the solution the partial desorption of the acceptor from the resin takes place as a result of electrostatic complex formation. This leads to the decrease of distribution acceptor's coefficient ($K_d$). Comparing $K_{d_o}$ and $K_d$ one can calculate the values of apparent acceptor-ligand association constants according to following equation:

$$K_{d_o} / K_d - 1 = k_1[B] + k_1k_2[B]^2 + \dots + k_1k_2\dots k_n[B]^n, \quad (*)$$

---

1) Institute of organoelement compounds of Academy of sciences of the USSR 117813 Moscow, Vavilova, 28, USSR.

where $K_{d_o}$ and $K_d$ - are resin-solution distribution coefficients of acceptor in the absence or in the presence of ligand B in the system,

[B] - is the concentration of free ligand,

$k_1, k_2, \dots k_n$ - are apparent association constants .

Polyampholytic nature of proteins and low charge density of their macromolecules practically exclude the possibility to employ the known types of ion-exchange resins in order to solve the problem in view. They didn't provide the reversibility and adsorption selectivity for acceptor. It was found that ion-exchange resins produced by immobilization of ligand possess the best properties. In order to study electrostatic complexation of A and B within the pH range 5-9, various types of ion-exchange resins were prepared: samples prepared by linking of the B with glutaric dialdehyde, or immobilization of B on activated aminoethylcellulose, or chemical modification of collagen.

The determination of $K_{d_o}$ and $K_d$ values was carried out by the following procedure. The certain quantity of the acceptor (A) and various quantities of the ligand (B) were added into the test-tubes to equal amounts of ion-exchange resin. The total volume of the system was constant. The necessary pH value was supported of by 5 mM phosphate buffer. After reaching the equilibrium by the shaking of the reaction for 4 hours and centrifugation of these mixtures the total quantity of A and B in supernatant was estimated. Since the ligand was not adsorbed by the resin, the adsorbed acceptor's quantity was estimated and $K_d$ value calculated. The $K_{d_o}$ value for the system without ligand was determined similarly from the acceptor's adsorbtion data.

Fig.1 illustrates the experimental curves of $K_{d_o}/K_d - 1$ as a function of mole ratios, P = ligand:acceptor. These curves characterise the process of the acceptor's desorbtion from the ion-exchange resin under electrostatic A-B complexation in the solution. In all the cases at $p < 1$ the curves had a linear character. This fact has given evidence to the formation of the only one type of soluble complexes in the system. By the method of approach to sedimentation equilibrium and turbidimetric titration B:A=1:1 composition of these complexes was determined [5]. For the case of equal concentrations of A and B associated in complex, the values of free concentrations of ligand (B) were calculated. This allowed to reconstruct the experimental plots yielded in co-ordinates $K_{d_o}/K_d - 1 = f[B]$ (Fig.2). According to these data and equation mentioned above (*), the values of apparent association constant $k_1$ in terms of the angular coefficient obtained from linear plots could be determined: for pH 6,8 in 5 mM phosphate buffer $k_1 = (4{,}95 \pm 0.37)\cdot 10^{-5}$M, for pH 5.5 in 5 mM phosphate buffer $k_1 = (4.00 \pm 0{,}28)\cdot 10^{-5}$M.

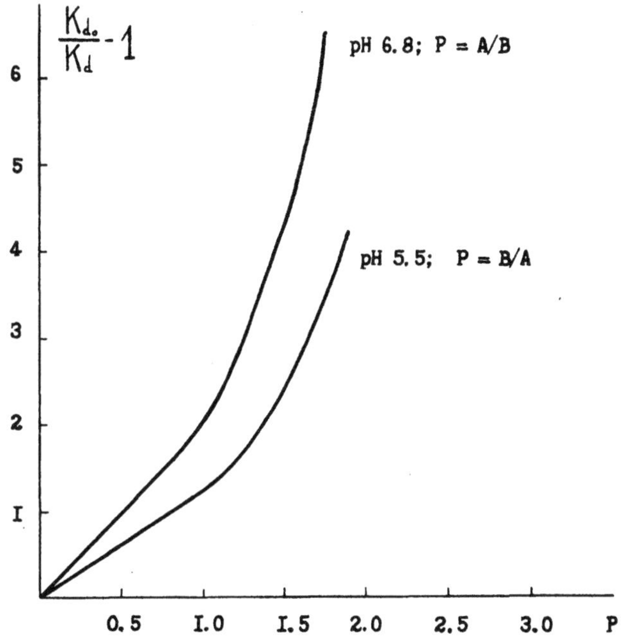


Fig.1. $K_{d_o}/K_d$ -1 versus mole ratios P= ligand : acceptor curves at different conditions (5 mM phosphate buffer, T=40°C).

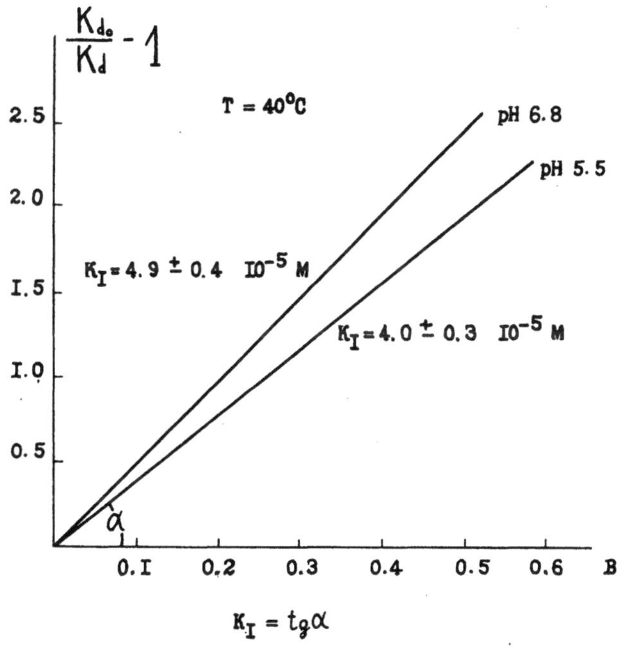


Fig.2. $K_{d_o}/K_d$ -1 versus free concentrations of ligand curves at different conditions (5 mM phosphate buffer, T=40°C).

Whithin the range of experimental mistake the variation of temperature from 20 to 40°C didn't practically affect the $k_1$ value, if the self-association of proteins under non-Coulombic forces had been suppressed by urea addition. The self-association process changed greatly the overall mechanism of electrostatic protein complexation as well as the values of association constants. As it is shown on Fig.1 the plots are rather curvilinear in the range of ligand concentrations higher than those of the acceptor ($P > 1$). This evidenced the formation of several types of protein complexes. The production and accumulation of neutral complexes ($AB_2$) led to their coagulation. The process of phase separation limited the application of the ion-exchange resin method for the investigation of A-B electrostatic interaction within the range of high mole ratio ligand:acceptor in the system.

Thus, ion-exchange resin method can be employed for the researching of electrostatic protein complexation and for the calculating of association constants in the initial stages only, when the process is determined by Coulombic forces.

The samples based on linked or immobilized ligands, when their ionogenic groups are less modificated, can be employed as most suitable ion-exchange resins.

REFERENCES

[1] Kurskaya E.A., E.S.Vainerman, S.V.Rogozhin: On complex formation of acid-process and alkaline-process gelatins. Nahrung. 26 (1979) 6,581-588.

[2] Vainerman E.S., W.Ya.Grinberg, W.B.Tolstogusov: Untersuchung der Wechselwirkung von Eiweissen mit Polysacchariden im Wassermedium. Kolloid Z. u. Z.Polymere. 250 (1972)10, 945-949.

[3] Nanninga L.B.: Formation constants and hydrolysis at 100° of calcium and magnesium complexes of adenosinetri-, di- and monophosphate. J.Phys.Chem. 61 (1957) 9, 1144-1149.

[4] Nakai C., W.Glinsmann: Interactions between polyamines and nucleotides. Biochemistry. 16 (1977) 25, 5636-5641.

[5] Kurskaya E.A., E.S.Vainerman, G.I.Timofeeva, S.V.Rogozhin. A study of soluble complexes of acid-process and alkaline-process gelatins by turbidimetric titration. Colloid polym.Sci. 258 (1980) 9, 1086-1091.

## HYDROPHOBICITY OF RYE AND WHEAT PROLAMINS DETERMINED BY SDS-BINDING

Noetzold, H. and E. Ludwig [1)]

### Introduction

The amphiphilic nature of proteins allows intra- and intermolecular hydrophobic interactions, which are responsible for many of their functional properties. A measure for such interactions is hydrophobicity, and attempts to predict properties of proteins from hydrophobicity have been made by a number of investigators. By experiment usually are only hydrophobic interactions of nonpolar amino acid residues on the surface of protein molecules approachabel. To determine a so-called surface hydrophobicity methods including fluorescence probe using cis-parinaric acid /3/ or 8-anilinnaphthosulfonic acid /1/, solubilisation of alkanes, hydrophobic partition method and hydrophobic chromatography /5/ are suitabel. Kato et al. /2/ suggest the determination of the surface hydrophobicity of proteins by using the dodecyl sulfate (SDS) binding method. According to the results of the above-mentioned authors, the SDS-binding capacity of proteins in the presence of extremely low concentration of SDS is proportional to the surface hydrophobicity determined by the fluorescence probe method using cis-parinaric acid.

### Objective

Since this method was suggested to be suitable for the determination of the surface hydrophobicity of insoluble proteins (protein systems) we attempted to determine the surface hydrophobicity of both rye and wheat prolamins and gluten by this method.

### Method according to Kato et al. /2/

Principle: In view of the interaction between SDS and protein, SDS was added to a protein solution (SDS-concentration $<$ critical micelle concentration). The SDS excess was removed and the bounded SDS was

---

1) Dresden University Technology, Dept. of Chemistry
DDR-8027 Dresden, Mommsenstr. 13

Table The nonmicellar SDS-protein binding by the method of Kato et al. /2/

| Protein | SDS-binding capacities (micrograms of SDS bound to 500µg of protein) | | |
|---|---|---|---|
| | SDS-binding in phosphate buffer published by Kato et al./2/ | SDS-binding in phosphate buffer own results | SDS-binding in 0.1N acetic acid own results |
| Ovalbumin 0.100% sol. | 1.4 | 0.5±0.2 | 4.3±0.3 |
| Ovalbumin 0.050% and 0.200% sol. | | 0.5±0.2 | |
| Ovalbumin 0,100% sol. heated 1°C/min from 20° to 80° | 3.1 | 2,3±0,3 | |
| ß-lactoglobulin 0,100% sol. | 6.0 | 5,9± 0.3 | 6,1±0,3 |
| ß-lactoglobulin 0.050% sol. | | 5.9±0.3 | |
| BSA 0,100% sol. | 9.7 | 10.0±0,3 | |
| BSA 0.050% and 0,025% sol. | | 13.5±0.4 | 16.6±0.4 |
| Rye prolamin Pluto/1985 0,10%, 0,20% | | 0,7±0.3 1) | 6.4±0.3 1) |
| Rye prolamin Pluto/1985 degreased 0,10%, 0,20% | | 0.6±0.3 1) | 6.2±0.3 1) |
| Rye prolamin flour usual in trade | | 0.8±0.3 1) | 6.8±0.3 1) |
| Gliadin Mironovskaja degreased | | 0,7±0.3 1) | |
| Gliadin Pilot degreased | | 0,7±0,3 1) | |
| Gluten Mironovskaja | | | 6.9±0.3 1) |
| Gluten Miranovskaja degreased | | | 6.7±0.3 1) |

1) no change after heating (1°C/min from 20° to 80°)

determined photometrically after reaction with methylene blue as a SDS-methylene blue complex.

## Results and discussion

The table shows the SDS-binding capacity of proteins investigated. For ß-Lactoglobulin, our values correspond to those of Kato et al. /2/ whereas those for BSA are somewhat greater and those for ovalbumin somewhat smaller.

We could show that the SDS-binding capacity under these experimental conditions is, in small limits, independent from the protein-SDS proportion.

The SDS-binding capacity of ovalbumin increased after heat denaturation. These results agree with those of Kato et al. /2/.

The SDS-binding capacities of the prolamins investigated are very small. There were no significant differences in the SDS-binding capacities of rye and wheat prolamins.

Changes in the SDS-binding capacities of prolamins during heat denaturation were not observed.

The method is well suitable for determining the SDS-binding capacities of proteins dissolved or homogenized in 0.1N acetic acid.

In the presence of 0.1N acetic acid the SDS-binding capacities increased with all proteins investigated, except ß-lactoglobulin.

In the presence of 0.1N acetic acid the SDS-binding capacities of rye prolamins, glutens and ß-lactoglobulin are approximately the same.

There were however, no significant differences in the SDS-binding capacities of rye prolamins, even in the presence of acetic acid.

There is no a reason to assume that the real surface hydrophobicity of prolamins in the presence of 0.1N acetic acid in comparison to phosphate buffer, pH 6.0, has greatly increased. For that reason we suppose that the interaction of prolamins with SDS in these experimental conditions is due to electrostatic bonds, too. Already Putnam and Neurath /4/ have studied the interactions between SDS and proteins. They observed that when small increments of SDS were added to solution of a pure protein the interaction was caused by electrostatic forces only.

Literature

/1/ Horiuchi, T., D.Fukushima, H.Sugimoto and T.Hattovi: Food Chem. 3 (1978), 35.

/2/ Kato, A., T.Matsuda, N.Matsudomi and K.Kobayashi: J. Agric. Food Chem. 32 (1984), 284.

/3/ Kato, A. and S.Nakai: Biochim. Biophysica Acta 624 (1980), 13.

/4/ Putnam, F.W. and H.Neurath: J. Biol. Chem. 159 (1945), 195.

/5/ Zawistowska, U., J.A.Bietz and W.Bushuk: Cereal Chem. 63 (1986), 414.

# FUNCTIONAL PROPERTIES AND CHEMICAL COMPOSITION OF CYTOPLASMATIC CONCENTRATES OBTAINED FROM ALFALFA JUICE

B. Baraniak, M. Bubicz and A. Baraniak[1]

The chloroplastic fraction of the proteins from alfalfa juice was coagulated with cation and anion flocculants (produced by Magnafloc). Cytoplasmatic proteins were obtained by the acid method in pH = 3.5. Protein content and its amino acid composition in cytoplasmatic preparation was dependent on the polyelectrolyte used in the process of fractionation of the juice. The protein in the examined preparation was rich in exogenous amino acids and was characterized by a high solubility in alkaline medium. The capacity for absorbing water in the obtained concentrates was high (150 - 200 %), whereas absorption of fats was low (30 - 40 %).

---

[1]Agricultural University, Dept. Chemistry and Biochemistry, 20-934 Lublin, ul. Akademicka 13, Poland

# DESIGNED PROTEIN MODIFICATION BY PROTEINASES

Gy. Hajós[1], A. Halász[1] and F. Békés[2]

The ability of proteinases to catalyse peptide bond synthesis has a historical background [1, 2] and has also awoke a great interest recently [3-7]. The enzymatic peptide modification (EPM ) proved to be a suitable enzymatic process to obtain protein product of designed amino acid composition. The reaction mechanism of this enzymatic process and the chemical nature of incorporation during EPM is, however, still not very clarified.

In this study methionine-enriched protein was produced from casein hydrolysate using an enzymatic peptide modification method. Methionine content of casein, casein-hydrolysate and product of the enzymatic peptide modification are summarised in Table 1. Methionine content in the EPM-product was found to be more than twice as much as that of the substrate protein.

Table 1: Methionine content of the samples

| Sample | Methionine (%)* |
|---|---|
| Casein | 2.3 |
| Casein hydrolysate | 2.2 |
| EPM | 4.8 |

* The methionine content of the samples is given as per cent of the total amino acid content

The structural changes in the products [8-10] were investigated in this work by SDS-polyacrylamide gel electrohoresis and by isoelectric focusing. For the evaluation of the electrophoretograms, a computer assisted method has been elaborated. Numerical comparison of distribution of protein fractions- i.e. the "homology" of samples- was done by a computer program. The term "homology" (H%) describes the differences in mobilities and intensities of each electrophoretic band

[1] Department of Biochemistry, Central Food Research Institute, Budapest, H-1525, Pf. 76
[2] Department of Food Technology and Biochemistry, Technical University of Budapest, Hungary

of the two samples compared:

$$H\% = \frac{2 \cdot \left( \sum_{i=1}^{k} D_i \right)}{N_1 + N_2} \cdot 100$$

where k = number of pairs of bands with a difference in mobility of smaller than ε. (For ε 0.5 % relative mobility was taken.)

$D_i$ = weighting factor which depends on the difference of intensities of the two homologue bands.

$N_1$, $N_2$ = number of bands in the two electrophoretograms compared.

Computer program was written in BASIC for IMB PC.

Besides the mentioned calculation a graphical evaluation was also carried out. Thus, the image of electrophoretic separation was depicted using the digitalised relative mobility and intensity data. The change in the number of peptide bonds was monitored by SDS gel electrophoresis. Since the average molecular mass remained practically unchanged during the EPM process, it means that the main force of this enzymatic reaction is neither a condensation nor a further hydrolysis.

The separation by net charge of protein fractions of the methionine enriched EPM-product was found to be different from that of the casein hydrolysate. It indicates that transpeptidation takes place in the enzymatic peptide modification.

Our recent results revealed the covalent nature of incorporation of the amino acids and transpeptidation in the course of EPM was also verified by using isoelectric focusing and computer analysis.

**Literature**


[1] Sawjalow, W.W. (1907) Z. Physiol. Chem., 54:119

[2] Wasteneys, H., Borsook, H. (1930) Physiol. Rev., 10:110-145

[3] Fujimaki, M., Arai, S., and Yamashita, M. (1977) Adv. in Chemistry Series, 160:156-184

[4] Sukan, G., and Andrews A.T. (1982) J. of Dairy Research, 49:265-278

[5] Aso, H., Kimura, H., Watanabe, M., and Arai, S. (1985) Agr. Biol. Chem. 49:1649-1654

[6] Ludwig, E., Krause, W., NÖtzold, H., and Tebling, F. (1981) Nahrung 25:K15-K17

[7] Ludwig, J., and Ludwig, E. (1985) Nahrung 29:949-955

[8] Hajós, Gy., and Halász, A. (1982) Acta Alimentaria 11:169-197

[9] Delincée, H., and Hajós, Gy. (1984) Acta Alimentaria 13:309-313

[10] Hajós, Gy. (1986) Nahrung 30:418-419

# PROTEASE INHIBITORS FROM POTATOES – PURIFICATION AND PROPERTIES

H. Schädlich[1], Ch. Flemming[1], A. Gabert[1] and A. Täufel[2]


## Introduction

It is well known, that potato tubers contain many different protease inhibitors. We report about the isolation and characterization of two inhibitors. The inhibition reactions were tested with trypsin, chymotrypsin, thermitase and subtilisin.

## Isolation and purification of the inhibitors

<u>Purification scheme</u>

**Potato tubers**
(species "Mariella")
↓
homogenization
↓
extraction with 0.1 N HCl
↓
lyophilization
↓
crude material (Fig. 1, Tab. 1)
↓
dialysis
↓
affinity chromatography on trypsin-sepharose 4 B (Fig. 2)

→ unbound fraction
→ elution pH 2.0 → **inhibitor I** (PI – I)

**unbound fraction**
↓
affinity chromatography on subtilisin-sepharose 4 B (Fig. 3)
↓
elution 4 M urea, pH 7.0 – 2.0
↓
separation with sephadex G 10
↓
**inhibitor II (peak I)**
(PI – II) (Fig. 4)

Table 1: Enzyme inhibition by material extracted from bands of PAGE
+ inhibition
- no inhibition

| Rf-value | thermitase | chymotrypsin | trypsin |
|---|---|---|---|
| 1 (0.11) | + | + | (+) |
| 2 (o.16) | – | – | – |
| 3 (0.22) | + | + | – |
| 4 (0.25) | + | + | + |
| 5 (0.30) | (+) | (+) | – |
| 6 (0.34) | + | ++ | + |
| 7 (0.41) | – | – | – |


[1]Institute of Biotechnology, Leipzig GDR
[2]Central Institute of Nutrition, Potsdam-Rehbrücke, GDR

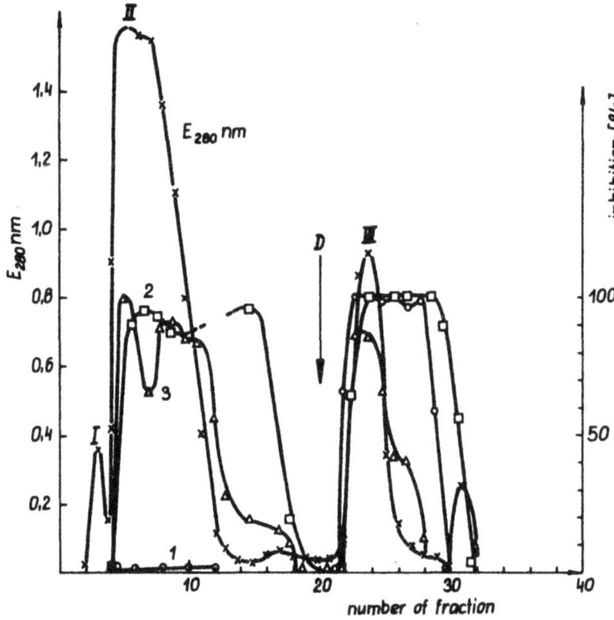


Figure 2: Activity against trypsin [1], chymotrypsin [2] and thermitase [3], D = desorption

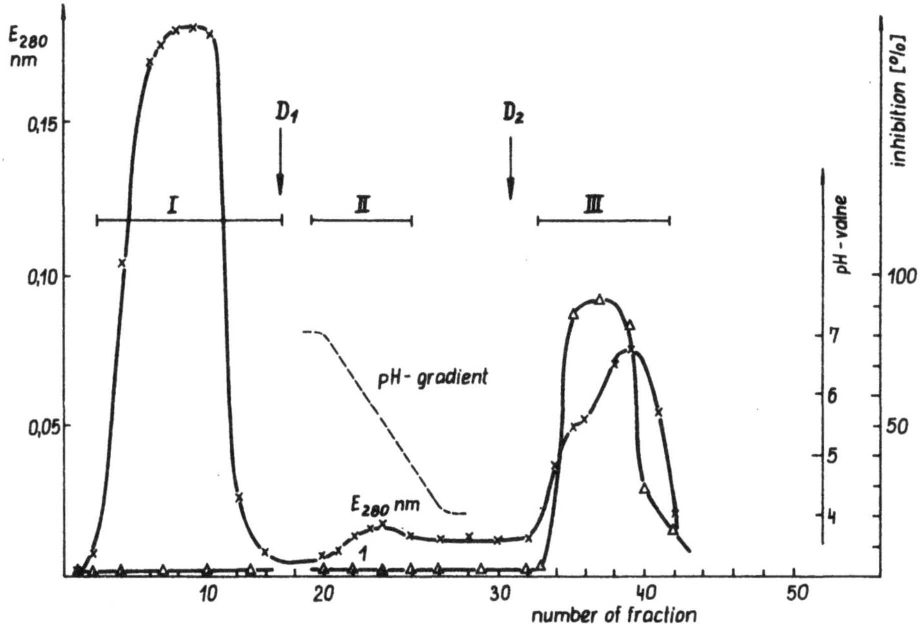


Figure 3: Activity against thermitase [1],
$D_1$: desorption with pH-gradient (7.0 - 4.0),
$D_2$: desorption with 4 M urea (0.1 M borate buffer, 5 mM Ca-acetate, pH 8.0)

Properties of the inhibitors

PI-I: It inactivates trypsin, chymotrypsin and thermitase competitively, Ki = $1.7 \cdot 10^{-8}$ [M] (thermitase)

PI-II: It inactivates chymotrypsin, thermitase and subtilisin in a competitive manner,

Ki = $6.5 \cdot 10^{-8}$ [M] (thermitase)

Ki = $1.7 \cdot 10^{-6}$ [M] (subtilisin)

MW 14 kD (SDS-PAGE), inhibits the esterolytical [1] and amidolytical [2] activity of thermitase completely, but the proteolytical activity [3] only partially (Fig. 5)

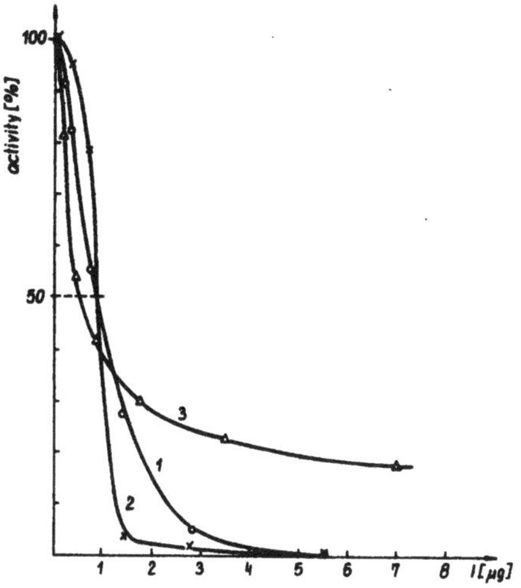


Figure 5: Inhibition of esterolysis [1], amidolysis [2] and proteolysis [3] of thermitase by PI-II,
substrate: N-Acetyl-L-tyrosine-ethylester [1], 4.8 micrograms/1 ml;
Succinyl-trialanyl-p-nitroanilide [2], 2.4 micrograms/0.22 ml;
Azo-casein [3], 0.48 micrograms/0.2 ml,
T = 55 °C , pH = 8.0

## Conclusions

Potato tubers contain only very small amounts of PI-I and PI-II. Both inhibitors are polyvalent. In contrast to inhibitors from soybean (STI), limabean (LBI) and egg white (OM), which were destroyed by the interaction with thermitase, the potato inhibitors inactivate thermitase permanently. Only by a combination of two affinity sorbents pure potato inhibitors are obtained.


## Acknowledgment

We thank Prof. R. Kleine for performing the PAGEs.

# SPECIFIC BINDING OF GLIADIN PEPTIDES TO INTESTINAL MUCOSA

M. Tschaikin (1), H.-J. Rühle (2), W. Mühle (1), F. Müller (1)

Gliadins - a group of wheat peptides - are known to cause the small intestinal mucosal damage in coeliac disease.The mechanisms of gliadin-induced injury have not been clearly established. Currently several hypotheses on the pathogenesis of coeliac disease are in discussion (peptidase deficiency, abnormal glycoprotein structure, virus infection). Specific binding of gliadin to enterocytes might be an initial reaction, independent of genetic mechanisms or additional exogenous factors. Data in the literature concerning specific gliadin binding (2,4,7,8,11,12) are contradictory.

The aim of the present paper was to study the existence of specific gliadin binding to fetal chicken intestine - a model system, where gliadin activity has been shown already (9). We used a soluble succinylated gliadin preparation as described by (10). A special proteolytical split product (PPG, Mr 12 400) of this succinylated gliadin was obtained after hydrolysis by an yet unidentified wheat protease contaminating the raw gliadin (1).

Binding was estimated by performing competitive displacement studies in presence of 125-I-labelled PPG 12 400 using homogenized fetal chicken intestine (prepared at the 12th day of fetal development).

An essential feature of specific binding is its hyperbolic dependence on tracer concentration (fig.1). Statistically significant binding was evident in concentration ranges of 10 to 400 nmol/l. Using the Hill-equation, KD value was 88 nmol/l, the binding capacity 275 pmol/g protein.

The specific binding is dependent on calcium concentration (up to 1.5 mmol/l).

---

(1) Department of Pathological Biochemistry, Karl Marx University, Liebigstraße 16, Leipzig, 7010, GDR.
(2) Department of Cell Biology and Regulation, Section of Biosciences, Karl Marx University, Talstraße 33, Leipzig, 7010, GDR.

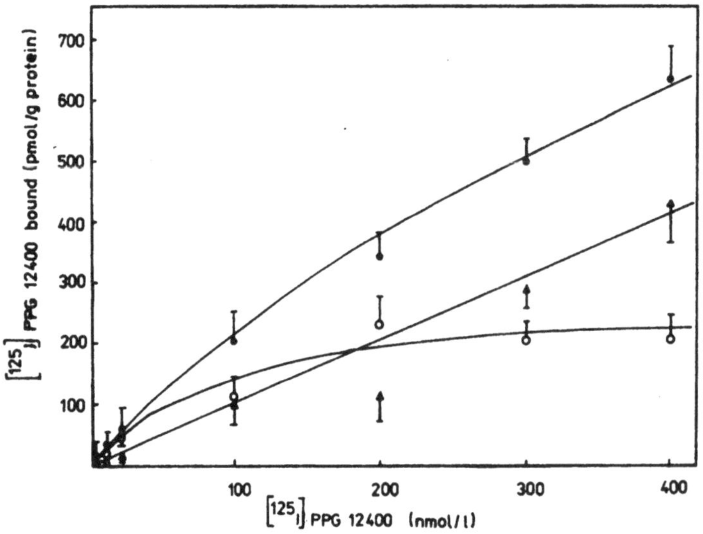


Fig. 1. Binding of 125-I-PPG 12 400 to fetal chicken intestine. Incubation time was 30 minutes, incubation temperature +4 °C, n = 5. (●) total binding, (Δ) nonspecific binding (in presence of 40 µmol/l unlabelled PPG 12 400) and (o) specific binding (obtained as difference of total and nonspecific binding).

For detecting the localization of specific binding sites an autoradiographic technique was used (suitable for localizing diffussible tracers; thaw-mount technique)(13).

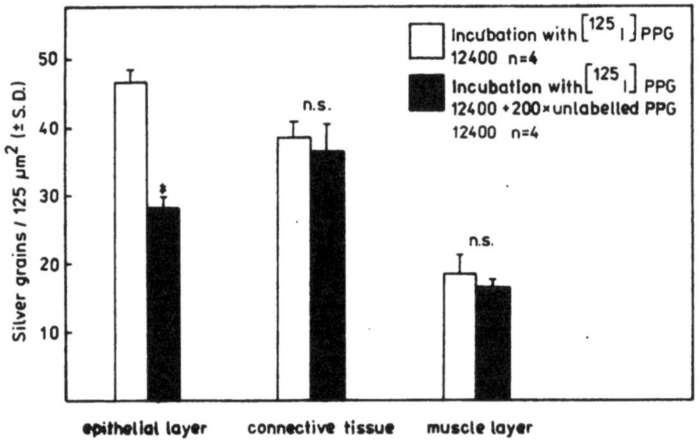


Fig. 2. Autoradiographic analysis of distribution of radioactivity in the different layers of fetal chicken intestine. (*) $p < 0.02$, n.s. = not significant.

Figure 2 describes the distribution of radioactivity in intestinal wall. Connective tissue and muscular layers were shown to contain 82.8 and 40.3 per cent, respectively, of the radioactivity found in the epithelium. After addition of an excess of unlabelled gliadin to the incubation medium, only the epithelial layer showed a significant decrease (39.3 per cent) of the silver grain density. Consequently, specific gliadin binding could be localized in the epithelial layer of chicken intestinum.

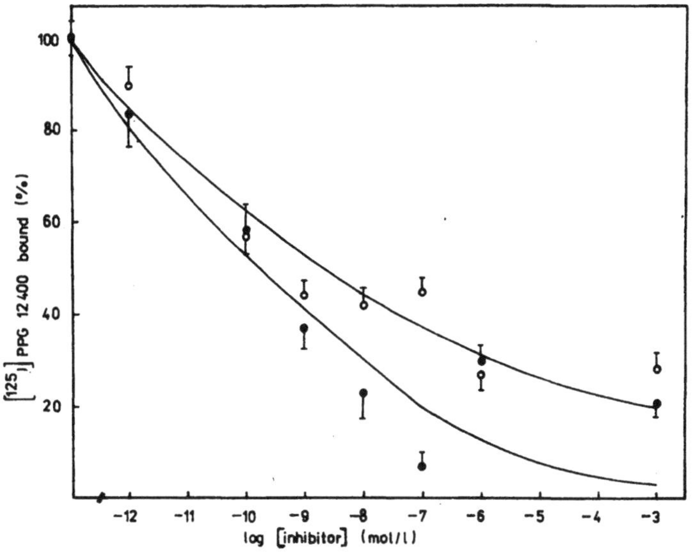


Fig. 3. Inhibition of 125-I-PPG 12 400 binding to fetal chicken intestine by morphine (o) and naloxone (•), n = 6.

According to literature isolated peptides from wheat gluten hydrolysates show a "high opiate-like activity" (5,6). Therefore studies were conducted to investigate the competition between gliadin and morphine (naloxone) for binding sites. Fig. 3 shows that morphine as well as naloxone competitively inhibit binding of 125-I-PPG 12 400 (KI = 3.44 nmol/l for morphine, KI = 0.22 nmol/l for naloxone). Because of these results gliadin may react with opiate binding sites.

From theoretical considerations (3,7) gliadin acts preferably with nondifferentiated cells. Therefore the dependence of gliadin binding on the stage of intestinal development was tested. A considerable specific binding rate was measured at the 12th day of embryonic period, whereas at the day 19 specific binding was no longer significant. This means that specific gliadin binding obviously depends on the stage of intestinal fetal development.

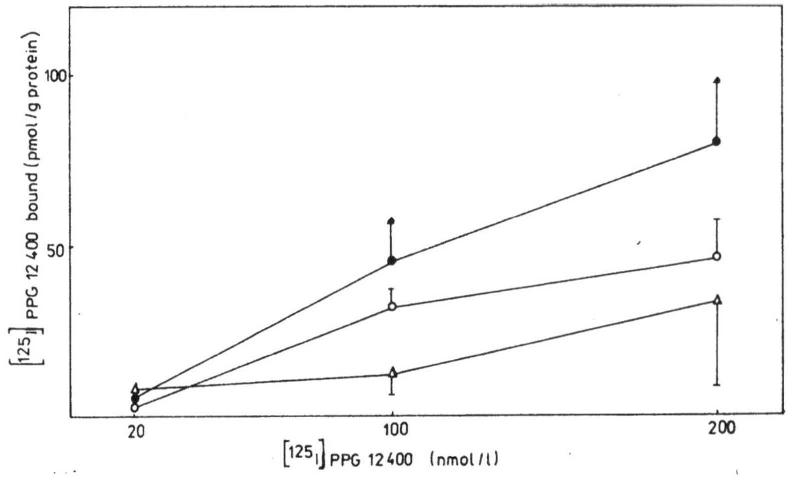


Fig. 4. Dependence of specific gliadin binding on intestinal development, n = 6. (●) 12th, (o) 15th, (▲) 19th day of fetal age.

Summerizing it can be concluded that a specific, calcium dependent binding exists between gliadin and the epithelial layer of fetal chicken intestine. The binding site is suggested to be an opiate receptor.

(1) Bönisch, G., W. Mühle and F. Richter: Wirtschaftpatent der DDR DD 236670 A1 WP 2585458.
(2) Colyer, Y., P. Y. Kumar, N.M. Waldron, M.L. Clark and M.J.G. Farthing: Clin. Sci. 72 (1987) 593-598.
(3) DeRitis, G., P. Occorsio, S. Auricchio, F. Gramenzi, G. Morisi and V. Silano: Pediat. Res. 13 (1979) 1255-1261.
(4) Douglas, A.P.: Clin. Chim. Acta 73 (1976) 357-361.
(5) Huebner, F.R., K.W. Lieberman, R.P. Rubino and J.S. Wall: Peptides 5 (1984) 1139-1147.
(6) Klee, W.A. and C. Zioudrou: in G. Hemmings (Ed.):The biochemistry of schizophrenia and addictions, MTP-Press 1980, 53-76.
(7) Köttgen, E., B. Volk, F. Kluge and W. Gerok: Biochem. Biophys. Res. Comm. 109 (1982) 168-173.
(8) Maury, C.P.I., A.-M. Teppo, M. Vuoristo, U. Turunen and I. Virtanen:Gut 27 (1986) 147-152.
(9) Mothes, Th., W. Mühle, F. Müller, W.T.J.M. Hekkens: Biol. Neonate 48 (1985) 59-64.
(10) Mühle, W., P. Walther, F. Richter and F. Müller: Z. med. Labor.-Diagn. 24 (1983) 41-46.
(11) Stern, M. and R. Dietrich: Eur. J. Pediat. 139 (1982) 13-17.
(12) Stern, M., B. Gellermann, H.-D. Belitz and H. Wieser: J. Ped. Gastroenterol. Nutr. 7 (1988) 122-127.
(13) Stumpf, W.E.: Acta Endocrin. Suppl. 153 (1971) 205-222.

# MOLECULAR BASIS OF FUNCTIONAL PROPERTIES OF MILK PROTEINS AND PRODUCTS OF THEIR DEGRADATION

J. Dziuba, H. Kostyra and A. Żbikowska[1]

## Introduction

The influence of molecular state of milk proteins on thermal stability susceptibility to coagulating enzymes action, as well as physical and sensory properties of milk peptide fractions were investigated. This kind of investigations may be significant for the estimation of milk quality and its technological value, and it may also contribute to better utilization of milk in the production of particular products.

## Experimental conditions

1. Cows selection: NBC breed, age 5 - 6 years, $3^{rd}$ - $4^{th}$ month of lactation, identical phenotype composition of proteins, clinical examinations eliminating mastitis;

2. Microbiological estimation of milk: total amount of microorganisms, acidifying microflors, psychrotrophes, E-coli, enterococcuses;

3. Description of molecular state of milk proteins and peptidelike nitrogen compounds: fractionation of micellar and soluble casein with ultracentrifugation method [1, 2], quantitative evaluation of milk proteins and fractionated casein with electrophoresis method in starch and polyacrylamide gel, separation of peptide fractions with ultrafiltration method on Sephadex G-25 gel, with thin layer chromatography (TLC) method and with high voltage electrophoresis, sensory evaluation of isolated peptide fractions [5];

4. Functional properties: thermal stability in pH range 6.4 - 7.0 [3], description of the enzymatic phase of coagulating enzymes action and the second phase of coagulation [4], proteins susceptibility to the action of coagulating enzymes on the basis of kinetic constants $K_M$ and V [4].

5. Establishing correlation between molecular state of milk proteins and investigated functional properties.

[1]Department of Physics and Food Chemistry
agricultural and technical academy, faculty of food technology
Olsztyn, Poland

**Results and Discussion**

All collected samples of milk were characterized by good microbiological quality. Total amount of bacteria in milk was ab. $2.2 \cdot 10^4$ cfu/cm$^3$.

Acidifying microflora made 29 - 64 % of the whole, while the contents of coli group bacteria and of enterococcuses were $1.5 \cdot 10^3$ and $2.1 \cdot 10^3$ cfu/cm$^3$, respectively.

Significant correlations dealing with molecular structure of milk proteins and its functional properties are presented in table 1.

Time of rennin coagulation depended significantly on the content of micellar casein but it did not depend on the micelle size. The size of micelles affected essentially the affinity of rennin to casein measured with the amount of released glycopeptides. The growth of large micelle parts in micellar casein was accompanied by the loss of released glycopeptides, while the growth of small micelle parts was related with the increase of released glycopeptides. Similar relations were found for the influence of the micelle size on thermal stability. Greater part of large micelles in micellar caseine was accompanied by lowered thermal stability, while the less one - in increased thermal stability.

The integration state of micellar caseine did not modify enzymatic phase of milk coagulation which was expressed in the lack of significant correlation among casein proteolysis constant $K_M$, the size of micelles and micellar casein content.

Table 1: Correlation coefficients of the investigated dependences

| Dependence | Linear coefficient r |
|---|---|
| Micellar casein content | |
| x thermal stability | - 0.721** |
| x rennin coagulation time | + 0.752** |
| Part of large micelles | |
| x thermal stability | - 0.856** |
| x affinity of rennin to casein | - 0.825** |
| Part of medium micelles | |
| x thermal stability | - 0.591* |
| Part of small micelles | |
| x thermal stability | + 0.886** |
| x affinity of rennin to casein | + 0.859 |
| Thermal stability | |
| x time of rennin coagulation | - 0.732** |
| x affinity of renninn to casein | + 0.713 |

*significant correlation
**highly significant correlation

As a result of quantitative separation of proteins and peptides solutions obtained after caseine precipitation in milk in pH 4.6 two or three fractions were obtained. By means of TLC they were found to contain 5 - 15 fractions reacting with ninhydrin. Sensory analysis of the fractions obtained from separating with Sephadex G-25 gel showed that they had butterish, slightly bitter-astringent or sweet-bitter taste.

## Conclusions

1. Functional properties of milk, such as susceptibility to rennin action and thermal stability, depend on the content of large and small micelles.

2. Integration degree of micellar casein does not modify enzymatic phase of milk coagulation.

3. Time of rennet coagulation of milk depends on the content of micellar casein, and not on the size of micelles.

4. Highly significant negative correlation between thermal stability of milk and time of rennet coagulation, as well as positive correlation between thermal stability and the amount of released glycopeptides can be used for the optimization of milk utilization in its processing.

## Literature

[1] Aoki, T., Y. Kahao;
Relation between micele size and formation of soluble casein on heating concentrated milk. J. Dairy Res. **50** (1983), 207 - 213

[2] Aoki, T., H. Suzuki and Z. Imamura;
Formation of soluble casein in whey protein-free milk heated at high temperature. Milchwiss. **29** (1974), 589 - 594

[3] Davies, D.T., J.C.D. White;
The stability of milk protein to heat. Subjective measurement of heat stability of milk. J. Dairy Res. **33** (1966), 67 - 81

[4] Dziuba, J.;
Inhibicja proteolizy kazeiny przez indukowany cieplnie kompleks k-kazeiny i ß-laktoglobuliny.
Zesz. nauk. ART Olszt, **4** (1975), 65 - 75

[5] Kostyra, H., W. Damicz;
Charakterystyka frakcji peptydowych mleka.
Zesz. nauk. ART Olszt. Technologia Zywnosci. **19** (1984), 79 - 87

# DENATURATION CHANGES IN PROTEIN STRUCTURE DURING THE HYDROTHERMAL TREATMENT OF RAPESEED

J. Fornal, D. Rotkiewicz, W. Giec, M. Piskula and H. Kozlowska[1]

## Introduction

Introducing double-improved rapeseed varieties to wide cultivation may develop a need for modification of oil extraction process mainly because of the inner seed structure different from that in the traditional varieties [1] and also different physical-chemical properties [2]. The aim of the modification should be maintaining the amount and quality of extracted fat as well as preserving high quality of protein.

Concerning above, hydrothermal treatment of whole seeds was suggested as the first unit operation of the technological process. The present work was aimed at investigation of the influence of hydrothermal treatment on proteins behaviour and fat extractivity.

## Materials

Seeds of four rapeseed varieties of various improvement degree were investigated: traditional Skrzeszowicki variety, the zeroerucic Beryl, and the double-zero BOH and Jantar.

Seeds of the first three varieties were steamed directly for 20 min at temp. 100°C. Meal for experiments was obtained from the seeds crushed in industrial devices and extracted with benzin. Samples of the Jantar variety rapeseed were collected after 3, 6, 9, 12, 15 and 20 min of steaming. Meal was obtained from the seeds crushed in a laboratory mill.

## Results and discussion

Total protein content in meals obtained from raw and steamed seeds of three varieties was similar (tab. 1).

Hydrothermal treatment for 20 min at 100°C caused significant decrease of soluble protein in the meals.

[1]Prof. Dr. H. Kozlowska, Dr. J. Fornal, Dr. D. Rotkiewicz,
M.S.M. Giec, M.S.M. Piskula,
University of Agriculture and Technology,
Institute of Food Engineering and Biotechnology,
10-745 Olsztyn-Kortowo, Poland

Table 1: Protein content in meals obtained from raw and steamed rapeseeds (% of dm)

| Sample | | Protein total | Protein soluble |
|---|---|---|---|
| Skrzeszowicki | raw | 43.0 | 25.1 |
| | steamed | 42.8 | 11.7 |
| Beryl | raw | 42.6 | 22.7 |
| | steamed | 42.7 | 13.8 |
| BOH | raw | 43.4 | 24.4 |
| | steamed | 42.7 | 12.7 |

Detailed analysis of protein solubility changes and myrosinase activity during the hydrothermal treatment for the double-zero Jantar variety seeds were shown on tab. 2.

Table 2: Protein content and myrosinase activity in rapeseed meals obtained from the Jantar variety during hydrothermal treatment (% of dm).

| Steaming time (min) | Protein total | Protein soluble | Decrease of myrosinase activity |
|---|---|---|---|
| 0 | 42.9 | 23.1 | 0 |
| 3 | 43.3 | 22.4 | 36 |
| 6 | 43.3 | 14.5 | 87 |
| 9 | 43.0 | 11.6 | 100 |
| 12 | 42.7 | 11.3 | 100 |
| 15 | 43.0 | 10.9 | 100 |
| 20 | 43.0 | 9.7 | 100 |

Denaturation changes are ilustrated on the microphotographs showing the image of the cotyledon cells of control seeds and 3 min steaming (phot. 1, 2).

Fat content in meals turned out to depend on both the rapeseed variety and hydrothermal treatment.

Table 3: Residual fat content in meals obtained from raw and steamed rapeseeds

| Sample | Skrzeszowicki raw | Skrzeszowicki steamed | Beryl raw | Beryl steamd | BOH raw | BOH steamed |
|---|---|---|---|---|---|---|
| Fat (% of dm) | 1.9 | 1.1 | 1.9 | 1.5 | 2.2 | 1.9 |

Steaming of the seeds resulted in a clear decrease of fat content in the meals of all investigated varieties. The greatest fat content was found to remain in meals of the improved rapeseed varieties. This confirms the information about the possibilities of various behaviour of the double-zero varieties during extraction due to the differences in structure.

The influence of hydrothermal treatment time on fat extraction from seeds of the Jantar variety is presented on fig. 1. It was observed that fat was extracted equally by all samples during first 20 min of extraction. We assume that it depends mainly on the amount of open cells, probably the same for each of the investigated samples. As extraction time was increased, there appeared considerable differences, e.g. extractivity grew significantly. Easier fat extraction from hydrothermally treated seeds may be result from decay of the membranes surrounding particular fat droplets under the action of heat and water, of their gathering into larger aggregates and cummulation near by the cell walls.

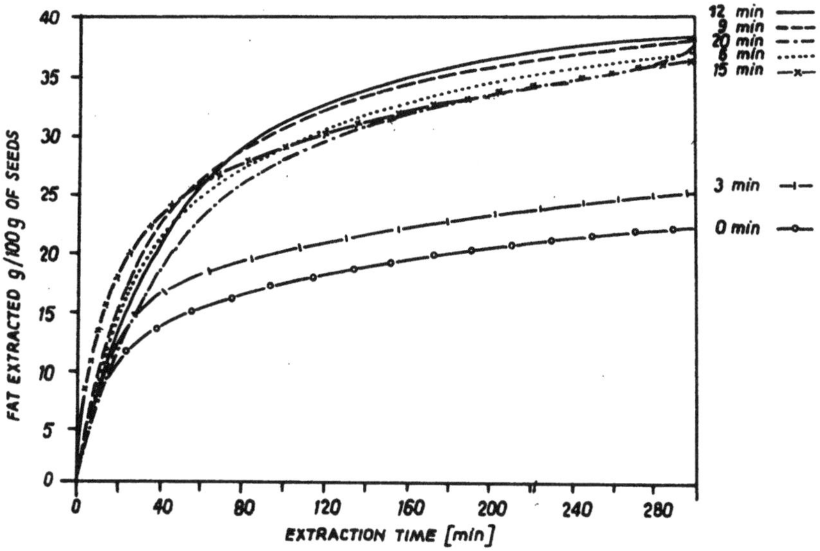


Figure 1: Fat extractivity on experimentally crushed samples of Jantar variety, extraction time 300 min

It is presented on the microphotogaphs of cotyledon cells of the Jantar variety seeds before (phot. 3) and after 9 min of steaming (phot. 4).

## Conclusions

1. Hydrothermal treatment of whole seeds results in the decrease of protein solubility, especially when steaming time exceeds 6 min.

2. Protein solubility changes are accompanied by considerable changes of microscopic image expressed by creating of protein conglomerates and their cummulating in the centre of cotyledon cells.

3. Decay of the membranes surrounding fat droplets and their gathering into larger aggregates can be observed which at the tendency to cummulate near by the cell walls makes fat extraction easier.

4. Degree of fat extraction and the structural changes of cotyledon cells depends on the time of heat and water action.

## References

1. Fornal, J.;
II Krajowe Sympozjum Chemii i Technologii Tluszczów, Gdansk, 1985

2. Fornal, J., H. Kozlowska and W. Giec;
7th Int. Rapeseed Congress, Poznan, 1987

# INFLUENCE OF FABA BEAN HYDROTHERMAL TREATMENT ON DENATURATION CHANGES IN PROTEIN

J. Fornal[1], J. Borowska[1], H. Kozlowska[1], Ch. Schneider[2] and H. Schmandke[2]

## Introduction

Former investigations showed that hydrothermal treatment is a simple and effective method of trypsin inhibitors inactivation in faba bean seeds [1]. Still this interesting process demands establishing of possibly the most advantageous conditions in which heat affects beans considering mainly the changes undergoing in proteins. The changes were determined by means of NSI, activity of trpysin inhibitors and through the observation of microstructure applying various parameters of hydrothermal treatment.

## Material and methods

Seeds of the Fribo faba bean variety were investigated. After dehulling cotyledons were treated hydrothermally under the following conditions

| Temperature (°C) | Time (min) |
|---|---|
| 100 | 2, 5, 10, 20 |
| 110 | 2, 5, 10 |
| 120 | 1, 2 |

Steamed cotyledons were dried at a temp. of 30°C to a moisture content of about 10 % and then grinded to granules of d = 0.2 mm. In thus prepared meal there were determined nitrogen solubility index (NSI) according to AOCS [3], trypsin inhibitors activity (TIA) acc. to Kakade et al. [2]; microscopic analysis was made with the scanning electronic microsope Tesla BS-300 at accelerating voltage 10 kV.

## Results

Hydrothermal treatment of faba bean cotyledons resulted in the lowering of nitrogen solubility, expressed by NSI (fig. 1 A).

[1]University of Agriculture and Technology, Institute of Food Engineering and Biotechnology, 10 - 957 Olsztyn, Building No. 43, Poland

[2]Central Institute of Nutrition, DDR - 1505 Bergholz-Rehbrücke, Arthur-Scheunert-Allee 114 - 116

The changes cleary depended on the temperature and time of steaming. The higher temperature was applied, the greater loss of nitrogen solubility was observed. Thus, steaming of the beans for 2 min at 100°C causes 12 % decrease of NSI, at 110°C - 27 % and 120°C - 41 %. The lowest NSI (11 %) was found for the beans steamed for 20 min. at 100°C. The decrease of nitrogen solubility was accompanied by lowering of trypsin inhibitors activity (fig. 1 B). It was rather the temperature than the time of steaming theat influenced TIA. Hence, total inactivation was obtained in the beans steamed for 10 min at 110°C, whereas extending of the steaming time to 20 min at 100°C caused only 64 % decrease of antitrypsin activity.

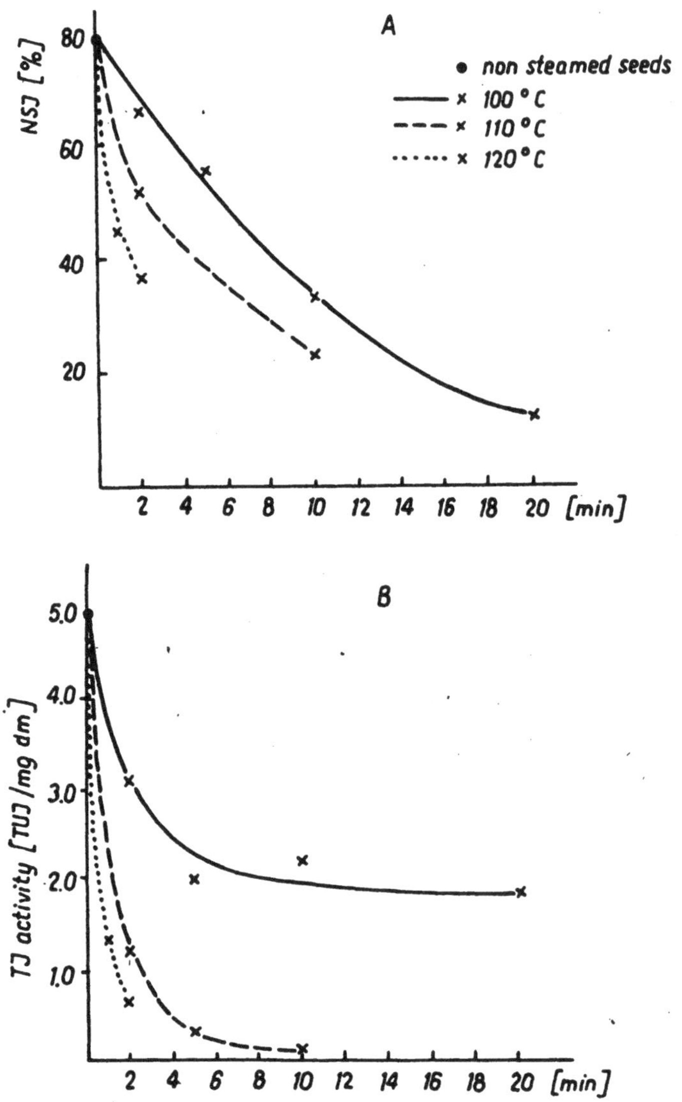


Figure 1: The influence of hydrothermal treatment on the NSI and TIB activity

Less solublitiy of faba bean proteins and the decrease of antitrypsin activity seem to be related with the changes of microscopic image of cotyledons (mainly of protein bodies).

Oval protein bodies of cotyledon cells in control beans (phot. 1) after steaming for 2 min at 100°C swell over their natural size and take spherical shape (phot. 2).

Hydrothermal treatment conducted for 5 min at 110°C caused more clear structural changes of protein substances (phot. 3). There was observed joining of protein bodies into larger conglomerates as well as deepening concavities on their surfaces resulting most probably from the destruction of protein structure. Microscopic image of cotyledon cells treated hydrothermally for 2 min at 120°C is presented on phot. 4. These parameters of the treatment brought about much more significant changes of proteins and starch which resulted in the creation of denatured protein mass and obvious starch gelatinization. It was accompanied by the quickest decrease of NSI and TI activity among all of investigated processes (fig. 1 A and B).

The present analysis of the influence of hydrothermal treatment on the changes of NSI, TIA and in faba bean cotyledon microstructure leads to the conclusion that a time of 2 min and a temperature of 110°C are optimal conditions in which obvious TIA decrease (75 %) was accompanied by relatively small NSI and cotyledon microstructure changes.

## Conclusions

1. Heat and moisture action on faba bean cotyledons resulted in lowered solubility of nitrogen compounds expressed as NSI and TIA; the temperature of steaming being of greater importance for the denaturation changes than the time of steaming.

2. Significant relation was found between decreasing of the NSI coefficient and TIA and the picture of protein bodies observed in the electronic microscope.

## References


[1] Borowska, J., D. Rotkiewicz, M. Piskula and Ch. Schneider; XVII Sesja Naukowa KTiChZ, Lodz 1986

[2] Kakade, M.L., J.J. Rackis, J.E. Mc Ghee and C. Puski; Cereal Chem., 51 (1974) 376 - 382

[3] Rutkowski, A. and H. Kozlowska; Preparaty zywnosciowe z bialka roslinnego WNT, W-wa 1981

# PREPARATION OF FUNCTIONAL RAPESEED PROTEINS BY ULTRAFILTRATION

J. Kroll[1], M. Kujawa[1] and W. Schnaak[1]

From commercial Rapeseed meal (var. Sollux) fractions with different protein content are prepared by extraction following different steps: isoelectric precipitation, ultrafiltration (UF), diafiltration (DF), drying (Flow sheet: Tab. 1). The albumin rich fractions obtained by UF and DF are excellent foamers (better than egg white; Tab. 2) and have a very good solubility (Fig. 1).
The globulin fractions prepared by isoelectric precipitation have no foaming properties (Tab. 2) and are comparatively less soluble (Fig. 1).
By UF and/or DF in contrast to other processes for protein producing it is possible to concentrate and clean all the solubilized proteins without losses (globulins and first of all albumins).
Following this you can observe an enrichment of proteins of dryed preparates (from 37.9 % to 78.1 %; Tab. 1) and simultaneously a drastic decrease of the content of toxic compounds (Progoitrin from 19 680 ppm to 1 040 ppm, butenyl-ITC from 13 980 ppm to 270 ppm, pentenyl-ITC from 2 390 ppm to 120 ppm, and phenylethyl-ITC from 500 ppm to 30 ppm; Tab. 3). The toxic compounds are mainly connected with the albumins. The phytate content of the fractions is not striking influenced by the described UF- and DF-conditions (Tab. 4).

(We are very much obliged to Mrs. R. Kroeck for preparing of the protein fractions and Mr. R. Mothes for estimation of phytate content).

[1] Central Institute of Nutrition, Potsdam-Rehbruecke, GDR

Tab. 3

Natural occuring toxic compounds in fractions prepared from Rapeseed meal (var. Soll ux)

| fractions | toxic compounds | | | | | | | | | |
|---|---|---|---|---|---|---|---|---|---|---|
| | VOT, free[1] | | Progoitrin[1] | | Glucosinolates as | | | | | |
| | | | | | Butenyl - ITC[2] | | Pentenyl - ITC[2] | | Phenyl - Ethyl - ITC[2] | |
| | [ppm] | [% rel.] | [ppm] | [% rel.] | [ppm] | [% rel.] | [ppm] | [% rel.] | [ppm] | [% rel.] |
| Rapeseed meal | 122 | – | 7200 | – | 6800 | – | 1700 | – | 370 | – |
| Extract 1, dried | 400 | 100 | 19680 | 100 | 13980 | 100 | 2370 | 100 | 500 | 100 |
| UF-Retentate 1, dried | 200 | 50 | 13680 | 70 | 6680 | 48 | 1670 | 70 | 250 | 50 |
| DF-Retentate 1, dried | 250 | 63 | 7250 | 37 | 4410 | 32 | 735 | 31 | 350 | 70 |
| DF-Retentate 2, dried | 190 | 48 | 1350 | 8 | 1160 | 8 | 170 | 7 | 90 | 18 |
| DF-Retentate 3, dried | 60 | 15 | 1040 | 5 | 270 | 2 | 120 | 5 | 30 | 6 |
| Globulin rich fraction | n.d. | – | 2520 | 13 | 1310 | 9 | 330 | 14 | 80 | 16 |
| Globulin fraction 1 | n.d. | – | 150 | 1 | 340 | 2 | 110 | 5 | 65 | 13 |
| Globulin fraction 2 | n.d. | – | 605 | 3 | 2480 | 18 | 830 | 35 | 370 | 74 |

1) estimated by HPLC according Schnaak et al.
2) estimated by GLC according Kujawa et al.

Tab. 4

Phytate[1] content of fractions from Rapeseed meal

| fractions | phytate content [mg phytic acid/g substance] | [mg phytic acid/g protein |
|---|---|---|
| Rapeseed meal | 40.9 | 128 |
| Extract 1, dried | 6.3 | 17 |
| UF-Retentate 1, dried | 10.1 | 18 |
| UF-Retentate 10:1, dried | 12.3 | 19 |
| DF-Retentate 1, dried | 15.6 | 24 |
| DF-Retentate 2, dried | 17.7 | 25 |
| DF-Retentate 3, dried | 21.4 | 27 |

1) estimated according RUTKOWSKA et al. in the modified form according MOTHES

Fig.1: Nitrogen solubility profiles of protein fractions from Rapeseed meal

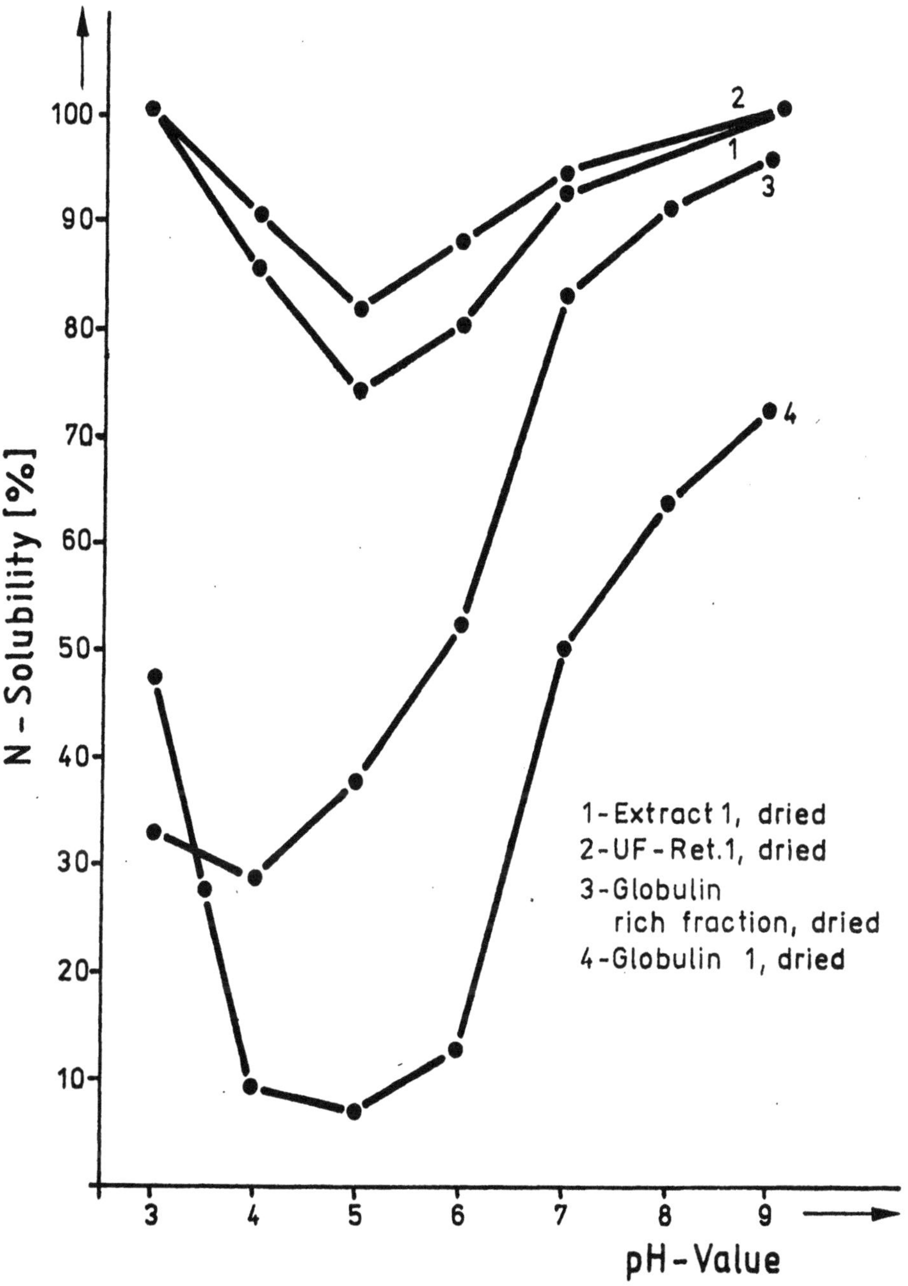

INFLUENCE OF THE INTERACTIONS OF PROTEINS WITH LIPIDS ON THE SURFACE PROPERTIES AND STABILITY OF EMULSIONS

E. Lange, J. Brückner u. G. Mieth [1)]

## INTRODUCTION

Lipidic emulsifiers have a long history in respect to their usage for formation and stabilization of emulsions [5]. During the last years proteins got increasing importance as emulsifiers and coemulsifiers due to their amphiphilic structure [3, 6].
Furthermore polyanionic hydrocolloids are also used to improve the emulsion stability by increasing the viscosity, by steric stabilization, and influencing the electric charge [1,2,7]. The level of knowledge about interactions between lipidic emulsifiers and stabilizers is low at present.

## AIMS

- Studies on the influence of lipidic emulsifiers and proteins on the interfacial tension decrease at the sunflower oil-water interface
- Effects of combinations of emulsifiers and stabilizers (proteins, hydrocolloids) on the interfacial tension decrease
- Influence of emulsifiers and stabilizers on the stability of thin aqueous films between two oil droplets (coalescence stability)
- Studies on the transferability of the results on emulsion systems

## MATERIALS

| | |
|---|---|
| Sunflower oil | - purified by treatment with $Al_2O_3$ |
| Emulsifier 1302 | - commercial monoglyceride emulsifier*, purified by recrystallization (monoglyceride content 98.4 %) |
| Soya phosphatide | - purified by washing with acetone and recrystallization |
| Faba bean isolate | - PI-0, produced by extraction with dist. water, isoelectric precipitation, spray drying (protein content 80 %) |
| | - PI-96, produced by acetylation, spray drying (acetyl. degree 96 %, protein content 74 %) |
| Pectin | - commercial products of the firm Herbstreith, BRD<br>Type NLG - esterif. degr. 50 %, pectin content 58 %<br>Type OM - " 32 % " 90 % |
| Water | - bidistilled |

## METHODS

Determination of
- the interfacial tension by the drop volume method, according to Tornberg [8]
- the coalescence stability by the method for the estimation of the stability of thin aqueous films, according to Müller and Kretzschmar [4]
- the emulsion stability by measuring the separated oil or water phase from the emulsion during certain time intervals

## RESULTS AND DISCUSSION

- The investigated lipidic emulsifiers, proteins and polyanionic hydrocolloids can be ordered in the following sequence according to their effectivity as interfacial tension depressors: pectins < monoglyceride < nonacetylated protein isolate < acetylated protein < phosphatide (Tab. 1).
- The time dependent rate of reduction of interfacial tension is different for the agents. The small and mobile monoglyceride molecule exhibits the fastest rate of interfacial tension reduction. The phospholipid and protein isolates require a longer time for reaching the equilibrium interfacial tension.
- The interfacial tension for protein isolates depends on the pH-value. The lowest equilibrium values are obtained in the range of the isoelectric point due to the more compactness and the lower electrical charge of the molecule at this pH-range.
- The combination of protein isolates with lipidic emulsifiers has synergistic effects on the interfacial tension decrease, whereas the combination of protein isolates with pectins shows antagonistic ones. The last mentioned is especially relevant for the acidic pH-range (Tab. 1).
- The combination of lipidic emulsifiers with pectins is only influenced (negatively) in the case of phospholipid-low esterified pectin.
- Especially efficient in the interfacial tension decrease is a combination of the two lipidic emulsifiers with pectin and protein isolate (Tab. 1).
- Referring to coalescence stability also synergistic and antagonistic effects are pointed out. With the monoglyceride in the combination with protein and pectin stable films are already obtained at concentrations at which the agents alone don't form stable films. In contrast to that, the stability of phosphatide films is reduced by combination with the stabilizers (Tab. 2).

- The concentration of emulsifiers and stabilizers deduced from the investigations on interfacial tensions and coalescence stability rendered as to low for making stable emulsions (≥60 minutes) of the W/O-or the O/W-type. The reason is that there are still other factors to take into consideration, like mechanical energy intake, the turbulence, the viscosity, the particle size distribution, and so on. Stable emulsions of a mixed type (O/W-W/O) are attained by combinations with a concentration of at least 0.2 % protein isolate, 0.05 % pectin and 0.02 % lipidic emulsifier (Tab. 3).

Table 1

Interfacial tension at the sunflower oil-water-interface as a function of concentration of emulsifiers and stabilizers and their combinations

| Agent | Concentration [mg/100 ml] | Interfacial tension [mNm⁻¹] |
|---|---|---|
| sunflower oil | - | 30,4 |
| pectin OM | 0,25 | 29,2 |
| | 0,50 | 28,5 |
| pectin NL | 0,25 | 29,0 |
| | 0,50 | 28,8 |
| PI-O | 0,05 | 16,5 |
| | 0,10 | 16,0 |
| | 0,25 | 15,5 |
| | 0,50 | 15,0 |
| PI-96 | 0,05 | 15,6 |
| | 0,10 | 14,0 |
| | 0,25 | 13,9 |
| | 0,50 | 13,8 |
| MG | 0,05 | 29.5 |
| | 0,10 | 26,3 |
| | 0,25 | 20,6 |
| | 0,50 | 16,3 |
| Phosphatide | 0,05 | 7,3 |
| | 0,10 | 6,0 |
| | 0,25 | 4,4 |
| | 0,50 | 1,0 |
| MG | 0,10 | 26,3 |
| + PI-O | 0,04 | 16,2 |
| + PI-O | 0,08 | 14,3 |
| + PI-O | 0,20 | 13,1 |
| MG | 0,25 | 20.6 |
| + PI-O | 0,04 | 14,9 |
| + PI-O | 0,08 | 12,7 |
| + PI-O | 0,20 | 11,8 |
| Phosphatide | 0,10 | 6,0 |
| + PI-O | 0,04 | 2,0 |
| + PI-O | 0,08 | 2,0 |
| + PI-O | 0,20 | 1,0 |
| Phosphatide | 0,25 | 4,5 |
| + PI-O | 0,04 | 1,0 |
| + PI-O | 0,08 | 1,0 |
| + PI-O | 0,20 | 1,0 |
| PI-O | 0,05 | 16,5 |
| + Pectin | 0.25 | 20.0 |
| PI-O | 0,10 | 16,0 |
| + Pectin | 0,25 | 17,1 |
| MG | 0,25 | |
| + Phosphatide | 0,25 | 4,2 |
| MG | 0,25 | |
| + Phosphatide | 0,25 | |
| + PI-O | 0,05 | 0,7 |
| MG | 0,25 | |
| + Phosphatide | 0,25 | |
| + Pectin NL | 0,25 | 5,3 |
| MG | 0,25 | |
| + Phosphatide | 0,25 | |
| + Pectin NL | 0,25 | |
| + PI-O | 0,05 | 0,8 |

Table 2

Lifetime[+] of thin aqueous films between two oil droplets in dependence on the addition of emulsifiers and stabilizers, pH 5.4 (180≙stable films)

| | | $H_2O$ | 0.05 % PI-0<br>69 | 0.01 % PI-96<br>98 |
|---|---|---|---|---|
| Phosphatide | 0.10 % | 107 | 52 | 180 |
| | 0.15 % | 180 | 78[x] | - |
| MG | 0.5 % | 21 | 180[x] | - |
| | 1.0 % | 23 | 31 | 140 |
| Pectin NL | 0.01 % | 110 | 117 | - |

[x] Pectin NL + in sec

Table 3

Emulsion stability for emulsions (50/50 v/v) of a mixed O/W-W/O-type, pH 5.4

| Agents | ES [%]<br>15 | 30 | 60 minutes |
|---|---|---|---|
| Control | 25 | 25 | 25 |
| 0.2 % PI-0 | 100 | 97 | 95 |
| 0.2 % PI-0+0,02 % MG | 100 | 97 | 97 |
| 0.2 % PI-0+0,05 % pectin NL | 100 | 100 | 97 |
| 0.2 % PI-0+0,05 % pectin NL+0,02 % MG | 100 | 100 | 100 |

LITERATURE


[1] Bergenstahl, B. in Phillips, G.O. et al (ed.) "Gums and Stabilizers for the food industry", Vol. 4, IRL Press, Oxford 1988.

[2] Dickinson, E. Proc. "Gums and Stabilizers for the Food industry", Wrexham 1987.

[3] Mc Watters, K. H., and Cherry, J.P. ACS-Symposium Series 147 (1981) 217 - 242.

[4] Müller, H.J., and G. Kretzschmar, Colloid Polymer Sci. 260 (1982) 2, 228 - 231

[5] Schuster, G. (ed.) "Emulgatoren für Lebensmittel", Akademie-Verlag, Berlin 1985.

[6] Parker, N.S., Crit. Rev. Food Sci. Nutrit. 25 (1987) 4, 285 - 315.

[7] Tolstoguzov, V.B., and Braudo, E.E. J. Dispersion Sci. Technol. 6 (1985) 5, 575 - 603

[8] Tornberg, E., J. Colloid Interface Sci. 64 (1978) 3, 391 - 402



1) Central Institute of Nutrition in Potsdam-Rehbrücke, Academy of Sciences of the GDR

# ENZYMATIC HYDROLYSIS OF CELL WALL PROTEIN

Th.Kreuter, H.Duwe and U.Lehwald [1)]

In search for novel protein sources for food we examined the enzymatic modification of microbial proteins.

Notwithstanding the sufficient biological value of the microbial protein there result partial hydrolysates of bitter taste in consequence of the enzymatic hydrolysis because of the hydrophobicity of the protein.

According to NEY /1/ the reason for the bitterness of protein partial hydrolysates is their hydrophobicity.

The hydrophobicity "Q" of the protein is calculated by addition of the specific hydrophobicity increments of all the amino acids, which are forming the protein molecule.

Q-values exceeding 5450 J/mol result in a bitter taste of the hydrolysates, while at lower Q-values no bitter peptides are appearing.

Common food proteins show the following Q-values:

| Protein source | Q-value (J/mol) |
|---|---|
| gelatin | 3322 |
| muscle meat | 5443 |
| casein | 6720 |
| baker's yeast: | |
| charge I | 5347 |
| charge II | 5753 |

The borderline character of the hydrophobicity of the yeast protein includes the possibility of the formation of bitter proteins in consequence of the enzymatically partial hydrolysis. Indeed we found bitter peptides from the total yeast protein if the degree of hydrolysis increased 10 % (determined by the method of LANGNER /2/ with trinitro-benzenesulfonic acid (TNBS).

The chain length of the peptides according to number of amino acid molecules as monomers is defined as follows:

$$\frac{\text{number of peptide bonds}}{(\text{number of peptide bonds}) + (\text{number of terminal amino groups})}$$

Approximately the mean of the chain length of protein partial hydrolysates is the reciprocal value of their relative degree of hydrolysis by the TNBS - method.

---

1) Institute of Biotechnology, Academie of Science of the G.D.R., Leipzig

Using not the total microbial protein but only the cell wall bound one for the enzymatic partial hydrolysis, we found in each case bitterfree hydrolysates. This fact opens various possibilities to introduce microbial protein partial hydrolysates into food. The utilisation of microbial cell wall residues for the production of protein partial hydrolysates for food may economize many processes for the production of other valuable preparations from single cells.
Fig 1. may demonstrate possible technical sources for proteinaceous cell wall residues:

Fig.1:

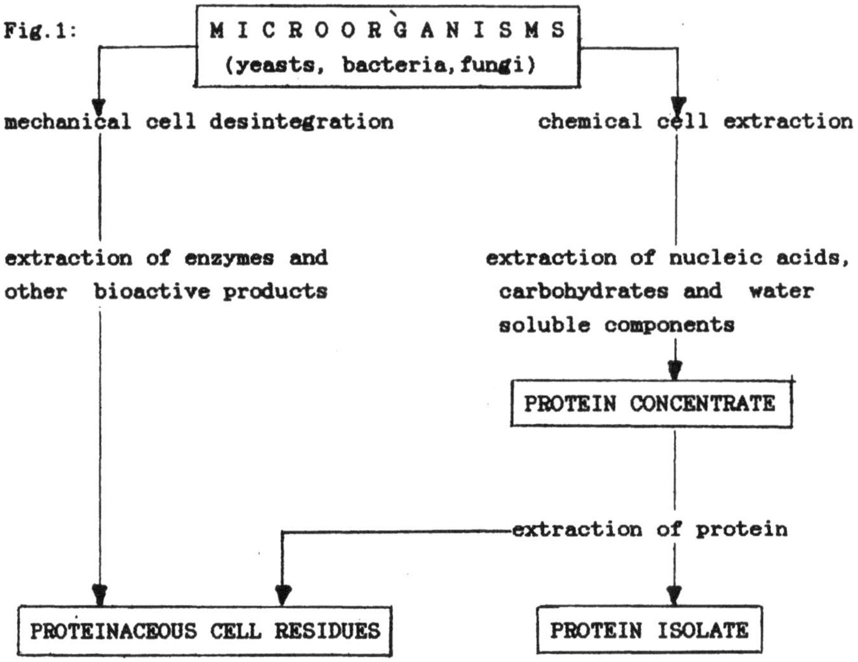


Figures 2, 3, and 4 show examples for the enzymatic protein partial hydrolysis of proteinaceous cell wall residues, protein isolate and protein concentrate, respectively. Only the product from cell wall residues was a bitterfree one.

Fig.2. Hydrolysis of cell wall residues:pH 8.0; 55°C; 120 min. 22 Tyrosine Units of thermitase / g true protein
x = sample no I;  N = 6.35 %
* = sample no II; N = 7.15 %

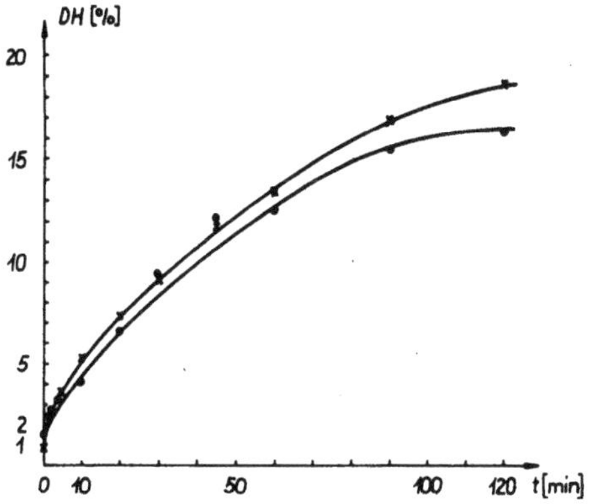


Fig.3. Hydrolysis of protein isolate: pH 8.0; 55°C; 150 min. 10 Tyrosine Units of Thermitase / g true protein
x = sample no III; N = 13.6 %
* = sample no IV; N = 14.1 %

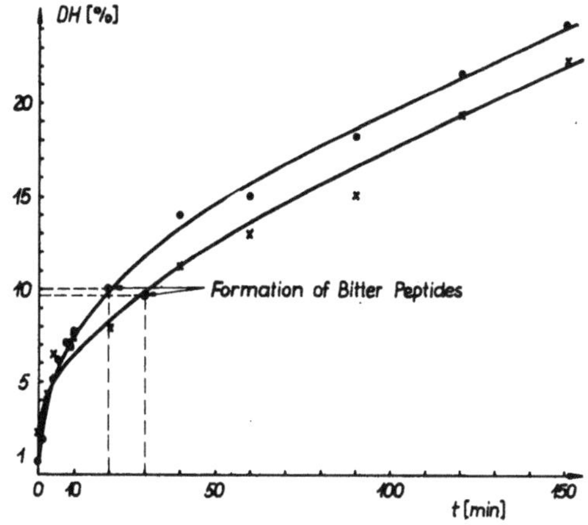


Fig.4. Hydrolysis of protein concentrate: pH 8.0; 55°C; 150 min. 22 Tyrosine Units of thermitase / g true protein
x = sample no V; N = 13.6 %
* = sample no VI; N = 12.8 %

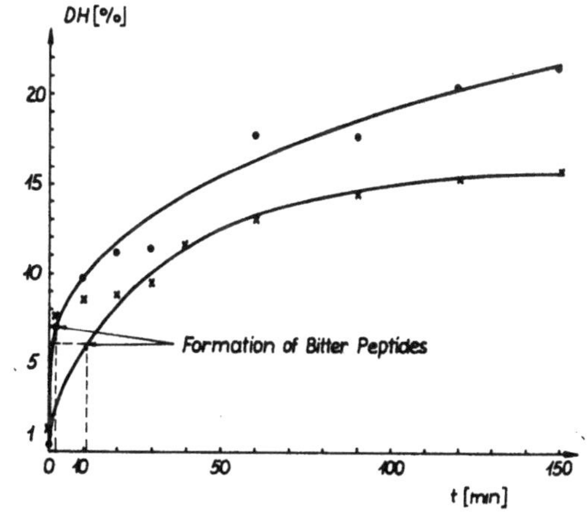


Literature:

/1/ NEY, K.H. Z. Lebensm.-Unters. und Forsch. 147(1971), pp. 64-68

/2/ LANGNER, J. Acta biol. med. german. 26(1971), pp. 935 - 951

**INVESTIGATION OF PRIMARY DEGRADATION PRODUCTS OF CASEIN IN DUTCH-TYPE CHEESE**

T. Sienkiewicz[1] and R. Schleusener[2]

**Introduction**

Proteolysis of cheese caseins is considered as the result of combined actions of primarily rennet, starter bacteria and original milk enzymes including as well heat-sensitive acidic and neutral proteinases as heat-resistant alkaline proteinases.

Proteolysis plays an important role in converting the calcium-paracaseinate curd into matured Dutch-type cheese, it affects both the flavour and the body of final product. Degradation products are also implicated in certain flavour defects, esspecially in bitterness. The present study concerning with hydrolysis of casein solutions is primarily directed to degradation of ß-casein. The used proteolytic enzymes are chymosin, bovine pepsin, a microbial rennet substitute, protease extract and Mucor mihei preparation "Fromase". Moreover the degradation niveau of both major casein components in a four week old Edam type cheese is investigated. A quantitative disc gel electrophoresis technique (PAFE) in connection with a densitometer-computer unit is used to investigate primary proteolysis in cheeses and model solutions.

**Results**

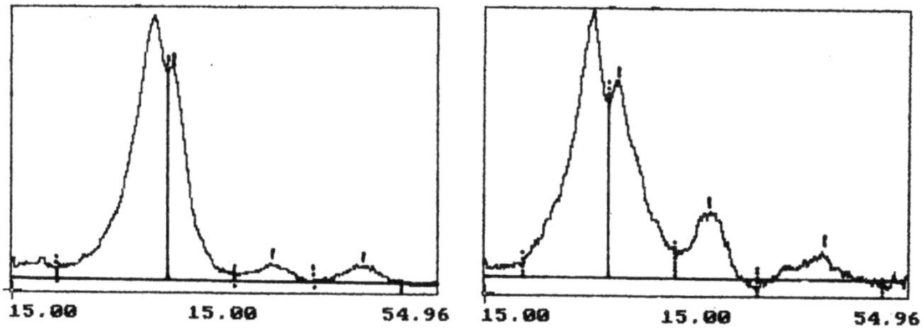


Figure 1: Densitogramms of ß-casein treated with a protease extract (0 hours and 45 hours)

[1]Humboldt-University of Berlin,
Department of Food Industry and Food Technology
[2]VEB Scientific-Technical-Economic Centre of Dairy Industry, GDR

Calculation using interpolation of protease extract

| No | 0 h Locn mm | 0 h Height AU | 0 h Area AU*mm | 0 h Rel ar % | 45 h Locn mm | 45 h Height AU | 45 h Area AU*mm | 45 h Rel ar % |
|---|---|---|---|---|---|---|---|---|
| 1 | 28.36 | 0.527 | 2.023 | 60.1 | 25.12 | 0.297 | 1.159 | 48.3 |
| 2 | 30.00 | 0.422 | 1.047 | 31.1 | 27.40 | 0.221 | 0.776 | 32.3 |
| 3 | 39.64 | 0.034 | 0.147 | 4.4 | 36.04 | 0.080 | 0.030 | 12.6 |
| 4 | 48.28 | 0.034 | 0.147 | 4.4 | 46.80 | 0.036 | 0.163 | 6.8 |

**Discussion**

Proteolysis in cheese

The results of electrophoretic experiments in figure 2 and table 1 showed a difference in breakdown between ß- and $\alpha_{s1}$-casein. After 4 weeks ripening five bands of breakdown products of ß- and six of $\alpha_{s1}$-casein were detected In table 1 the residual amounts of undecomposed $\alpha_{s1}$- and ß-casein representing appearently 45 to 50 % of the original quantity are calculated from the densitograms.

The residual proportions of $\alpha_{s1}$-and ß-casein of our investigations are not similar to the average values for Gouda cheese. Several workers (VISSER et al., 1977; CREAMER, 1974) have reported that in hard cheese (Dutch type) $\alpha_{s1}$-casein is degraded more easily (primairly to $\alpha_{s1}$-I) than is ß-casein. Within a period of 4 weeks only a faint zone remains, representing 7 - 10 % of the original $\alpha_{s1}$-casein. About 80 % of ß-casein being unattacked for up to 1 month (VISSER et al., 1977). According to our resultes the $\alpha_{s1}$-I-casein is not the only degradation product of $\alpha_{s1}$-casein after four weeks. The sum of the other $\alpha_{s1}$-casein degradation products exceeds the portion of the $\alpha_{s1}$-I-component. A big part of the $\alpha_{s1}$-casein is also not degraded.

The degradation of ß-casein to products with slow electrophoretical mobility γ-caseins which is stronger than is reported in the literature points to the effect of alkaline proteinases in our cheese probes.

Model experiments

The electrophoretical comparison of the attack of the different enzymes on ß- and $\alpha_{s1}$-casein showed characteristic differences in the degradation of caseins in a model solution.

An accelerated degradation was found both on application of microbial rennet (experimental preparation) and on ß-casein as at $\alpha_{s1}$-casein, too. In this case the ß-casein was nearly completly degraded without forming of ß-casein I and ß-casein II degradation products although the clotting strength in the Formagraph experiment corresponded to chymosin (fig. 3).

Table 1: Relative proportions of unattacked $\alpha_{s1}$− and β-Casein and of degradation products in four weeks ripened Edam cheese.
Gel scan XL laser densitometer LKB Sweden; Calculation of peaks area using interpolation

| | Fraction of casein | $\gamma_3$ | $\gamma_2$ | $\gamma_1$ | β | $\alpha_{s2}$ | $\alpha_{s1}$ | ? | $\alpha_{s1}$-I | $\alpha_{s1}$VI+V | $\alpha_{s1}$II | $\alpha_{s1}$III | $\alpha_{s1}$IV |
|---|---|---|---|---|---|---|---|---|---|---|---|---|---|
| Charge Edam cheese 4 weeks old | Number of band on the PAGE pattern | 3 | 4 | 5 | 6 | 7-9 | 10 | 11 | 12 | 13 | 14 | 15 | 16 |
| d 2 | | 5.0 | 4.0 | 6.2 | 20.5 | 5.4 | 23.3 | 5.2 | 9.3 | 8.3 | 3.8 | 3.0 | 0.9 |
| d 3 | | 5.0 | 4.4 | 5.4 | 18.8 | 10.2 | 24.3 | 4.9 | 7.9 | 7.2 | 3.6 | 1.9 | 1.2 |
| d 4 | | 5.1 | 4.8 | 5.9 | 19.1 | 11.1 | 20.1 | 5.1 | 7.6 | 8.1 | 3.2 | 2.5 | 2.1 |
| d 5 | | 5.0 | 4.8 | 5.0 | 18.2 | 9.5 | 21.6 | 4.8 | 8.3 | 8.6 | 3.6 | 2.9 | 2.2 |
| d 6 | | 4.7 | 4.5 | 5.6 | 18.1 | 9.7 | 19.9 | 5.7 | 10.2 | 8.4 | 2.0 | 3.8 | 2.8 |
| d 7 | | 4.6 | 5.0 | 5.7 | 17.7 | 10.8 | 22.9 | 5.4 | 8.9 | 6.6 | 2.0 | 2.9 | 2.2 |
| d 8 | | 4.8 | 4.7 | 5.3 | 22.1 | 12.8 | 25.5 | 4.7 | 5.2 | 7.5 | 3.2 | 2.8 | 2.3 |
| d 9 | | 6.6 | 5.4 | 6.0 | 22.0 | 8.3 | 22.2 | 4.2 | 7.1 | 6.5 | 1.9 | 2.8 | 2.4 |
| d 10 | | 6.8 | 5.0 | 6.2 | 23.1 | 7.7 | 19.9 | 3.9 | 8.9 | 7.3 | 1.6 | 3.1 | 2.0 |
| d 11 | | 4.0 | 4.2 | 5.3 | 20.9 | 10.5 | 22.8 | 4.6 | 9.3 | 7.5 | 1.7 | 3.5 | 1.8 |
| d 12 | | 4.8 | 4.4 | 7.4 | 26.6 | 5.5 | 20.0 | 4.5 | 9.3 | 8.7 | 1.5 | 3.3 | 0.0 |
| d 13 | | 4.5 | 5.0 | 6.3 | 21.1 | 10.5 | 20.2 | 4.4 | 10.2 | 6.7 | 1.6 | 2.8 | 2.2 |
| No 2 d 1 | | 3.4 | 4.4 | 4.7 | 22.8 | 11.5 | 26.6 | 3.6 | 10.8 | 6.0 | 1.3 | 1.9 | 1.8 |
| No 2 d 2 | | 3.9 | 4.0 | 5.2 | 21.8 | 13.2 | 28.0 | 3.8 | 5.0 | 5.1 | 3.1 | 2.0 | 1.4 |
| Mean $\bar{x}$ | | 4.87 | 4.62 | 5.76 | 20.91 | 9.77 | 22.66 | 4.63 | 8.98 | 7.49 | 2.44 | 2.80 | 2.03 |
| S. Dev SD | | 0.92 | 0.41 | 0.70 | 2.44 | 2.35 | 2.65 | 0.62 | 1.11 | 0.88 | 0.92 | 0.57 | 0.43 |
| Variance % | | 18.8 | 8.9 | 12.1 | 11.7 | 24.0 | 11.7 | 13.3 | 12.4 | 11.8 | 37.5 | 20.9 | 21.7 |
| Sum | | 68.2 | 64.6 | 74.9 | 292.8 | 136.8 | 317.3 | 64.8 | 107.8 | 97.4 | 34.1 | 39.2 | 24.4 |

Fromase 46 TL had the biggest clotting strength in the chosen dilution but it effected a slower degradation of the ß-casein than the microbial rennet but a quicker degradation than chymosin and bovine pepsin. The rapid formation of ß-casein II (after 8 h) and the residual amounts of ß-casein (after 48 h) are characteristic for this process (fig. 4).

Chymosin and bovine pepsin produced a band tightly under the band of ß-casein. After 48 h bovine pepsin produced ß-casein II in contrast to Proteinase which are extracted from S. cremoris after modification of the method of HUGENHOLZ et al. (1984) after 45 h shows a clearly visible degradation of the ß-casein to ß-casein I and ß-casein II.
In the same time a band tightly under the band of ß-casein is formed similar to the effect of chymosin and bovine pepsin.
According to figure 1 a three times higher amount of ß-casein I than ß-casein II formed the S. cremoris protease.
The $\alpha_{s1}$-casein was degraded by the experimental preparation of microbial rennet already after 60 min and formed $\alpha_{s1}$-I-casein.
There was a distinct increasing of $\alpha_{s1}$-I-casein.
In a model solution the action of Fromase 46 TL, chymosin and bovine pepsin to $\alpha_{s1}$-casein showed on the PAGE no detectable degradation products.

## Literature


[1] Creamer, L.K.; Proc. 19th Int. Dairy Congr. 1 D

[2] Hugenholz, K., F. Exterkate and W.N. Konings; Appl. Environ. Microbiol. **48** (1984) 1105 - 1110

[3] Schleusener, R., E. Kirst and T. Sienkiewicz; Milchforschung - Milchpraxis **24** (1982) 4, 94 - 96

[4] Visser, S.M.W. and A.E.A. Groot-Mostert; Neth. Milk Dairy J. **31** (1977) 247 - 264

EFFECT OF FROZEN STORAGE ON THE STRUCTURE, THE FUNCTIONALITY AND BIOGENIC AMINE CONTENT OF MUSCLE PROTEINS

Mietsch, F.[1)], Baráth, Á.[1)], Éliás, I.[1)], Fehér, J.[1)], Halász, A.[1)], Merész, P.[2)]

In the literature a lot of authors study the changes which proceed in meats during frozen storage. Among other things the experiments concern with structural changes, organoleptic properties, functional properties or how to get rid of certain unfavourable changes.
An important problem of long-term storage of foods is the emergence of biogenic amines. These agents are produced when specific amino acids undergo decarboxylation usually catalyzed by specific decarboxylase enzymes produced by microorganisms. Biologically active amines have important physiological effects in humans, generally either psychoactive or vasoactive.
In the present work the structural changes of muscle proteins were investigated during a some-month long storage, SDS-PAGE technique was applied to determine these changes.
Besides certain functional properties (emulsifying activity, emulsion stability, water absorption capacity, oil absorption capacity) were measured. The content of biogenic amines was determined by ionexchange chromatography.

## Materials and methods

Our experiments were carried out with fresh pork obtained from the slaughter-house. The pork was kept frozen at -20 degrees centigrade for 6 months.
Emulsifying activity and emulsion stability were determined by the method of PEARCE and KINSELLA (1978) and KATO et al. (1981). The determination of water and oil absorption capacity were carried out according to LIN, HUMBERT and SOSULSKI (1974).
Biogenic amines were extracted from meat by the method of GEHRKE et al. (1977) and finally detected with an amino acid analyzer (Biotronik, FRG).

---

1) Central Food Research Institute, 1525 Budapest, P.O.Box 76, Hungary
2) Technical University of Budapest, Institute of Biochemistry and Foodtechnology, 1111. Budapest, Müegyetem rkp. 3, Hungary

For SDS-PAGE samples were prepared as follows:
Ten-gram samples were homogenized in 90 ml of cooled 0.6 M KCl solution with an ULTRA-TURRAX T 18/10 (JAHNKE & KUNKEL IKA Werk, FRG) for ten seconds four times. After homogenizing the samples were centrifuged (30 min. at 6000 rpm) and the supernatant was used for the SDS-PAGE which was carried out by a PHARMACIA equipment (Sweden). The chromatograms were evaluated by a Labor MIM densitometer (Hungary) and an on-line computer (Commodore-64).

## Results and discussion

The data of water and oil absorption capacity, emulsifying activity and emulsion stability are shown in table 1. and table 2.

Table 1: Water and oil absorption capacity of pork in dependence of storage time at -20°C

| months | oil absorption capacity (%) | water absorption capacity (%) |
|---|---|---|
| 0 | 212.21 ± 11.82 | 266.18 ± 5.32 |
| 1 | 225.99 ± 14.53 | 242.42 ± 13.06 |
| 2 | 220.29 ± 3.69 | 249.89 ± 5.94 |
| 3 | 223.87 ± 10.24 | 245.35 ± 11.63 |
| 6 | 231.03 ± 5.70 | 236.83 ± 5.59 |

Table 2: Emulsifying activity and emulsion stability of pork in dependence of storage time at -20°C

| months | emulsifying activity ($m^2/g$) | emulsion stability (minutes) |
|---|---|---|
| 0 | 109.86 ± 5.36 | 1.05 ± 0.23 |
| 1 | 111.82 ± 6.34 | 1.05 ± 0.17 |
| 2 | 116.53 ± 7.03 | 1.21 ± 0.08 |
| 3 | 117.52 ± 3.73 | 1.17 ± 0.06 |
| 6 | 118.57 ± 6.00 | 1.03 ± 0.09 |

The statistical evaluation of the results shows that there is no significant difference in dependence on storage time (water absorption capacity: $F_{calc.} = 2.64$, $F_{tab.} = 3.63$, $P = 5$ %; oil absorption capacity: $F_{calc.} = 1.24$, $F_{tab.} = 3.63$, $P = 5$ %; emulsifying activity: $F_{calc.} = 0,86$, $F_{tab.} = 5.19$, $P = 5$ %; emulsion stability: $F_{calc.} = 1.13$, $F_{tab.} = 5.19$, $P = 5$ %). On the basis of the SDS-PAGE chromatograms we can say that during the six-month storage time the structure of the investigated muscle proteins didn't change extremely (figure 1).

Figure 1: SDS-PAGE chromatograms of pork in dependence of storage time at $-20^{0}C$

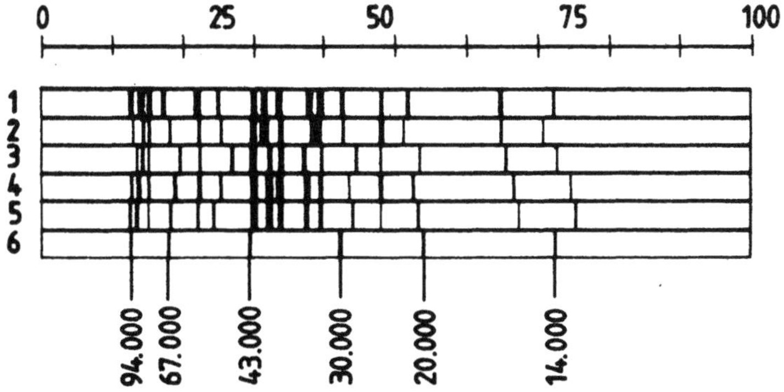


1: 0.month; 2: 1.month; 3: 2.month; 4: 3.month; 5: 6.month; 6: standard

These results are similar to those observed by HAMM et al. (1982). HAMM et al. couldn't observe any changes in protein structure during frozen storage of meat. In addition, they didn't observe changes in water-holding capacity either.
Some authors say that protein denaturation occurs only after an at least one-year frozen storage period. Our results seem to support their investigations.
In our work we investigated the change in the content of five biogenic amines (putrescine, histamine, cadaverine, spermidine, spermine), too. The separation of a standard mixture is shown in figure 2.

Figure 2: Separation of a biogenic amine standard

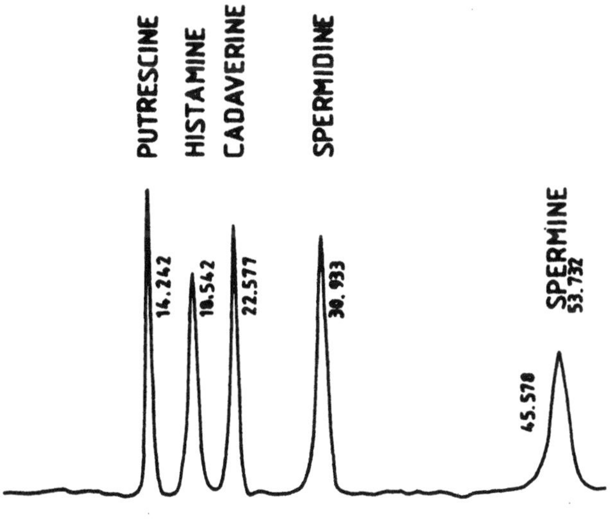

Results and Discussion

The described prosedure leads in the case of FWF to a marked muscle like anisotropic structure. Horse mackerel gives also a certain degree of structurization, but not to the same extent as fresh water fish does.
The additives rapeseed oil, potato starch, FBPI, and pectin influence structure and texture in different manner dependent on species of fish, content of the respective additive and composition of the system. In the following some selected examples of the crest-line analyses are given showing tendencies of influence on structure and texture.

| | FWF | Horse mackerel |
|---|---|---|
| Visible | Higher concentrations of rapeseed oil and low concentrations of pectin have a positive influence on the structurization, whereas starch has nearly no influence. High concentrations of FBPI give less structure. (Fig. 1) | Higher concentrations of rapeseed oil have a negative influence on the structure, whereas starch shows nearly no influence on the degree of structurization. (Fig. 2) |
| Firmness | To reach the desirable firmness it is recommended, to add rapeseed oil and starch at a medium level, pectin at a high level and FBPI at a very low level. As in the case of structure no influence of the concentration of starch is detectable. | To reach the desirable firmness it is recommended to add all four additives at a medium level. low levels of pectin and FBPI lead to firmer products. |
| Penetration values | The penetration values increase with increasing concentrations of rapeseed oil, pectin and starch, whereas increasing concentrations of FBPI decrease the penetration values. | The penetration values in dependence on the additives show similar tendencies as shown for FWF. |

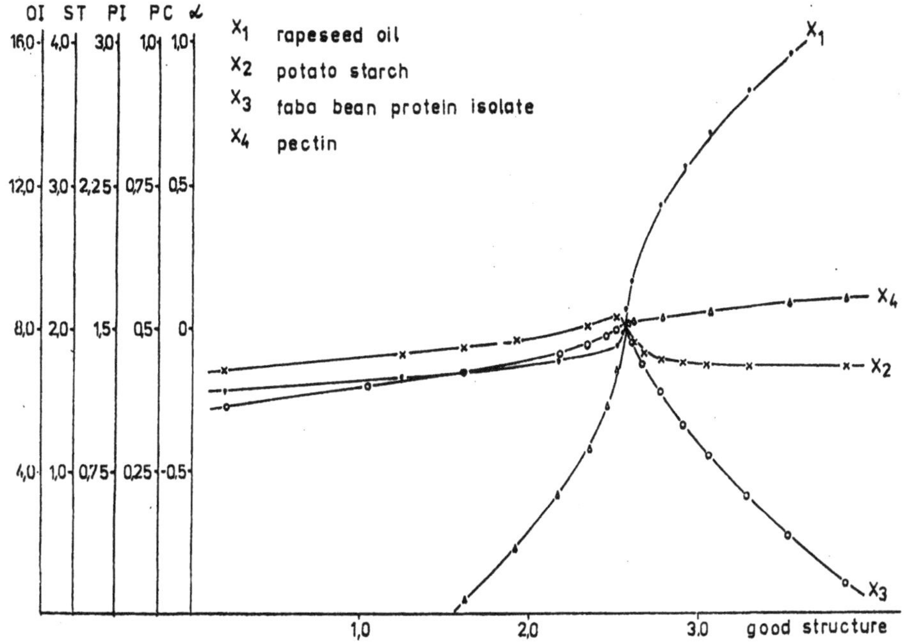


Fig. 1: Crest - line analysis for the structurization of minced fresh water fishes
(degree of structurization)

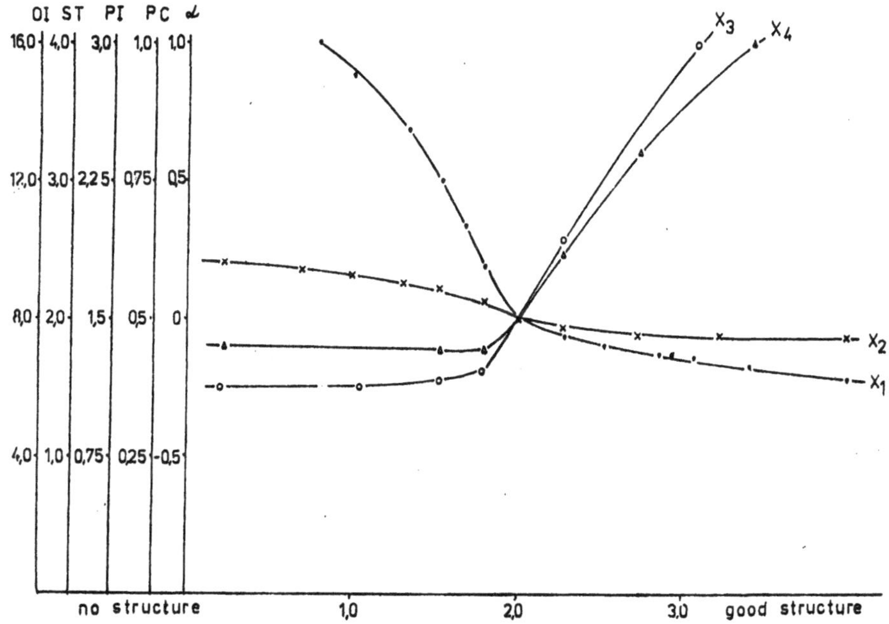


Fig. 2: Crest - line analysis for the structurization of minced horse mackerels
(degree of structurization)

## Conclusions

- Using cryostructurization it is possible to create muscle like structures in comminuted fish flesh.
- With the aid of the used additives texture and structure of the products can be modified.
- The species of fish influences the degree of structurization.
- The results show the necessity for further investigations dealing with a deeper understanding of the mechanism of the structurization especially in relation to the role of additives.

## Literature


/1/ Consolacion, F. J. and P. Jelen, Freeze Texturization of Proteins: Effect of the Alkali, Acid and Freezing Treatments on Texture Formation, Food Microstructure 5 (1986),1 33 - 39

/2/ Lawrence, R., F. Consolacion and P. Jelen, Formation of Structured Protein Foods by Freeze Texturization, Food Technol. 40 (1986) 3, 77 - 82, 90

INFLUENCE OF FABA BEAN PROTEIN ISOLATE-PECTIN-MIXTURES ON O/W-SYSTEMS

M. Schultz and G. Schmidt[1)]

## INTRODUCTION

Recently in our working group an extented fundamental study is in progress, to investigate the influence of unmodified or acetylated faba bean proteins, alone or in combination with pectins at different pH-values, kind and strength of ionic environment on the internal structure, rheological behaviour and long term stability of o/w-emulsions. Here are represented first results dealing with effects of different concentrations of faba bean protein isolates and different concentration of pectin on an o/w-emulsion with 30 weight per cent of the oil phase.

## MATERIALS AND METHODS

- Faba bean protein isolate, unmodified and acetylated (acetylation degree 97 %), concentration range in the emulsions 0.1 to 3.0 %.
- Sunflower oil, purified with $Al_2O_3$.
- Pectin, low-esterified (degree of esterification 38 %), concentration range in the emulsions 0 to 0.5 %.
- Preparation of emulsions (o/w-type with a 30/70 weight ratio of oil and aqueous phase, initial pH of the aqueous phase 7.0) was carried out by sonification with a laboratory ultrasonic disintegrator under controlled conditions (50 °C, 3 x 1 min, 400 W).
- Rheological measurements were carried out with the rotating viscosimeter Rheotest 2 (VEB MLW Medingen) with a gap of 1 mm. They includes measuring of viscosity at a shear rate of 437.4 $s^{-1}$ and calculation of basic flow properties within a shear rate range of 9.0 to 729 $s^{-1}$ after preshearing at shear rate of 729 $s^{-1}$ for 45 min. The flow curves were exploited mathematically according to Ostwald de Waele.
- pH-determination in dependence on storage time (1 to 6 days).
- Stability evaluation is carried out with a laboratory centrifuge at 3 000 x g, measuring the separated volume of the aqueous phase after different times of centrifugation.

1) Central Institute of Nutrition of the Academy of Sciences of the GDR Potsdam-Rehbrücke

## RESULTS AND DISCUSSION

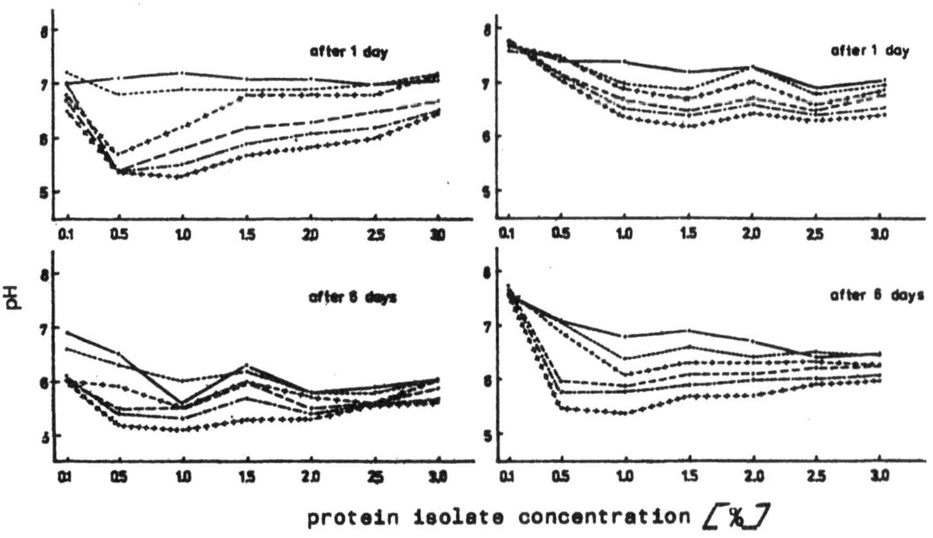


Fig. 1 The influence of the pectin on the pH-value of fresh and aged emulsions (A = unmodified protein, B = acetylated protein)[1)]

Fig. 1 A and B show that at given protein concentration the pH-value decreases with increasing pectin concentration. A more pronounced influence of the pH-value is observed in case of unmodified protein isolate compared with the acetylated isolate. Within the observed storage time (up to 6 days) a continuing change of the pH-value is observed. Fig. 2 A and B show that the apparent viscosity increases with increasing protein concentration nearly linearly in case of acetylated protein isolate but not linearly in case of unmodified protein isolate. With increasing pectin concentration the apparent viscosity increases in particular at higher protein concentrations. In case of unmodified protein isolate the increase of the viscosity is more pronounced. The emulsions with lower contents of protein and pectin show a nearly Newtonian flow behaviour. With increasing contents of protein and pectin the emulsions show an increasing pseodoplastic flow behaviour. Within the investigated range all emulsions do not show yield value.

1) In all figures means:

| | | | |
|---|---|---|---|
| ——— | without pectin | — — — | 0.3 % pectin |
| ------- | 0.1 % pectin | -·-·-· | 0.4 % pectin |
| -+-+-+- | 0.2 % pectin | ++++++++ | 0.5 % pectin |

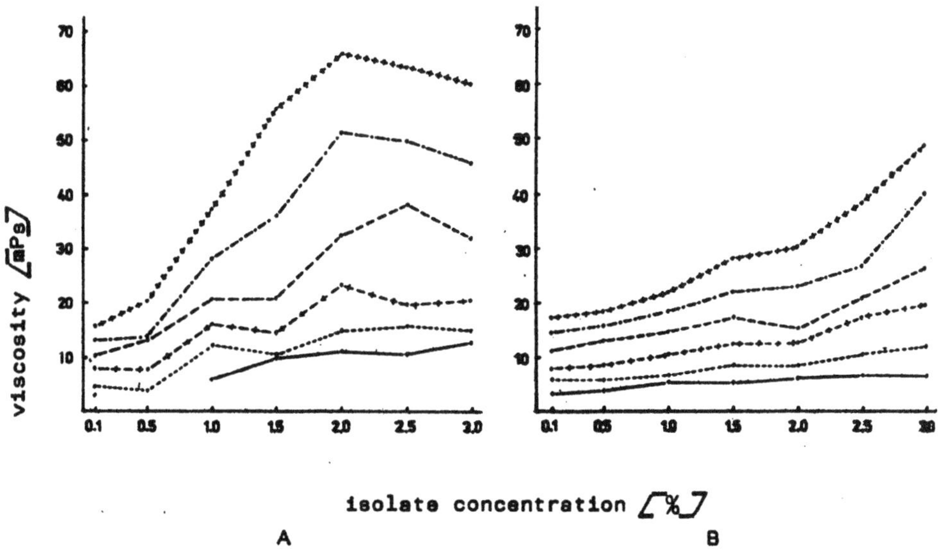


Fig. 2 The influence of the pectin content on the apparent viscosity of the emulsions (A = unmodified protein, B = acetylated protein)

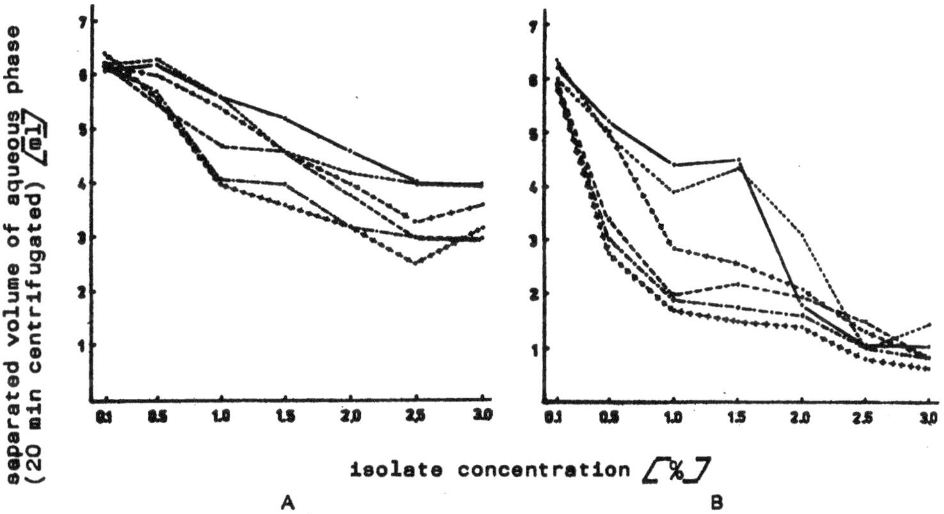


Fig. 3 The influence of the pectin content on the centrifugal stability (CS) of the emulsions (A = unmodified protein, B = acetylated protein)

has been determined. Calculation:

$$FBC = \frac{(m_1 + m_o - m_2) \cdot 100}{\rho_{oil} (m_2 - m_o)}$$

If about 50 mg of protein are used for FBC determination the variation coefficient is 5-10%. Compared with similar methods FBC values are low because physically bound oil seems to be removed to a large extent (table 1). Numerous publications do not take in consideration that usually more oil is bound by capillary forces than by hydrophobic interactions. There is a streng correlation between bulk density of a protein sample and FBC values (figure 1). In the case of above described procedure correlation coefficient is -0.8.

Table 1. FBC values of proteins

| protein | origin | bulk density /g/ml/ | FBC - values /ml/100g/ from VOUTSINAS & NAKAI by | | LUDWIG et al. by | |
|---|---|---|---|---|---|---|
| | | | macromethod acc. to (3) | micromethod acc. to (7) | modified macromethod acc. to (3) | presented micromethod |
| ovalbumin | Sigma | unknown | 560.0 | 37.7 | | |
| | Serva | 0.07 | | | 435 | 265 |
| | Serva | 0.22 | | | 196 | 98 |
| bovine serum albumin | Sigma | unknown | 340.0 | 25.0 | | |
| | Serva | 0.38 | | | | 60 |
| | Serumwerk Dessau | 0.21 | | | 297 | 98 |
| | | 0.34 | | | 149 | 48 |
| ß-lactoglobulin | Sigma | unknown | 210 | 4.2 | | |
| | prep.(1) | 0.34 | | | 97 | 66 |
| casein | prepared | unknown | 95.0 | 10.1 | | |
| | prepared | 0.38 | | | 154 | |
| | prepared | 0.52 | | | 105 | 46 |
| faba bean protein | Paulinaue | 0.59 | | | 43 | 42 |
| ...... | | | | | | |
| silicagel | Merck | 0.36 | | | 172 | 103 |

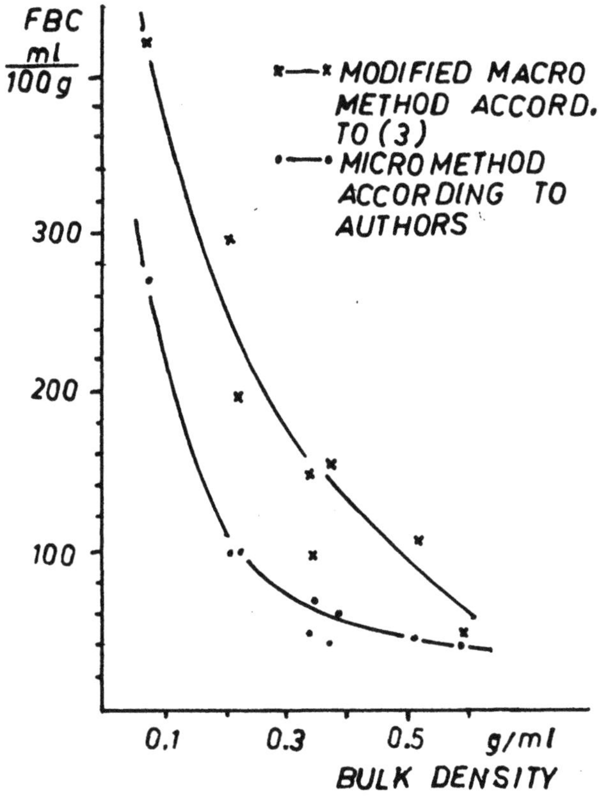


Figure 1. Dependence of the FBC determined by two methods on the bulk density

References


/1/ Aschaffenburg, R. and J. Drewry: Arch. Biochem. Biophys. 65 (1957) 273

/2/ Kinsella, J.E.: CRC Crit. Rev. Food Sci. Nutr. 7 (1976), 219

/3/ Lin, M.J.Y., E.S. Humbert and F.W. Sosulski: J. Food Sci. 39 (1974), 368

/4/ Nakai, S.: J. Agric. Food Chem. 31 (1983), 676

/5/ Schwenke, K.D., L. Prahl, E. Rauschal, S. Gwiazda, K. Dabrowski and A. Rutkowski: Nahrung 25 (1981), 59

/6/ Sosulski, F., E.S. Humbert and K. Bui: J. Food Sci. 41 (1976), 1349

/7/ Voutsinas, L.P. and S. Nakai: J. Agric. Food Chem. 31 (1983), 58

/8/ Wang, C.J. and J.E. Kinsella: J. Food Sci. 41 (1976), 286

# DETERMINATION OF VERY SMALL Ki-VALUES IN ENZYME-INHIBITOR INTERACTING SYSTEMS

Ch. Flemming, H. Schaedlich, H. Wand [1)]

## Introduction

Since the sixthties several japanese research groups isolated and characterized a dozen and more protease inhibitors from different microbial strains. Plasminostreptin, one of these inhibitors, was described by Kakinuma et al. /1/ at first. It is a macromolecular protease inhibitor, produced by a streptomyces strain and inhibits trypsin, subtilisin and thermitase among others. Common to all these inhibitors and also to plasminostreptin are strong interactions with enzymes. As for all inhibitors with inhibition constants of $< 10^{-6}$ M it is difficult to determine the Ki-values with the known graphic methods.

By modification of these methods we tried to determine the Ki-values of trypsin, thermitase and subtilisin.

## Determination of the Ki-values

The titration of the enzymes trypsin, thermitase and subtilisin with plasminostreptin (Fig. 1 a, b) reflects the strong interaction of the reactants. The enzyme activity decreases linearly to a degree of 90 % in the case of trypsin and nearly to 100 % inhibition in the case of subtilisin. In contrast, at Ki-values $\geq 10^{-6}$ M there is a more or less asymtotical approach of the titration curve to the abscissa.

By using the unmodified Dixon plot in the case of the inhibition of trypsin we obtain an apparently nonlinear inhibition of a noncompetitive type (Fig. 2).

The modification taken by us consists in substituting the concentration of the total inhibitor $/I_{total}/$ by the concentration of the free inhibitor $/I_{free}/$. $/I_{free}/$ has to be calculated from the equations 1 to 4.

$$\frac{V_I}{V_{max}} = \frac{/ES/}{/E_{total}/} \qquad 1$$

$$\frac{K_M}{S} = \frac{/E_{free}/}{/ES/} \qquad 2$$

[1)] Institute of Biotechnology GDR-7050 Leipzig, Permoserstraße 15

$$/E_{total}/ = /E_{free}/ + /EI/ + /ES/ \quad 3$$

$$/I_{total}/ = /I_{free}/ + /EI/ \quad 4$$

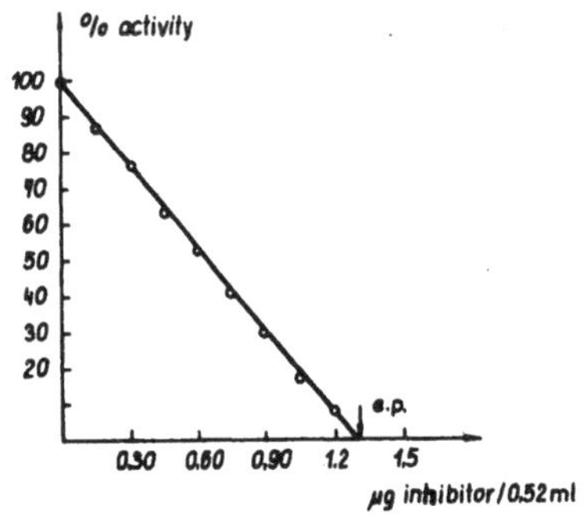


Fig. 1 a: Titration of trypsin with plasminostreptin
$/E/ = 3.3x10^{-7}$ M
$/S/ = 5.77x10^{-4}$ M

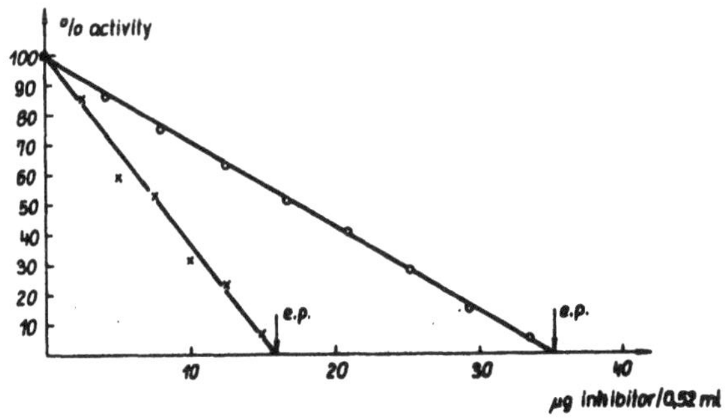


Fig. 1 b: Titration of subtilisin and thermitase with plasminostreptin
subtilisin
$/E/ = 7.49x10^{-6}$ M
$/S/ = 5.0\ x10^{-4}$ M (o — o)
thermitase
$/E/ = 1.5x10^{-6}$ M
$/S/ = 4.8x10^{-4}$ M (x — x)

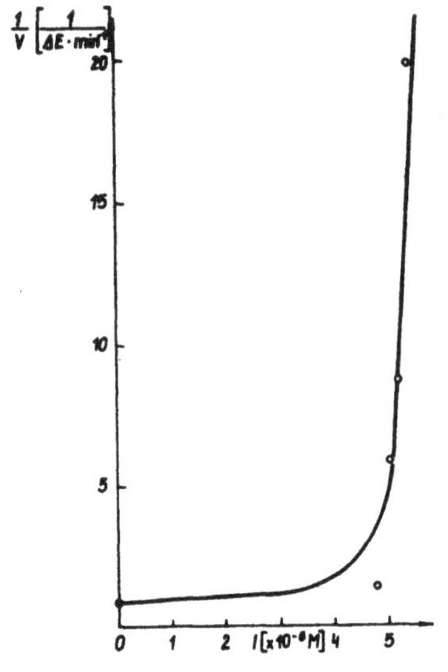

Fig. 2: Unmodified DIXON plot of the inhibition of trypsin by plasminostreptin
$/E/ = 2.5 \times 10^{-6}$ M
$/S/ = 4.8 \times 10^{-4}$ M

$V_I$ denotes the enzyme activity remaining after the addition of the inhibitor and has to be measured.
By increasing the enzyme concentration 5 to 10 times in comparison with the standard conditions and reaction times up to 2 hours it was possible to get valid results. By this modification in the case of trypsin we determined a Ki-value of $0.83 \times 10^{-9}$ M and a competitive inhibition (Fig. 3 a, b).
With the Steck-Wallach plot /2/ we determined a slightly different Ki-value of $1.13 \times 10^{-9}$ M (Fig. 4).

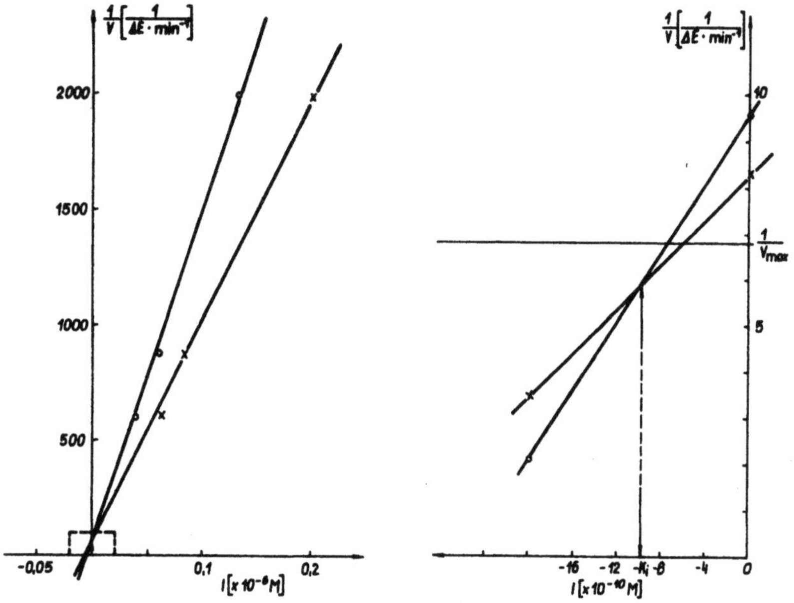


Fig. 3: Determination of inhibition type and Ki-value

a) $/S_1/ = 4.8 \times 10^{-6}$ M (o —— o)

$/S_2/ = 9.6 \times 10^{-4}$ M (x —— x)

$/I_{free}/$ was calculated

b) detail enlargement

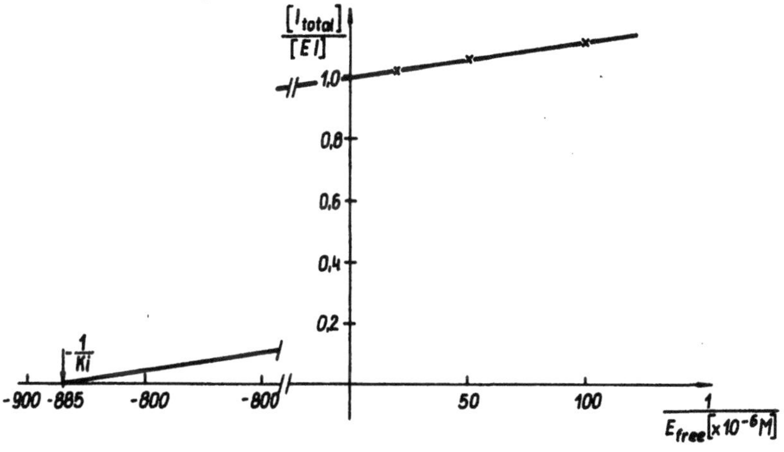


Fig. 4: Determination of the Ki-value of the inhibition of trypsin by plasminostreptin by the method of STECK-WALLACH

## Conclusions

The problem of determining low Ki-values has been solved at least partially by application of modified graphical methods.
The reaction of subtilisin with plasminostreptin with a Ki-value of about $10^{-12}$ M we estimated only denotes a limit we could'nt overcome.

## Literature


/1/ Kakinuma, A.; Sugimo, H.; Moriya, N.; Isono, M.: J. Biol. Chem. 293 (1978) 1529

/2/ Steck, Th.; Wallach, D.: Biochem. Biophys. Acta 97 (1965) 510

# LIPOPROTEIN COMPLEXES IN INFANT MILK FORMULAS AND MILK POWDER

Z. Zbikowski[1], S. Ziajka[1], A. Zbikowska[2] and K. Bature[1]

## Introduction

Mechanisms of the formation of lipoprotein complexes in milk concentrates are rather complicated. Interaction between lipids and proteins can take place in form of covalent bonds, van der Waals forces, ionic or hydrophobic interactions, hydrogen bridges or the combination of these /3, 4/. The level of these complexes may increase in course of the drying of food products, this is due to a transformation of the lipoprotein complexes into strongly bounded forms. Formation of the lipoprotein complexes is usually accompanied by polymerization phenomena which also decrease the quality of the product /2/.

## Material

Studies were made on commercial milk formulas for infants (Lactovit 0 and Bebiko 1) and on whole milk powder.

## Methods

Lipoprotein complexes were extracted with a mixture of chloroform and methanol (2 : 1) and with petroleum benzin, according to Pokorny et al. /3/.

## Results and discussion

The products under study differed slightly as regards the amount of lipoprotein complexes (1.1 - 1.3 g/100 g). More pronounced differences were observed with respect to fat content (74.4 - 80.7 %, Table 1). An increase of the amount of the complexes under study took place during sample storage at 18 °C for 6 months, to the level of 2.1 - 2.8 g/100 g. On the other hand, fat content decreased to 71.6 - 72.9 %.

[1]Institute of Dairy Technology, University of Agriculture and Technology Olsztyn, Poland

[2]Institute of Physics and Food Chemistry, University of Agriculture and Technology, Olsztyn, Poland

Table 1: The content of fat fractions which were obtained by step-wise selective extraction from insoluble parts of infant milk formula and milk powder

| Kind of sample | Content of | | | Content of fat /in %/ extracted by | | |
|---|---|---|---|---|---|---|
| | fat % | lipoprotein complexes g/100g | fat in lipoprotein complexes % | petrol benzin | chloroform and methanol | petrol benzin hydrolisis |
| **Fresh product** | | | | | | |
| Lactovit O[x] | 36.9 | 3.42 | 78.0 | 70.1 | 15.8 | 14.1 |
| Bebiko I[x] | 35.8 | 3.56 | 77.2 | 67.8 | 15.6 | 16.6 |
| Milk powder | 36.9 | 3.52 | 72.1 | 69.3 | 19.9 | 10.8 |
| **After 6 months storage at 18°C** | | | | | | |
| Lactovit O[x] | 38.5 | 5.69 | 67.1 | 63.8 | 17.2 | 18.9 |
| Bebiko I[x] | 37.4 | 5.81 | 67.2 | 60.1 | 16.3 | 23.6 |
| Milk powder | 38.7 | 5.73 | 67.4 | 63.0 | 21.5 | 15.6 |

x - infant milk formula

Table 2: The content of fat fractions which were obtained by step-wise selective extraction from infant milk formula and milk powder

| Kind of sample | Content of | | | Content of fat /in %/ extracted by | | | |
|---|---|---|---|---|---|---|---|
| | fat /%/ | lipoprotein complexes /g/100g/ | fat in lipoprotein complexes /%/ | petrol benzin | Chloroform | methanol | petrol benzin after acid hydrolysis |
| **Fresh product** | | | | | | | |
| Lactovit $0^x$ | 20.1 | 1.14 | 80.7 | 43.4 | 27.1 | 24.9 | 4.6 |
| Bebiko $I^x$ | 16.5 | 1.12 | 80.4 | 36.1 | 32.8 | 25.6 | 5.5 |
| Milk powder | 25.1 | 1.31 | 74.4 | 35.5 | 27.8 | 28.9 | 3.9 |
| **After 6 months storage at 18°C** | | | | | | | |
| Lactovit $0^x$ | 20.1 | 2.14 | 72.9 | 48.1 | 25.6 | 18.5 | 7.8 |
| Bebiko $I^x$ | 16.5 | 2.06 | 72.5 | 39.2 | 31.1 | 20.9 | 8.8 |
| Milk powder | 25.1 | 2.78 | 71.6 | 42.6 | 26.5 | 22.9 | 8.0 |

x - infant milk formula

EINHORN, Ulrike
Humboldt-Univ. Berlin, Sect. NGW/LMT, Pflugstr. 6 b, Berlin, DDR-1040

FLEMMING, Christian
Acad. Sci. GDR, Inst. Biotechnol., Permoserstr. 15, Leipzig, DDR-7050

GAST, Klaus
Acad. Sci. GDR, Central Inst. Molecular Biol., Berlin-Buch, DDR-1115

GRUNERT, Siegfried
Humboldt-Univ. Berlin, Sect. Chem., Dep. Food Chem., Goethestr. 54, Berlin, DDR-1120

HARWARDT, Irene
Inst. Deep-Sea-Fishery and Fish Processing, Rostock-Marienehe, DDR-2510

KOPPERSCHLÄGER, Gerhard
Karl-Marx-Univ. Leipzig, Inst. Biochem., Liebigstr. 16, Leipzig, DDR-7010

KRAUSE, Wolfgang
Tech. Univ. Dresden, Dep. Food Chem. Tech. Biochem., Mommsenstr. 13, Dresden, DDR-8027

KRETSCHMAR, Utta
Humboldt-Univ. Berlin, Sect. NGW/LMT, Pflugstr. 6 b, Berlin, DDR-1040

KROH, Lothar
Humboldt-Univ. Berlin, Sect. NGW/LMT, Invalidenstr. 42, Berlin, DDR-1040

KROLL, Jürgen
Acad. Sci. GDR, Central Inst. Nutr., Bergholz-Rehbrücke, DDR-1505

LANGE, Erika
Acad. Sci. GDR, Central Inst. Nutr., Bergholz-Rehbrücke, DDR-1505

LEHWALD, Ulrike
Acad. Sci. GDR, Inst. Biotechnol,. Permoserstr. 15, Leipzig, DDR-7050

LIPPERT, Eberhard
Humboldt-Univ. Berlin, Sect. NGW/LMT, Pflugstr. 6 b, Berlin, DDR-1040

LUDWIG, Eberhard
Tech. Univ. Dresden, Dep. Food Chem. Tech. Biochem.,
Mommsenstr. 13, Dresden, DDR-8027

LUDWIG, Ingeborg
Tech. Univ. Dresden, Dep. Food Chem. Tech. Biochem.,
Mommsenstr. 13, Dresden, DDR-8027

MIETH, Gerhard
Acad. Sci. GDR, Central Inst. Nutr., Bergholz-Rehbrücke, DDR-1505

MOTHES, Ralf
Acad. Sci. GDR, Central Inst. Nutr., Bergholz-Rehbrücke, DDR-1505

MUSCHIOLIK, Gerald
Acad. Sci. GDR, Central Inst. Nutr., Bergholz-Rehbrücke, DDR-1505

NOETZOLD, Horst
Tech. Univ. Dresden, Dep. Food Chem. Tech. Biochem.,
Mommsenstr. 13, Dresden, DDR-8027

PÄHTZ, Wilma
Acad. Sci. GDR, Central Inst. Nutr., Bergholz-Rehbrücke, DDR-1505

RAAB, Barbara
Acad. Sci. GDR, Central Inst. Nutr., Bergholz-Rehbrücke, DDR-1505

ROTHER, Gudrun
Acad. Sci. GDR, Inst. Polymer Chem., Teltow-Seehof, DDR-1530

SCHÄDLICH, Hiltrud
Acad. Sci. GDR, Inst. Biotechnol., Permoserstr. 15, Leipzig,
DDR-7050

SCHMANDKE, Horst
Acad. Sci. GDR, Central Inst. Nutr., Bergholz-Rehbrücke, DDR-1505

SCHLEUSENER, Reinhard
VEB WTÖZ Dairy Industry, Sachsenhausener Str. 7, Oranienburg,
DDR-1400

SCHNEIDER, Christoph
Acad. Sci. GDR, Central Inst. Nutr., Bergholz-Rehbrücke, DDR-1505

SCHULTZ, Manfred
Acad. Sci. GDR, Central Inst. Nutr., Bergholz-Rehbrücke, DDR-1505

SCHWENKE, Klaus Dieter
Acad. Sci. GDR, Central Inst. Nutr., Bergholz-Rehbrücke, DDR-1505

SIENKIEWICZ, Tadeusz
Humboldt-Univ. Berlin, Dep. Food Industry Food Technol.,
Invalidenstr. 42, Berlin, DDR-1040

TÄUFEL, Alfred
Acad. Sci. GDR. Central Inst. Nutr., Bergholz-Rehbrücke, DDR-1505

TSCHAIKIN, Marion
Karl-Marx-Univ. Leipzig, Inst. Pathol. Bioche., Liebigstr. 16,
Leipzig, DDR-7010

TULSNER, Manfred
Humboldt-Univ. Berlin, Sect. Chem. Dep. Food Chem.,
Goethestr. 54, Berlin, DDR-1120

WAND, Manfred
Acad. Sci. GDR, Inst. Biotechnol., Permoserstr. 15, Leipzig,
DDR-7050

WESTPHAL, Günter
Humboldt-Univ. Berlin, Sect. NGW/LMT, Indvalidenstr. 42, Berlin,
DDR-1040

WIENHOLD, Klaus
Acad. Sci. GDR, Research Cent. Chem. Toxicol., Permoserstr. 15,
Leipzig, DDR-7050

ZIRWER, Dietrich
Acad. Sci. GDR, Central Inst. Molecular Biol., Berlin-Buch,
DDR-1115

**Hungary**

BARÁTH, Ágnes
Central Food Res. Inst., 1022 Budapest II, Herman Ottó út 15

GÁBOR, Elisabeth
Univ. Horticulture Food Industry, Coll. Fac. Food Industry,
Szeged, Marx 7, H-6727

HAJÓS, Gyöngyi
Central Food Res. Inst., 1022 Budapest II, Herman Ottó út 15

LÁSZTITY, Radomir
Tech. Univ. Budapest, Dep. Biochem. Food Technol. H-1502
Budapest, Pf. 91

MIETSCH, Frank
Central Food Res. Inst., 1022 Budapest II, Herman Ottó út 15

**India**

PRAKASH, Vishweshwariah
Central Food Technol. Res., Dep. Food Chem. Biophys. Chem. Sec., Mysore-570013

**Italy**

CERLETTI, Paolo
Univ. Milan, Inst. Biochem. Chem., Via Celoria 2, 20133 Milano

**Japan**

KATO, Akio
Yamaguchi Univ., Dep. Agric. Chem., Yamaguchi 753

**Poland**

BUBICZ, Maria
Agric. Univ., 20-934 Lublin, ul. Akademicka 13

DABROWSKI, Kazimierz
Agric. Univ. Warsaw, 03-849 Warszawa, Grochowska 272

GWIAZDA, Stanislaw
Agric. Univ. Warsaw, 03-849 Warszawa, Grochowska 272

JANKIEWICZ, M.
Acad. Agric., Inst. Food Technol. Plant Origin, ul. Wojska Polskiego 31, 60-624 Poznan

KACZKOWSKI, Jerzy
Agric. Univ. Warsaw, Dep. Biochem., 02-528 Warszawa, Rakowiecka 26/30

KEDZIOR, Zenon Marek
Acad. Agric., Inst. Food Technol. Plant Origin, ul. Wojska Polskiego 31, 60-624 Poznan

KOSTYRA, Henryk
Univ. Agric. Technol. Inst. Physics and Food Chem., 10-957 Olsztyn 5

KOZLOWSKA, Halina
Univ. Agric. Technol. Inst. Food Eng. Biotechnol., 10-957 Olsztyn 5

ROTKIEWICZ, Daniela
Univ. Agric. Technol. Inst. Food Eng. Biotechnol.,
10-957 Olsztyn 5

ŻBIKOWSKI, Zdzislaw
Univ. Agric. Technol. Inst. Dairy Technol., 10-957 Olsztyn 5

**Soviet Union**

TOLSTOGUSOV, Vladimir
Inst. Organoelement. Comp., Acad. Sci. USSR, Moscow 117312,
Vavilova 28

VAINERMAN, Efim
Inst. Organoelement. Comp., Acad. Sci. USSR, Moscow 117312,
Vavilova 28

VAINTRAUB, Josif
State Univ. Kishinev, Sadovaya 60, Kishinev 277014

**United Kingdom**

HARDING, Stephen
Univ. Nottingham, Dep. Appl. Biochem. Food Sci.,
Sutton Bonington, Loughborough, LE12 5RD

**United States of America**

SWANSON, Barry, G.
Washington State Univ., Dep. Food Sci. and Human Nutrition,
Pullman, Washington 99164-6330

Subject Index

# APPENDIX

ISMOND, M. A. H., S. D. ARNTFIELD and E. D. MURRAY
Surface properties in relation to the self-association (micellization) of an isolated fababean (Vicia Faba) protein

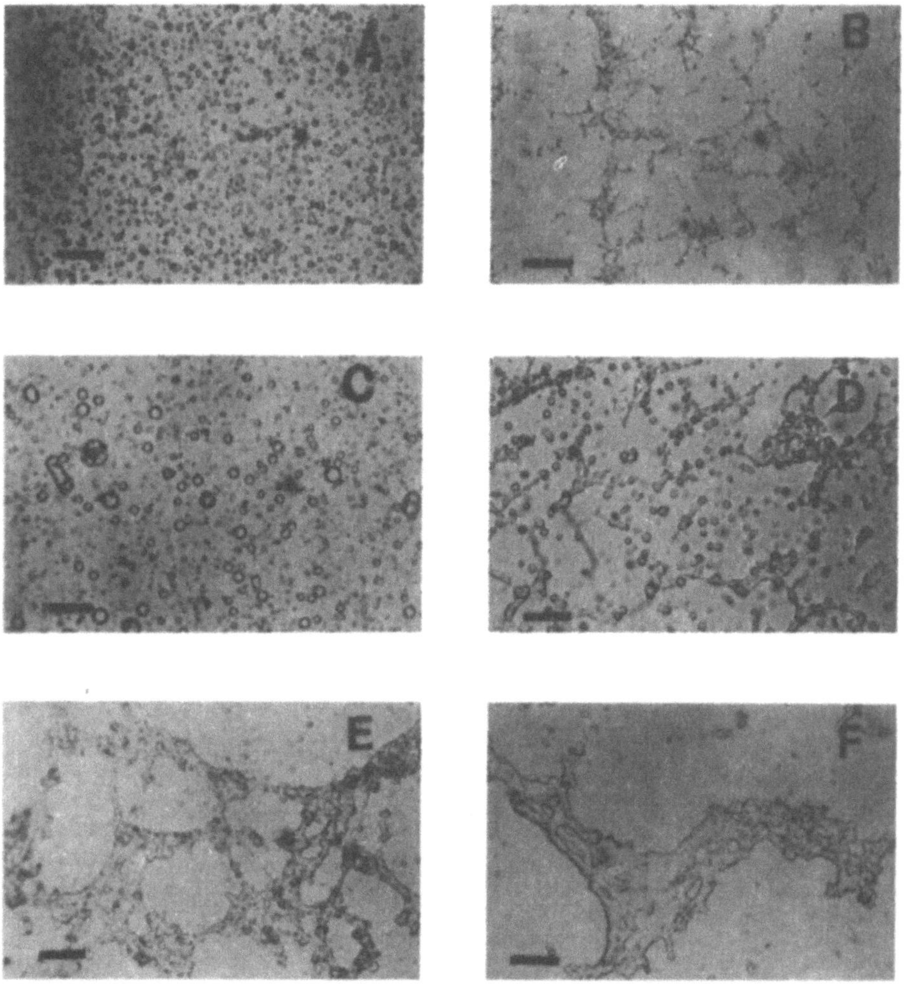


Figure 2:
Photomicrographs of micelle responses obtained with vicilin in a variety of environments. Bar represents 25 µm. Each response has been assigned a numerical value representing the micelle rating. A. Rating 1 – small micelles (< 2 µm in diameter); B. Rating 2 – small micelles in aggregates, possible granular network; C. Rating 3 – small, intermediate and large yet discrete micelles (2–20 µm in diameter); D. Rating 4 – all sized micelles, some coalescence; E. F. Rating 5 – extensive coalescence to give networks (E) or protein sheets (F). [4]

Zu S. 147

MARION, D., C. LeROUX, C. TELLIER, S. AKOKA, D. GALLANT, J. GUEGUEN, V. POPINEAU and J. P. COMPOINT
Lipid-protein interactions in wheat gluten: a renewal

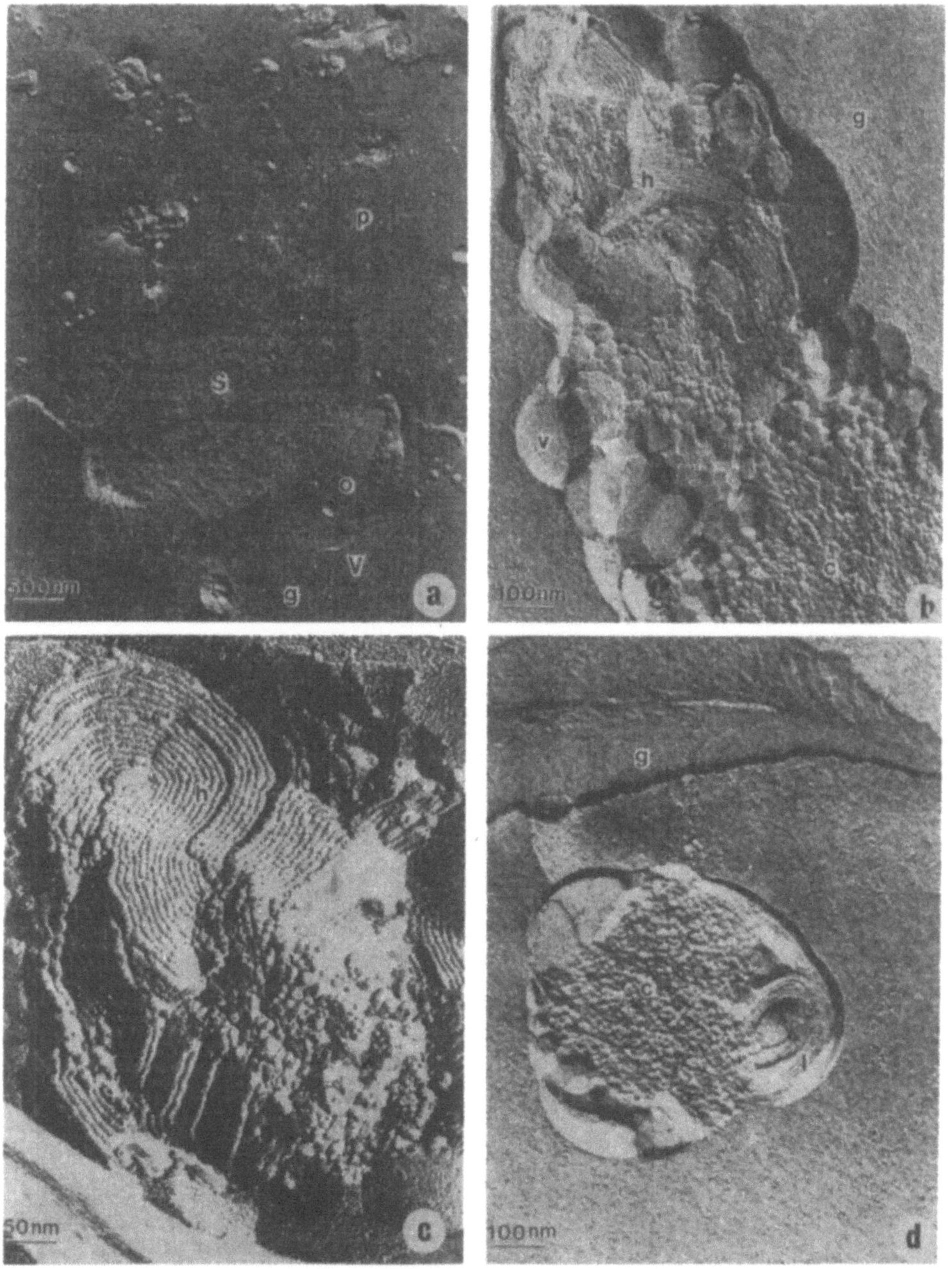


Figure 1. Freeze-fracture electron microscopy of wheat flour dispersed in pure glycerol (see text for explanations). Protein network (p); starch granule (s); glycerol area (g); hexagonal liquid-crystalline lipid phase (h); lamellar liquid-crystalline lipid phase forming multilamellar (l) or single vesicles (v); cubic liquid-crystalline lipid phase (c); oil globule (o)

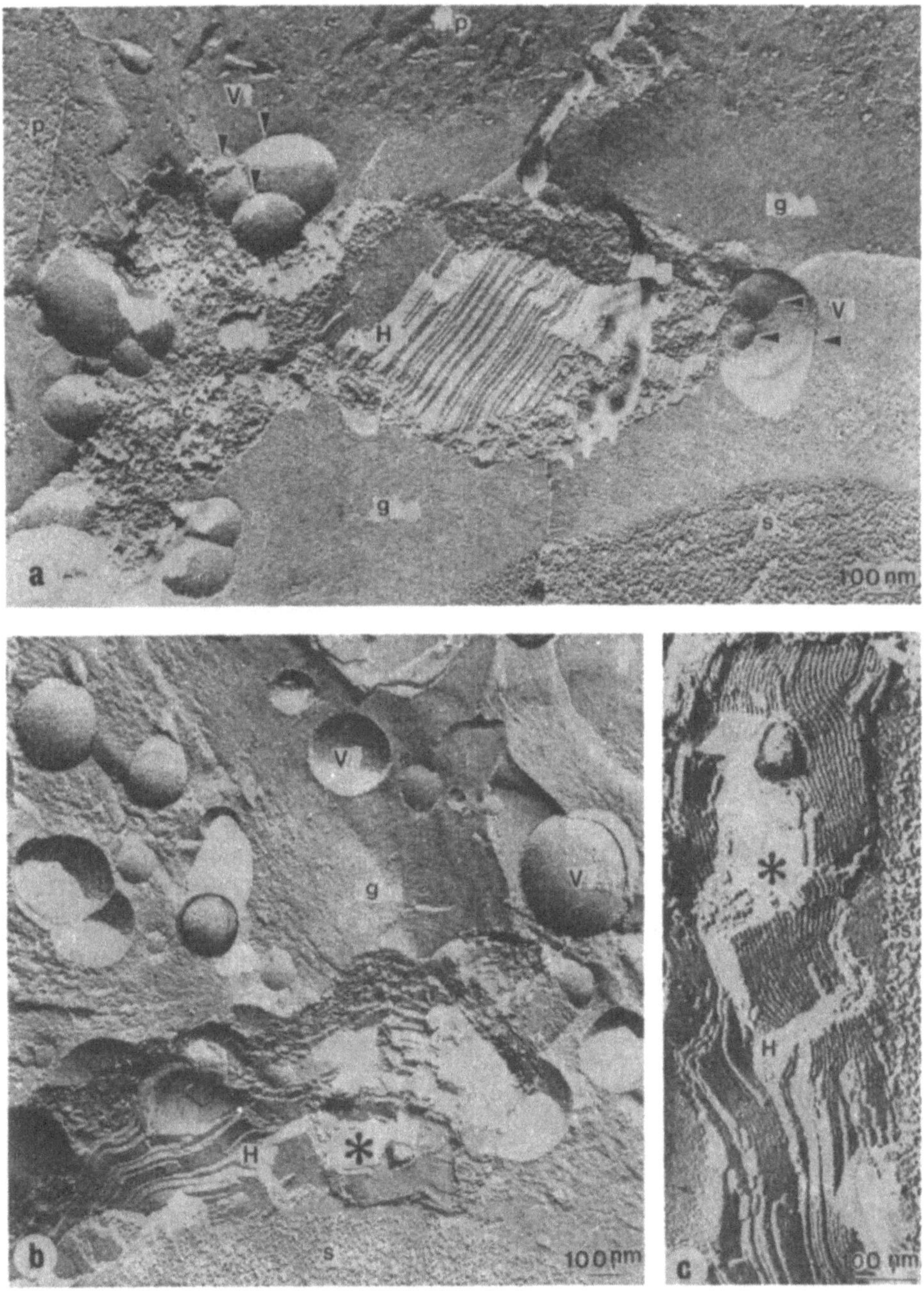


Figure 2. Freeze-fracture electron microscopy of wheat endosperm embedded in pure glycerol (see text for explanations). Abbreviations as in figure 1.

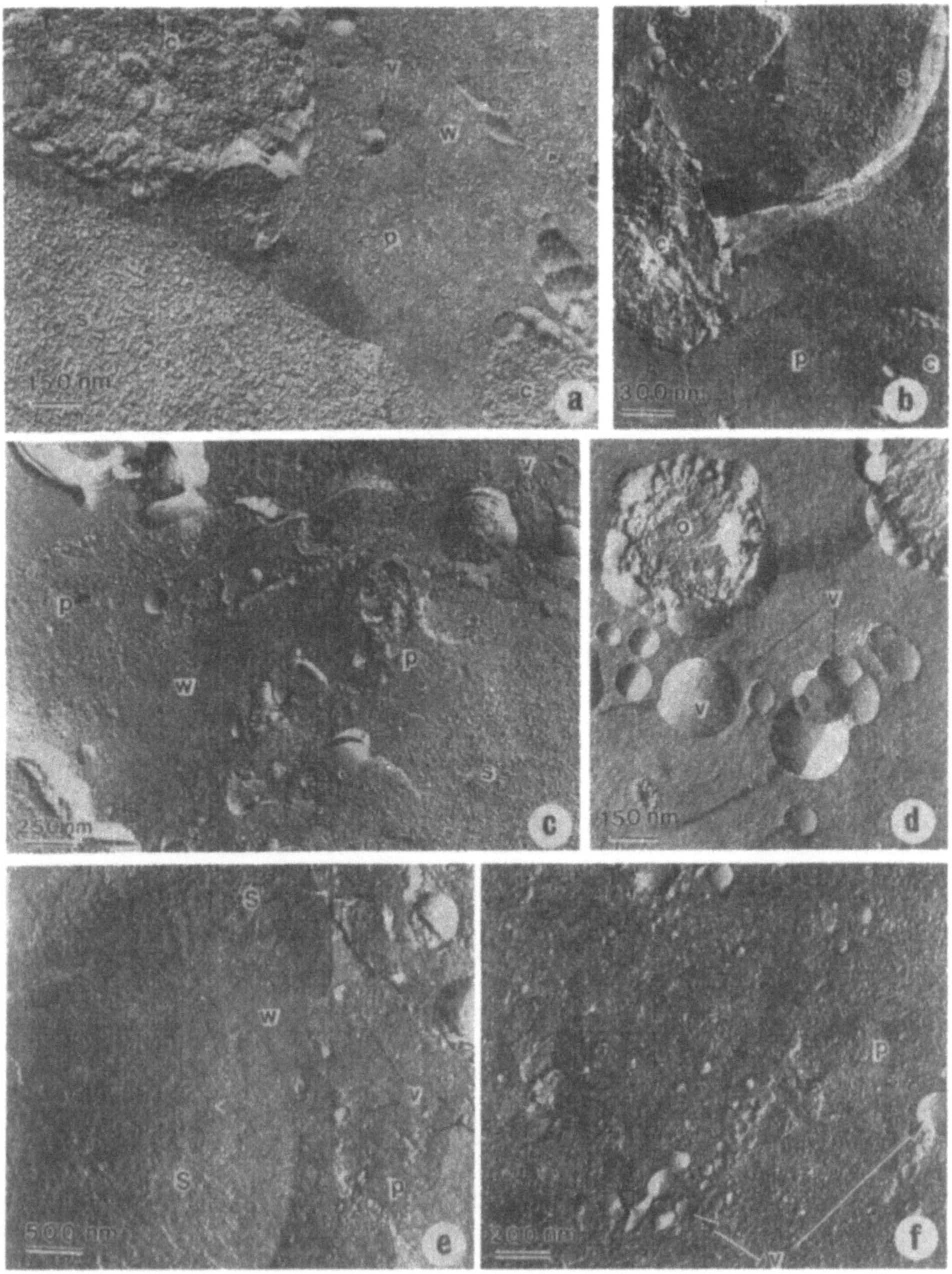


Figure 3. Freeze-fracture electron microscopy of wheat doughs and gluten. Wheat flour doughs with 30 (a–b) and 60% (c–d) water content; Wheat flour dough with 30% water content and a resting time of 2 hr (e); extracted wheat gluten (f); water area (w); other abbreviations as in figure 1.

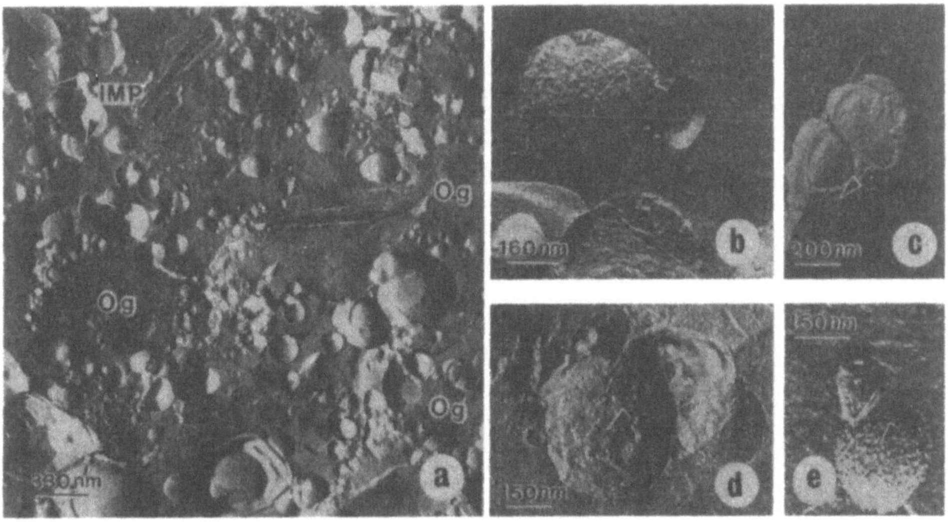


Figure 4. Freeze-fracture electron microscopy of lipid vesicles extracted from wheat flour by flotation ultracentrifugation on sucrose medium. Isolated lipid vesicles (a) exhibiting oil globule (Og) and vesicles with intramembrane particles (IMP); details of vesicles with IMP (b–e).

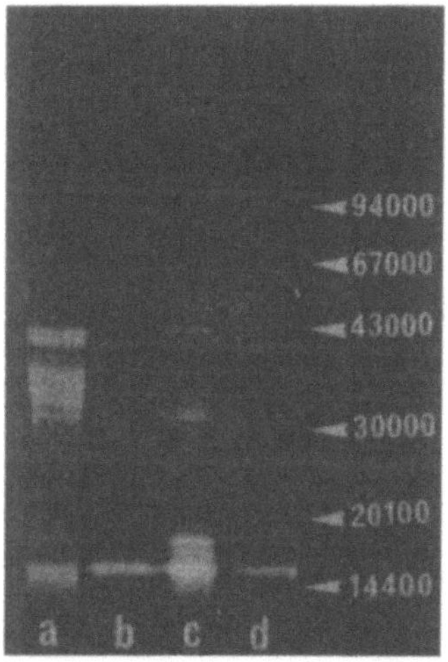


Figure 5. SDS-PAGE (10–20%) of reduced proteins associated with lipid vesicles. Total wheat flour proteins extracted with Tris-HCl 0.1 M pH 7.5 SDS 2% β-mercaptoethanol 2% (a); reduced proteins associated with FI (b) and FII (c) membrane fractions floatting on 20 and 40% sucrose medium, respectively; 16500 molecular weight protein purified by gel filtration on Superose 6 B (FPLC) in Tris-HCl 0.1 M pH 7 SDS 1% (c).

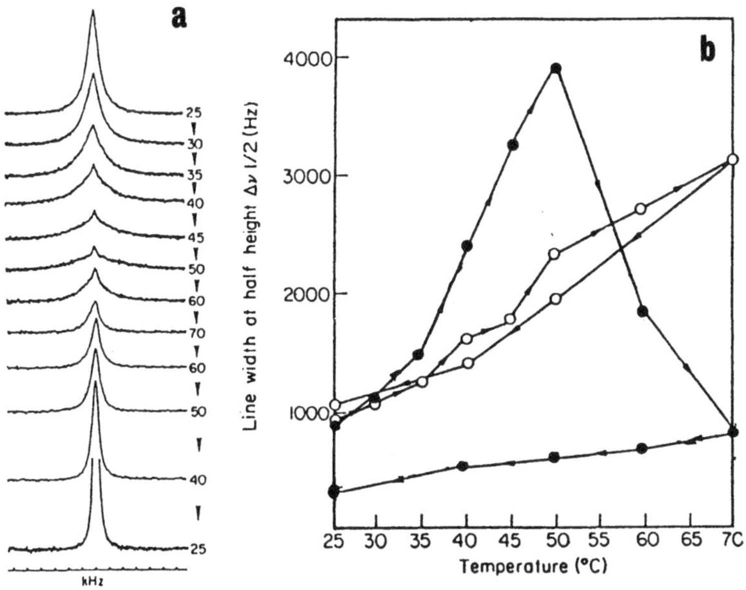


**Figure 6.** Phosphorus nuclear magnetic resonance spectroscopy of extracted wheat gluten during a heating-cooling cycle. Spectra obtained during a heating-cooling cycle (a); line width at half height of the NMR signal (b) during a heating-cooling cycle of fresh (●) and reduced gluten (○) see ref 11 for details of NMR measurements.

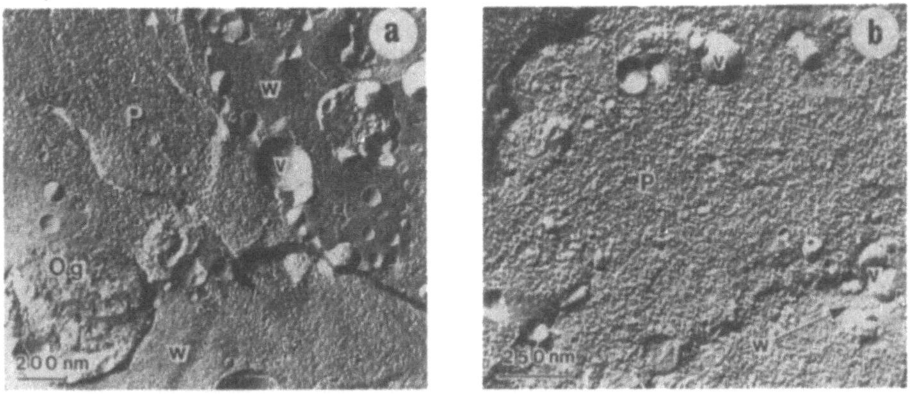


**Figure 7.** Freeze-Fracture electron microscopy of fresh (a) and reduced gluten (b) after a heating-cooling cycle. Abbreviations as in figure 1.

Zu S. 189

CERLETTI, P., M. DURANTI, D. GIANI and N. GUERRIERI

The legumin-like storage protein system in lupin seed and its regulation by proteolytic enzymes

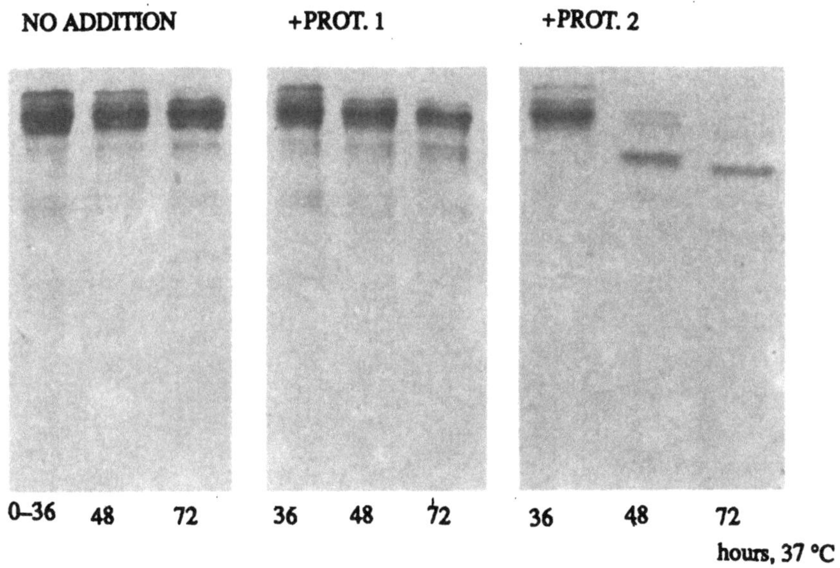


Figure 3. Degradation of globulin 8 by proteinase 1 and 2
Globulin 8 (0.5 mg/ml) was incubated at 37 °C in 50 mM Pi pH 8.0 containing 0.15 M NaCl with or without added proteinase 1 (10 μg/mg) or proteinase 2 (20 μg/mg). At the indicated times aliquots of 7 μg protein were analyzed by SDS-PAGE under non reducing conditions.

Zu S. 283

SCHÄDLICH, H., CH. FLEMMING, A. GABERT and A. TÄUFEL
Protease inhibitors from potatoes – purification and properties

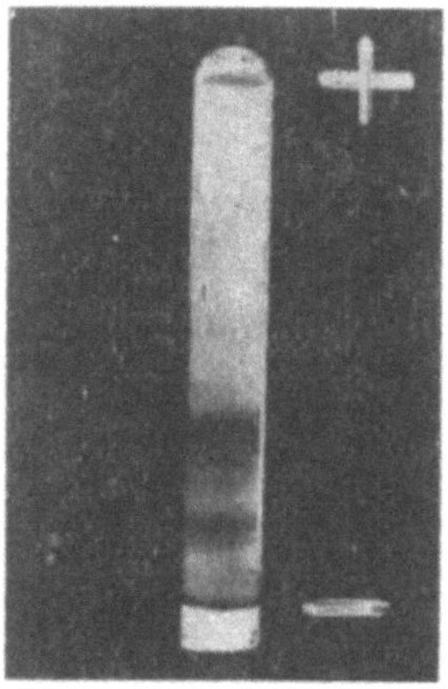


Figure 1. PAGE of the crude material of the inhibitor, sample load: 0.2 mg, development time: 110 min at 3.4 mA

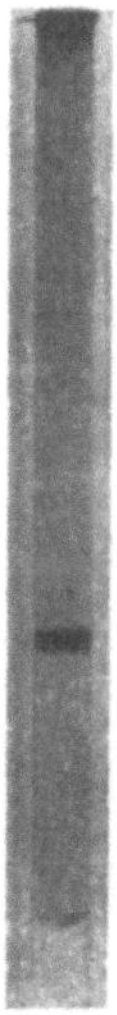

Figure 4. PAGE of PI–II, sample load: 0.56 mg/0.1 ml, development time: 105 min at 4 mA

Zu S. 295

FORNAL, J., D. ROTKIEWICZ, W. GIEC, M. PISKULA and H. KOZLOWSKA
Denaturation changes in protein structure during the hydrothermal treatment of rapeseed

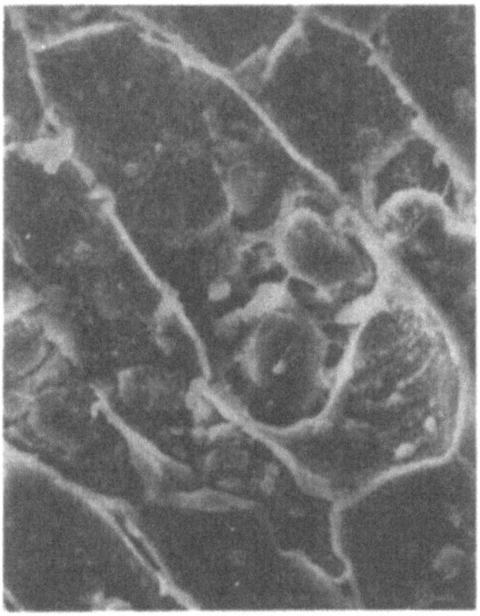

Phot. 1

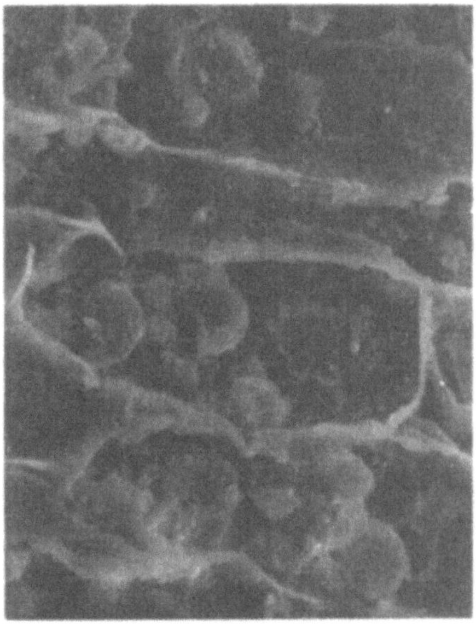

Phot. 2

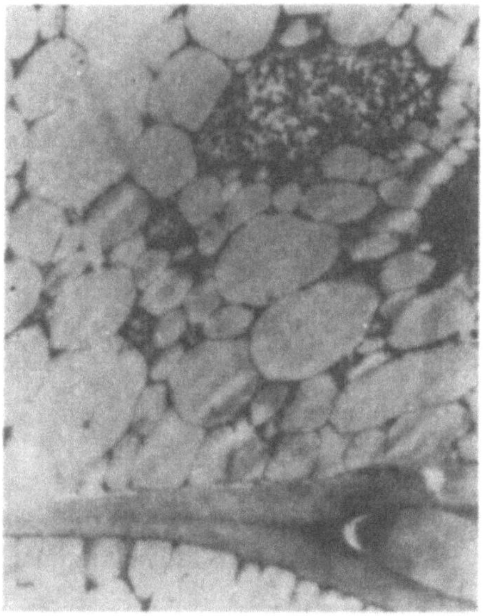

Phot. 3

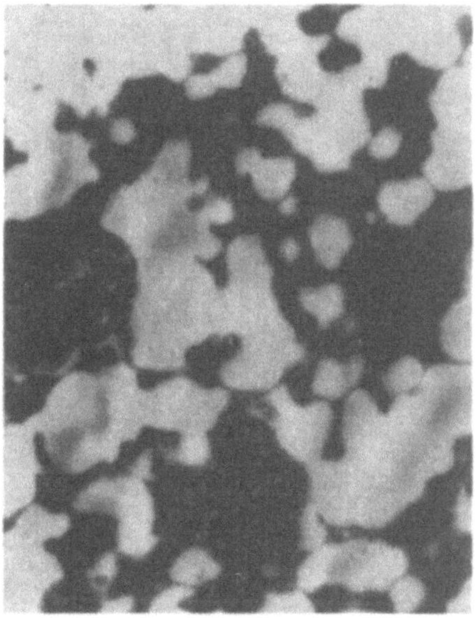

Phot. 4

Zu S. 299

FORNAL, J., J. BOROWSKA, H. KOZLOWSKA, CH. SCHNEIDER and H. SCHMANDKE
Influence of faba bean hydrothermal treatment of denaturation changes in protein

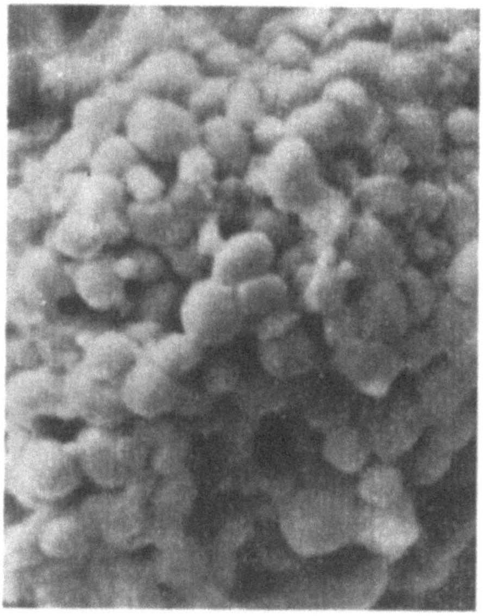

Phot. 1
control

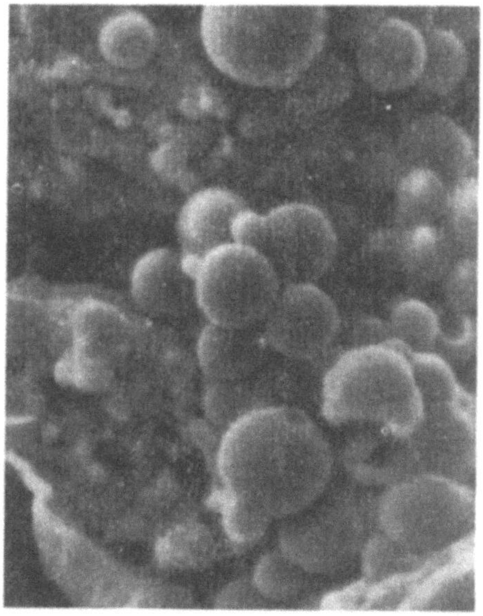

Phot. 2
heated 100 °C/2 min

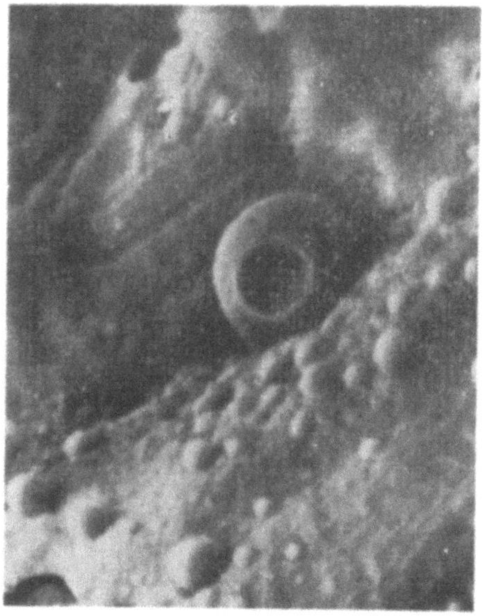

Phot. 3
heated 110 °C/5 min

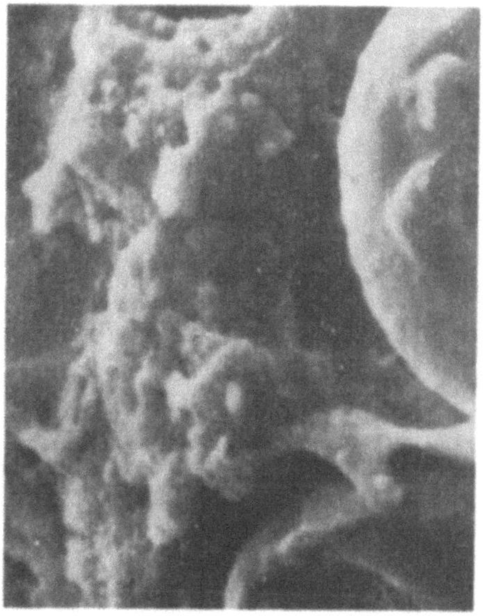

Phot. 4
heated 120 °C/2 min

SIENKIEWICZ, T., and R. SCHLEUSENER
Investigatiion of primary degradation products of casein in dutch-type cheese

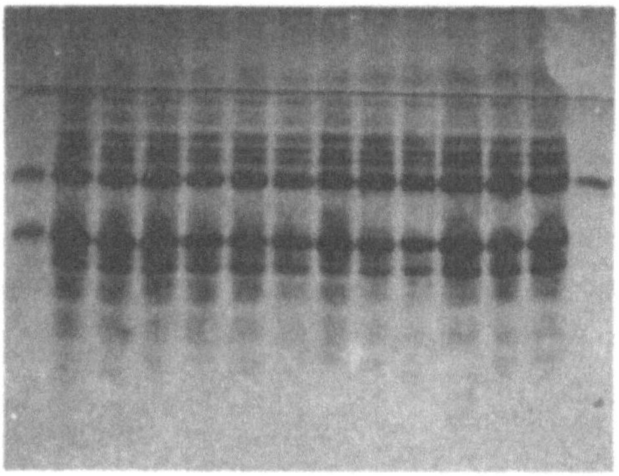

Figure 2. The PAGE patterns of an 4. weeks ripened twelve Edam type cheese charges from left to right: rennet casein, 2–13 cheese samples β-casein. Sample application 20 µl; 0.25% cheese in 8 M urea. PAGE 10% acrylamide, 4.5 urea, pH 8.3/Tris/Glycine/Tris/HCl buffer, Protein staining in gel with coomassie brilliant blue R-250 in 12.5% trichloracetic acid (SCHLEUSENER et al., 1982)

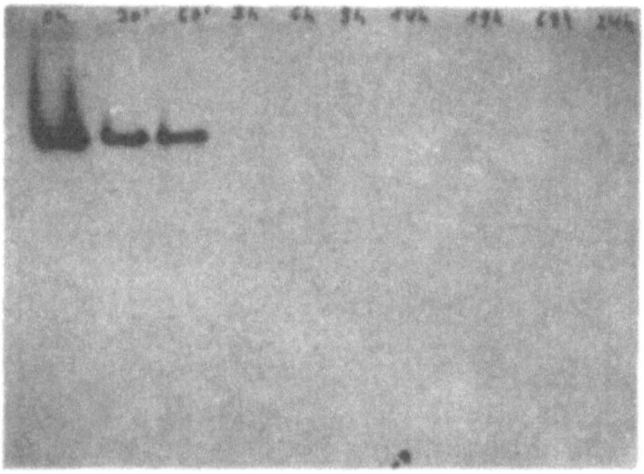

Figure 3. Electrophoresis gel of β-casein treated with microbial rennet substitute 8experimental preparation) as a function of time, PAGE, 12.5% acrylamide, 4.5 M urea and other conditions as Figure 1

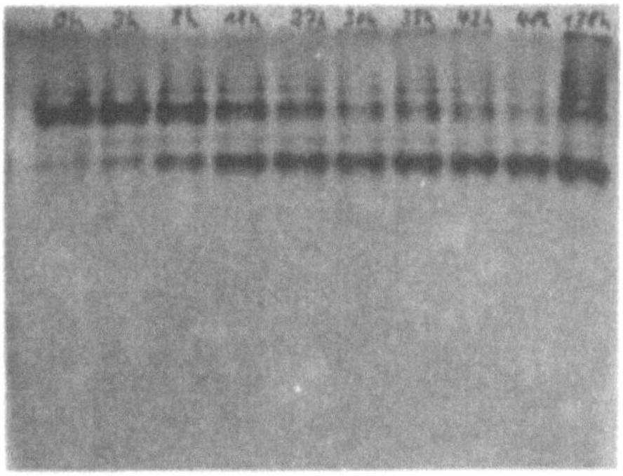

Figure 4. Electrophoresis gel of β-casein treated with Fromase 46 TL as a function of time, PAGE; 12.5% acrylamide, 4.5 M urea and other conditions as Figure 1